Children in a
Changing Health System

The Johns Hopkins Series in Contemporary Medicine and Public Health

Consulting Editors:

Martin D. Abeloff, M.D.
Samuel H. Boyer IV, M.D.
Gareth M. Green, M.D.
Richard T. Johnson, M.D.
Paul R. McHugh, M.D.
Edmond A. Murphy, M.D.
Edyth H. Schoenrich, M.D., M.P.H.
Jerry L. Spivak, M.D.
Barbara H. Starfield, M.D., M.P.H.

Also of Interest in This Series:

Carl Eisdorfer, David A. Kessler, and Abby N. Spector, eds., *Caring for the Elderly: Reshaping Health Policy*
Madelon Lubin Finkel, ed., *Surgical Care in the United States: A Policy Perspective*
Ann Barry Flood and W. Richard Scott, *Hospital Structure and Performance*
Merwyn R. Greenlick, Donald K. Freeborn, and Clyde R. Pope, eds., *Health Care Research in an HMO: Two Decades of Discovery*
Janet D. Perloff, Phillip R. Kletke, and Kathryn M. Neckerman, *Medicaid and Pediatric Primary Care*
Barbara Starfield and Others, *The Effectiveness of Medical Care: Validating Clinical Wisdom*
David W. Young and Richard B. Saltman, *The Hospital Power Equilibrium: Physician Behavior and Cost Control*

Children in a Changing Health System
Assessments and Proposals for Reform

edited by

Mark J. Schlesinger, Ph.D.
Center for Health and Human Resources Policy
John F. Kennedy School of Government
Harvard University
and Department of Social Medicine
Harvard Medical School

and

Leon Eisenberg, M.D.
Chairman, Department of Social Medicine
Harvard Medical School

The Johns Hopkins University Press
Baltimore and London

© 1990 The Johns Hopkins University Press
All rights reserved
Printed in the United States of America

The Johns Hopkins University Press, 701 West 40th Street, Baltimore, Maryland 21211
The Johns Hopkins Press Ltd., London

The paper used in this publication meets the minimum requirements of American National Standard for Information Sciences—Permanence of Paper for Printed Library Materials, ANSI Z39.48-1984.

Library of Congress Cataloging-in-Publication Data

Children in a changing health system: assessments and proposals for reform/edited by Mark J. Schlesinger and Leon Eisenberg.
    p.   cm.—(The Johns Hopkins series in contemporary medicine and public health.)
  Includes bibliographical references.
  ISBN 0-8018-3973-4 (alk. paper)
  1. Child health services—United States. 2. Child health services—Government policy—United States. I. Schlesinger, Mark Jeffrey. II. Eisenberg, Leon, 1922– . III. Series.
  [DNLM: 1. Child Health Services—United States. 2. Health Policy—United States. WA 320 C53652]
RJ102.C487   1990
362.1'9892'00973—dc20
DNLM/DLC
for Library of Congress   89-24406
                                                                                    CIP

*To the memory of our friend and colleague
John Allington Butler,
who conceived of this book,
selected its authors, and inspired us to complete it*

Contents

Contributors   ix
Foreword   xi
    Julius Richmond
Acknowledgments   xiii
Introduction   xv

I Children's Health Needs, Health Status, and Legal Rights

1. Children's Health Status, Health Risks, and Use of Health Services   3
   Barbara Starfield and Paul Newacheck
2. Health Care for Children with Special Needs   27
   Ann B. Taylor, Susan G. Epstein, and Allen C. Crocker
3. Legal Issues in Children's Health Care   49
   Gary Melton, Ira M. Schwartz, and Michael D. Resnick

II Changes in the Financing of Health Services and Their Effects on Children's Health Care

4. A Children's Health Care Budget   67
   Mary Jo Larson
5. Children and Private Health Insurance   89
   Sara Rosenbaum
6. Medicaid as Public Health Insurance for Children   131
   Margaret A. McManus and Stephen M. Davidson
7. Provider Payment and Children's Health Care   158
   Constance M. Horgan and Samuel S. Flint

III Changes in the Organization of Service Providers and Their Effects on Children's Health Care

8. Private Medical Providers and Children's Health Care   183
   Mark J. Schlesinger
9. The Role of the Public Sector in Providing Children's Health Care   215
   Lorraine V. Klerman and Kyle L. Grazier, with Kathleen C. Thomas
10. The Health Care Implications of Early Childhood Group Care Programs   243
    Judith S. Palfrey and Alix Handelsman

11 Children's Health Care and the Schools   265
    Deborah Klein Walker, John A. Butler, and Annette Bender

IV Integrating Funding and Services for Children

12 The Evolution and Future Role of Title V   297
    Bernard Guyer
13 Little People in a Big Policy World: Lasting Questions and New Directions in Health Policy for Children   325
    Mark J. Schlesinger and Leon Eisenberg

Index   361

Contributors

Annette Bender, M.S., Independent Health Consultant (formerly at Department of Behavioral Sciences, School of Public Health, Harvard University)

John Butler, Ed.D., Children's Hospital, Boston, Massachusetts (deceased)

Allen C. Crocker, M.D., Director, Developmental Evaluation Clinic, Children's Hospital, Boston, Massachusetts

Stephen M. Davidson, Ph.D., Director Health Management Programs, Boston University School of Management

Susan G. Epstein, M.S.W., Co-Director, Project SERVE, Boston, Massachusetts

Samuel S. Flint, Ph.D., Director, Department of Child Health Care Financing and Organization, American Academy of Pediatrics, Elk Grove Village, Illinois

Kyle L. Grazier, Dr.P.H., Associate Professor, School of Public Health, University of California, Berkeley

Bernard Guyer, M.D., M.P.H., Department of Maternal and Child Health, School of Public Health, Harvard University

Alix Handelsman, M.D., Fellow, Division of Ambulatory Pediatrics, Children's Hospital, Boston, Massachusetts

Constance M. Horgan, Sc.D., Research Associate, Bigel Institute for Health Policy, Heller School, Brandeis University

Lorraine V. Klerman, Dr.P.H., Professor, Department of Epidemiology and Public Health, Yale University School of Medicine

Mary Jo Larson, M.P.A., Research Associate, Bigel Institute for Health Policy, Heller School, Brandeis University

Margaret McManus, M.H.S., McManus Health Policy, Inc., Washington, D.C.

Gary Melton, Ph.D., Professor and Director, Law/Psychology Program, Department of Psychology, University of Nebraska

Paul Newacheck, Dr.P.H., Institute for Health Policy Studies, School of Medicine, University of California, San Francisco

Judith S. Palfrey, M.D., Chief, Division of Ambulatory Pediatrics, Children's Hospital, Boston, Massachusetts

Michael D. Resnick, Ph.D., Associate Professor and Director of Research, Adolescent Health Program, University of Minnesota, Minneapolis

Julius Richmond, M.D., Director, Division of Health Policy Research and Education, Harvard Medical School

Sara Rosenbaum, J.D., Director of Programs and Policy, Children's Defense Fund, Washington, D.C.

Ira Schwartz, M.S.W., Professor and Director, Center for Study of Youth Policy, University of Michigan School of Social Work, Ann Arbor

Barbara Starfield, M.D., M.P.H., Professor and Head, Division of Health Policy, Department of Health Policy and Management, Johns Hopkins University School of Hygiene and Public Health

Ann B. Taylor, Ed.D., Co-Director, Project SERVE, Boston, Massachusetts

Kathleen C. Thomas, B.A., Research Assistant, Department of Epidemiology and Public Health, Yale University School of Medicine

Deborah Klein Walker, Ed.D., Assistant Commissioner, Bureau of Parent, Child, and Adolescent Health, Massachusetts Department of Public Health (formerly Associate Professor, Department of Behavioral Sciences, Harvard School of Public Health)

Foreword

This volume presents a most timely analysis of the child health issues facing the nation. If it is true that a nation can be judged by how well it treats its children, our recent record is distinctly mixed. The disturbing news is that over the past decade children have been slipping into poverty at about the same rate the elderly have been emerging from poverty. Concomitantly, the decline in the infant mortality rate has slowed, immunization rates for poor children have declined, fewer children have a primary source of care, and more children are uninsured for health services.

The infrastructure for public health services on which poor families depend heavily has been eroding, according to a recent report of the Institute of Medicine. The maternal and child health programs, established by the Social Security Act in 1936 and administered by the states, experienced significant reductions in inflation-adjusted funding in the early 1980s.

The good news has been that in the long perspective the child health record of the nation has improved. The acute infectious diseases no longer rank among the first five causes of death in children, although the emergence of AIDS poses a new threat of childhood mortality. As a consequence, the congenital disorders, low birthweight, developmental disabilities, accidental injuries, and the complicated issues of drug abuse, suicide, homicide, and child abuse are more prominent concerns in child health. These introduce new complexities and emphasize the interrelatedness of child health issues with social, economic, and educational factors in the development of the child and the family.

Simultaneous with the increase in complexity of health problems has come an increase in the complexity of the organization and financing of child health services. Medicaid (Title 19 of the Social Security Act) is the primary federal-state program for financing health service for families of low income and is basically fifty different programs. Eligibility and administration can vary considerably from state to state. If we add to this the program for children with special needs that is administered through departments of education, developmental disabilities programs, as well as the Women, Infant, and Children Supplemental Nutrition Program (WIC) administered by the Department of Agriculture, we can gain some insights into how large a challenge complexity poses for providing child health services comprehensively and with equity.

These issues are presented not in despair, for these various public programs have effective track records in serving the medical and health-related needs of children and their families. However, we are at a crossroads. If we are to assure comprehensive, continuing health services of high quality to all children in need, we must shift our policy-making focus toward improving the organization and financing of services. This will involve a reconsideration of the long-term drift toward fragmented, highly specialized, discontinuous services. Making comprehensive services accessible, financially and geographically, may also require rethinking the current public and private roles in the financing and delivery of health services.

The analyses and proposals presented in this volume should facilitate this process. We are fortunate in having gone through a process of consciousness-raising concerning the plight of children and their families in recent years. We certainly have the best educated and trained health professionals in the world. We cannot afford to squander the resources, to allow our system to drift without direction and without the guidance it needs to help it reach those who would otherwise be overlooked. This nation has the resources to commit to the futures of its children. We need to chart the course and demonstrate the political will to fulfill our commitment.

> Julius B. Richmond, M.D.
> Director, Division of Health Policy Research
>   and Education
> Harvard Medical School
> Former Surgeon General of the United States

Acknowledgments

This project has been long in development. More than four years ago, it began with an observation: that amidst the welter of change and innovation in the health care system, little attention was being paid to the well-being of children, who could not articulate their needs and had few reliable agents to act in their behalf. This was John Butler's observation, and he asked us to work with him to help call attention and look for more constructive responses to this issue. This task was to lead us down a complicated path, one much shaped by John's vision of how children's health needs are met through the interaction of a complex network of medical, social, and educational services.

To help us explore this complexity, we called upon a talented collection of authors, drawn from a variety of settings and diverse academic disciplines. We asked a good deal of them, because we envisioned this project producing a collective, and not just a collected, volume of work. To this end, the authors met in a pre-writing conference, reworked their outlines in light of their colleagues' comments, rewrote their papers following the general conference at which they were first presented, and rewrote them yet again after several rounds of editing. Authorship has its own (somewhat limited) rewards, but the authors included in this volume went (more or less willingly) far beyond the usual call of duty.

Many people, not credited here as authors, made important substantive contributions to this effort. From the inception of this project, Julius Richmond lent guidance and wisdom to our efforts. His understanding of (and participation in) much of this nation's child and family policy over the past three decades was a constant source of insight. Lisbeth Schorr acted as rapporteur at the conference where these papers were first presented. She did a truly remarkable job of summarizing and synthesizing the proceedings. This synthesis informed our work on the final chapter of the book, and Lee graciously allowed us to borrow some of her more felicitous phrasings in writing that chapter. A number of scholars—Karen Davis, Robert Blendon, George Masnick, Susan Meisner, William Bithoney, Lori Diprete, Harold Richman, and Matthew Stagner—contributed papers to the conference that were not, due to space limitations, included in this volume. An even larger number of people served as discussants at the conference: Peter Budetti, Peter Edleman, Barry Ensminger, Christine Ferguson, Sam Flint, Florence Frucher, Betty Hamburg, Michael Stoto, Suzanne Mulstein, Donald Muse, Anne Rosewater, Katherine Swartz, Louise Trubeck, and Julie Wilson. Their remarks—which would have merited publication in their own right had we a book twice the length of this one—improved all the chapters included here, but made particularly important contributions to the final chapter.

Funding for this entire enterprise was provided by the Division of Maternal and Child Health in the Department of Health and Human Resources. Vince Hutchins and Merle McPherson of the Division were generous in their advice as well as financial support and showed great patience throughout the book's long gestation.

A number of people worked long and diligently to convert the rough drafts of papers into more finished products. Pamela Brown Drumheller and Lori Diprete made important editorial contributions; Mathew Myercheck word processed many of the chapters; Kathleen Grathwol and Kathleen Flynn aided in preparing the manuscript as well as in the final editing. Once in manuscript form, the volume came into good hands at the Johns Hopkins University Press. A critique by George Silver, who served as reviewer for the Press, further improved all the chapters. The inevitably lengthy process of multiple reviews and reediting was greatly facilitated by the guidance (and occasional gentle prodding) of Wendy Harris, science editor at the Press. A more gracious and charming editor would be hard to find.

On November 25, 1988, John Butler passed away, far too young at age 45. His thoughts had shaped the beginnings of this project, his spirit its fruition. John devoted his life to calling people's attention to children's welfare, so often the subject of benign neglect. Without his voice to carry this message, we must raise ours to fill the silence. It is to this end, and in John's memory, that we dedicate this book.

Introduction

Americans have traditionally taken much the same attitude toward government that they have toward their neighborhood handyman: government gets called in when there's a problem. People are never particularly happy about making the call—in fact, they put it off as long as possible. They tolerate the repairs as long as the bills don't seem excessive, but are always ready to doubt both the competence and the integrity of the work. To hold down costs, the handyman is expected to patch and mend, not to suggest that the whole system be scrapped and a new one installed.

These expectations have left an important legacy, one that shapes how we relate to government as well as limiting the effectiveness of public policy making. One aspect can be seen by contrasting the handyman model to our relationship with another service provider, the auto mechanic. We expect to bring our cars in to the mechanic periodically and are advised to do so for regular preventive maintenance. But, apart from a limited number of routinely reported statistics, there is no comparable process for assessing how well our social institutions are performing. Nor do we regularly pull those institutions in for a "tune-up" under governmental auspices.

In the absence of mechanisms to review and assess societal performance, public policy responds to problems only when they are actively placed on the political agenda—when some agrieved constituent makes the call for some repairs. A significant industry of lobbyists, political action groups, and related organizations has emerged to do this. But for many Americans, that call will come late or will be indistinct, obscured by static. Children are one such group. Their direct political voice is weak. Despite the efforts of groups like the Children's Defense Fund or the House Select Committee on Children, Youth and Families, they have relatively few representatives to carry their message, so policymakers often only poorly understand their needs.

When we began the project embodied in this volume, it was our sense that this was precisely the situation facing the health care of America's children. Over the past decade, the U.S. health care system has been transformed at a rate that few had anticipated. The ways in which health care providers are organized and paid, the relative roles of public and private sectors, the influence of market forces on the delivery of services, the nature of health insurance, have all been significantly altered. These have had important, though often unrecognized, effects on children's health care. At the same time, other seemingly unrelated societal trends have changed children's health care needs and their access to health services. Some have had largely negative effects, including changes in family composition and workforce participation as well as the reduced availability of jobs with fringe benefits such as health insurance. Other changes have had more positive consequences, such as emerging new legal rights for children to various services, including education for the handicapped.

Some of these changes reflect broad societal trends and are largely outside the influence of policy makers. But many are the result of explicit governmental policies designed to meet other goals. Unfortunately, most have been adopted with little thought for or understanding about their consequences for children. In part, this is because children's interests are less effectively voiced in political arenas. In part, it is an outgrowth of an era when policy makers have narrowed their vision of health policy to a concern for costs. Under these circumstances, children become that much easier to ignore, since they represent only about 10 percent of the national health care bill.

This volume is intended to reintroduce a concern for children into the policy debate—to identify more clearly the failings of an increasingly stressed health care system and to design more effective "repairs" to serve children's needs. It touches on a variety of ongoing efforts to reform the health care system, as well as policies involving related social institutions that have important consequences for children's health and well-being. To this end, the book speaks to two audiences. The first are those in the policy-making community who have had little exposure to issues involving children but whose actions have a significant impact on children's welfare. The second includes those who have focused their concern and professional activities on children's health but who may not fully appreciate the extent to which broader trends and policies affect and circumscribe their efforts.

The structure and content of the book reflect this dual focus. The first part, and the first chapter of the second, are intended to acquaint readers with important aspects of children's health care needs as well as with the ways in which health-related services for children are financed and delivered. The issues discussed in these chapters will be familiar to most child health professionals, though the discussion of the emerging importance of various nonmedical influences on health may still offer some useful insights to such readers. Parts II and III begin with a review of broad trends in health care financing and delivery—trends familiar to most policy makers concerned with health issues—but go on to explore their often-overlooked consequences for children. Part IV examines ways in which these various trends and needs interact with existing programs for children, such as Title V and in terms of a more comprehensive conceptual framework for health policy making.

Many of these chapters were presented initially as papers at a conference held at Harvard University in November 1986 (though all have been updated by the authors to reflect changes in conditions and public policies through early 1988). The book thus shares some characteristics with virtually all multi-authored volumes. Although the authors met collectively to discuss both the overall purpose of the book and the content of their individual chapters, each author, in the end, speaks with his or her own voice, reflecting the particular concerns and values that he or she brings to these issues. We believe that this diversity of perspectives is an important asset. But it also means that the policy recommendations presented in each chapter do not in themselves add up to a coherent whole.

We have tried to address the need for a broader, more consistent, conceptual framework for children's health policy in the final chapter of the book. In formulating this discussion, we drew on the issues, concerns, and assessments provided in the earlier chapter. In that sense, the final chapter represents an integration of the material presented throughout the book. But it is an integration that was very much shaped by our own values, values that may not be shared by all readers, nor indeed by all the chapter authors. The proposals that we offer in the final chapter represent one consistent—and, we hope, reasonably compelling—way to respond to the emerging health policy needs of America's children. But they are not the only way of doing so. The last chapter can usefully be read as a summary of the issues that must be addressed in constructing a consistent framework for policy making, as well as a set of specific recommendations for reform.

Inevitable with multi-authored works, there emerge gaps in content that are apparent only after the book nears completion. A number of topics, including prenatal care, child abuse, mental illness, AIDS, and the relationship between health care and welfare reform, received less attention than many would feel they merit (though all are discussed in more than one chapter). In some cases, this represented an explicit decision on our part to narrow the focus of the volume. Such choices are always difficult, but they are also unavoidable. From the perspective of this book, there is little unique about these omitted services—they are shaped by the trends and forces that are described throughout the book. The issues involved in infants with AIDS are virtually identical to those discussed more generally in the chapters on multiple risk children, children with chronic illness, and public providers of children's health services: the absence of private insurance for high-cost illnesses, the need to coordinate a complex array of services, and the continued requirement for an effective public delivery system to provide for the health needs of these children. The availability and adequacy of mental health or prenatal care are affected by the same factors—increased competition and consolidation among health care providers—that are altering the delivery of other health care services.

Some special features of the policy-making process that are related to children, though not unique to health care, do merit some additional discussion. Virtually every observer who has studied policy making in the United States, as it involves children, has concluded that it is in some sense biased against their interests. A review of these concerns will provide a useful context for further thinking about what is feasible and desirable in child health policy.

Over the past decade, a number of authors have examined the effectiveness of American public policy designed to further the interests of children (Steiner, 1981; Grubb and Lazerson, 1982; Pizzo, 1983; Richman and Stagner, 1986; Longman, 1987; Gould and Palmer, 1988). Noting the high rate of poverty, poor access to health and human services, and growing indices of problems among children in the United States compared to other countries, these authors concluded that U.S. policies affecting children have a number of serious failings (Gould and Palmer, 1988). These have been variously attributed to concerns for preserving family autonomy at the expense of children's welfare (Steiner, 1981; Gould and Palmer, 1988), ambivalent attitudes toward children from different ethnicities, races, or social classes (Grubb and Lazerson, 1982; Richman and Stagner, 1986), or difficulties in effectively presenting children's needs in the political arena (Pizzo, 1983; Longman, 1987).

Proposed solutions have varied as much as these diagnoses. Some argue for providing children with more effective advocates (Ross, 1983). Others focus on the structure of public programs. One side contends that children would benefit from being placed in separate programs with earmarked financing, while equally thoughtful observers argue with equal fervor that children are better included in universal entitlement programs, like Social Security or Medicare (Grubb and Lazerson, 1982; Richman and Stagner, 1986). Still others argue that children should be "sold" as a societal investment, necessary for securing our nation's economic future (Committee for Economic Development, 1987; Schorr, 1988).

Each of these perspectives on policy making is reflected in the recommendations of one or more of the chapters in this book. Each viewpoint is plausible and has its supporters. All of these perspectives can and undoubtedly will continue to coexist—public policy making in this country has never shown a strong need for consistency nor an emphasis on developing consensus around the motives for reform. But even if we do not try to identify a single "best" approach to policy making in the interests of children, it is becoming increasingly apparent that we must consider more carefully how these various perspectives on children's policy interact and to some extent compete with one another.

Different approaches to reform of the policy-making process embody, and legitimate, very different standards of societal equity. Those that focus on better advocacy, whether by the Children's Defense Fund, Title V agencies, or some newly created office in the federal Department of Health and Human Services, implicitly accept interest-group competition as the basis for allocating public resources. Those that cast the debate in terms of societal investment must rest their case on a benefit-cost calculation—computed in whatever terms they prefer—that shows that the nation reaps a higher return on its investment for children than for other citizens. Those that emphasize participation in common programs, such as Social Security, assume that "equal treatment" can adequately be adapted to meet children's special needs.

With so many alternative standards of equity, it is easy to imagine health policy reforms (or those for any other set of services) for children foundering in a debate over whether the particular proposal suitably advances a broader societal standard of justice or more adequately protects the general interests of children. This could easily lead to policy inertia, with children's advocates warring among themselves or conveying to policy makers seriously conflicting messages.

Because representation of children's interests in political arenas is so tenuous, because the nation's track record in protecting those interests is so uninspiring, we can ill-afford such political stalemates. We therefore conclude that, as difficult as it will be, we must begin building a consensus about the appropriate basis for policy making involving children. It is our hope that the perspectives, issues, and recommendations presented in this volume represent a first step in this direction for U.S. health policy.

References

Committee on Economic Development. 1988. *Children in Need: Investment Strategies for the Educationally Disadvantaged*. New York.
Gould, Stephanie and John Palmer, 1988. Outcomes, Interpretations and Policy Implications. In *The Vulnerable*, ed. John Palmer, Timothy Smeeding, and Barbara Boyle Torrey, 413–442. Washington, D.C.: Urban Institute Press.
Grubb, W. Norton and Marvin Lazerson. 1981. *Broken Promises: How Americans Fail Their Children*. New York: Basic Books.
Longman, Phillip. 1987. *Born to Pay: The New Politics of Aging in America*. Boston: Houghton Mifflin.
Pizzo, Peggy. 1983. Slouching toward Bethlehem: American Federal Policy Perspectives on Children and Their Families. In *Children, Families and Government:*

Perspectives on American Social Policy, ed. Edward Zigler, Sharon Kagan and Edgar Klugman, 10–43. New York: Cambridge University Press.

Richman, Harold and Mathew Stagner. 1986. Children: Treasured Resource or Forgotten Minority? In *Our Aging Society: Paradox and Promise*, ed. Alan Pifer and Lydia Bronte, 161–79. New York: W. W. Norton.

Ross, Catherine. 1983. Advocacy Movements in the Century of the Child. In *Children, Families and Government: Perspectives on American Social Policy*, ed. Edward Zigler, Sharon Kagan and Edgar Klugman, 165–76. New York: Cambridge University Press.

Schorr, Lisbeth. 1988. *Within Our Reach: Breaking the Cycle of Disadvantage.* New York: Anchor Press.

Steiner, Gilbert. 1981. *The Futility of Family Policy*. Washington, D.C.: Brookings Institution.

I

Children's Health Needs, Health Status, and Legal Rights

1
Children's Health Status, Health Risks, and Use of Health Services

Barbara Starfield, M.D., M.P.H., and Paul Newacheck, Dr.P.H.

By traditional standards, children are relatively healthy, especially when compared to adults. With the exception of the first year of life, death rates are much lower and few problems recur frequently enough to command the attention given to adult conditions, such as coronary artery disease, cancer, hypertension, or Alzheimer's disease. By other criteria, however, children may be much more disadvantaged than is commonly recognized.

The Changing Health Problems of Children

Death rates in infancy and childhood have declined markedly during the twentieth century. Mortality rates in childhood (to age 15) declined 20–30 percent from 1975 to 1982 alone. The decline has been most noticeable in the case of infectious causes of death (Starfield, 1985a), but has also been recorded for injuries and poisonings, cancer, and respiratory conditions. Rates of hospitalization, average lengths of stay, and total days spent in the hospital have declined, although to a lesser degree (12 percent, 4 percent, and 15 percent, respectively, between 1980 and 1984; Table 1.1). These declines in inpatient rates, because they occurred entirely between 1980 and 1984, could well have been the result of several recent changes in the health care system (including the introduction of prospective hospital payment systems, the expansion of alternative forms of medical care organizations such as HMOs, as well as reductions in Medicaid eligibility for poor children) as much as a result of possible declines in morbidity.

Despite these declines, some health problems have increased in frequency. Death rates associated with homicide and suicide are now higher than they were in the mid-1970s. Hospitalization rates associated with asthma, perinatal problems, and mental health problems have been increasing. Even though lengths of stay for almost all types of problems (except mental problems) have declined, the total number of days spent in the hospital has increased for asthma, perinatal problems, and mental

Table 1.1 Hospitalizations, U.S. Children Ages 0–14, 1971–1985

Item	1971	1975	1980	1984	1985
Patients discharged per 10,000 children	702.3	714.9	717.6	620.1	571.9
Average length of stay (days)	4.7	4.6	4.4	4.5	4.6
Total days	3300.8	3288.5	3157.4	2790.5	2630.7

Source: Advance data from National Center for Health Statistics, Series 13, Nos. 16, 35, 74, 84.

Note: Excludes newborns.

illness (calculations from National Center for Health Statistics Series 13, Nos. 15, 35, 74, 84).

Accompanying the decline in mortality and morbidity due to acute illnesses has been an increase in chronic illness among children. A number of chronic conditions are prevalent among children (Table 1.2). Newacheck and colleagues (1984, 1986) documented an increase in the proportion of children with limitation of activity associated with chronic conditions, as reported by parents in the National Health Interview Survey. Rates of limitation of activity have doubled since 1960, as has the proportion of children with *major* limitation of activity.

Thus, although death rates have been declining and continue to decline at a marked rate, there is considerable cause for concern about the high frequency of many different types of problems experienced by children and about possible interactions between acute and chronic ailments in individual children.

The Frequency and Distribution of Health Problems in Children

Despite the increasing complexity of morbidity in children, the methods of measuring child health in use now are essentially the same as those used several decades ago (Starfield, 1985a). These methods ascertain the prevalence of conditions rather than the state of health of children, who may have varying numbers and types of conditions.

Table 1.2 indicates the major categories of conditions ranked in order of their frequency among deaths, hospitalizations, and abnormal physical examinations. The relative importance of particular conditions, at least in terms of their frequency, differs among these sources of information. This suggests that either a combination of methods or a new way of ascertaining information about morbidity is required to accurately characterize child health.

Table 1.3 indicates the approximate frequency of selected conditions in children as reported by a variety of health interview surveys. Only conditions with a frequency of more than one per thousand are

Table 1.2 Comparative Rank Orders According to Frequency of Child Health Conditions, United States

Deaths	Hospitalizations	Physical Examinations
1. Injuries/poisoning, incl. homicides	Respiratory problems	Dental problems
2. Cancer	Injuries/poisonings	Skin pathology
3. Congenital anomalies	Neurological problems	Ear problems
4. Respiratory problems	Infections	Eye problems
5. Circulatory problems	Congenital anomalies	Neuromuscular/joint problems
6. Infections	Genitourinary problems	Musculoskeletal problems
7. Ill-defined conditions	Ill-defined conditions	Cardiovascular problems
8. Mental problems, incl. suicides	Conditions of perinatal origin	
9. Neurological problems incl. meningitis	Skin/subcutaneous tissue problems	
10. Genitourinary problems	Musculoskeletal problems	

Sources: Deaths: U.S. Vital Statistics, Monthly Vital Statistic Reports (various years). Hospitalizations: U.S. Hospital Discharge Survey, Vital and Health Statistics, Series 13, various years. *Physical Examination:* U.S. Health Examination Surveys and U.S. Health and Nutrition Examination Survey, as summarized in Starfield and Budetti, 1985.

Note: Deaths age 1–14. Hospitalizations age 0–15, but excluding newborns. Rankings are approximate due to differences in ascertainment across the age groups (1–5, 6–11, 12–17) within childhood.

included, and common acute conditions (such as "colds," ear infections, and the "flu") are excluded. The sum of these individual frequencies is well over 500 per thousand, or one in every two children. As most children are in fact free of any of these conditions, it is clear that some children have more than one, and probably several. Although the extent of such clustering of health problems in the population of children is unknown, recent work is beginning to shed light on this phenomenon; new data show that health problems, even those not ordinarily thought of as genetic or congenital, tend to be concentrated in subgroups of children rather than distributed randomly throughout the population.

This concentration of health problems was illustrated by a study of children enrolled for extended periods of time in "prepaid" medical plans (Starfield et al., 1984). Over time, different types of illnesses tended to cluster in a relatively small proportion (about 30 percent) of children. Children with the most acute illnesses were also those who were most likely to experience the other types of morbidity. In addition, they contributed heavily to the use of health services. More than half (54 percent) of the children with constantly high use (in the top third of the distribution in each of two three-year periods) had a wide range of acute and chronic conditions (rather than specific chronic illnesses or conditions), as compared with only 25 percent of children whose use was not constantly high (Starfield et al., 1985d).

Table 1.3 Estimates of Prevalence of Selected Conditions per 1,000 Children Elicited by Various Surveys and the National Health Interview Survey (1979–81), United States

Condition	Various Surveys	Health Interview Survey
Mental/behavioral problems	100–150	N/A*
Elevated blood lead (above 25 microgm/dl)	90	N/A
Hay fever/seasonal allergy	36–40	54.9
Asthma	35	37.9
Visual problems with usual correction	30–40	9.6
Sinusitis	30	51.1
Orthopedic problems	28	19.8
Mental retardation	25	N/A
Hearing problems	10–16	16.7
Congenital health conditions	6	3.4
Seizures	3–4	3.1
Other chronic medical conditions		
Eczema, dermatitis, urticaria		39.1
Chronic bronchitis		37.5
Hypertrophied tonsils/adenoids		29.1
Diseases of sebaceous glands		22.8
Heart conditions		19.6
Speech impairment		15.9
Anemia		7.9
Other inflammation of skin		7.9
Urinary diseases		7.3
Migraine		5.6
Diseases of nail		4.8
Frequent constipation		4.6
Chronic enteritis/colitis		4.1
Umbilical hernia		3.2
Arthritis		3.1
Other skin diseases		2.8
Chronic laryngitis		2.6
Functional upper gastrointestinal disorder		2.2
Osteomyelitis		2.0
Nasal polyp		1.7

Sources: Gortmaker (1984); Starfield and Budetti (1985); Hankin and Starfield (1986); NCHS, August 1984. For Health Interview Survey, 1979–81: National Center for Health Statistics (1986).

*Not assessed.

Health Status and the Use of Health Services

Few national surveys have been directed at collecting information specifically about child health status. Most current national data sets were originally designed to collect information on adults or, at best, the population as a whole. This orientation has resulted in generally less reliable or useful data for children. In 1981, for the first time, a large national survey was conducted specifically to provide an information base on children's health status and use of medical services. This survey, the Child Health Supplement to the National Health Interview Survey, contained an extensive questionnaire entirely devoted to measuring the health of the U.S. noninstitutionalized population under age 18 (National Center for Health Statistics, 1982). The survey is described in more detail in the Appendix to this chapter.

Based on a checklist of child health problems included in the survey, it is estimated that 42 percent of all noninstitutionalized children under 18 years old had conditions in one or more of the morbidity categories shown in Figure 1.1 during the year before the interview. The leading morbidity category was *allergies,* which affected 12 percent of all children during the year before the interview. Following allergies, the most prevalent conditions included *chronic specialty problems, symptoms and signs, repeated ear infection,* and *chronic medical conditions.* The least prevalent morbidity categories included *dermatologic conditions, acute likely-to-recur conditions,* and *acute self-limited conditions.* Prevalence for the latter two morbidity categories is much lower than other information would suggest, due to the fact that many mild acute conditions were intentionally excluded from the checklist.

Results from prior research in specific clinical settings indicate that children can be clustered in groups with low, moderate, and high levels of morbidity. Analysis of child health supplement data explores the extent of such clustering in a general population over the year before the interview. As shown in Table 1.4, 58 percent of the children had no reported checklist conditions; 27 percent had reported conditions in only one morbidity category; 10 percent had reported conditions in two

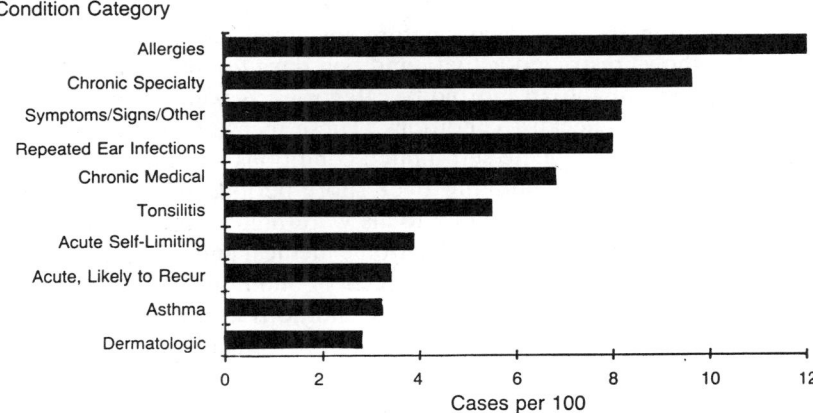

Figure 1.1 The prevalence of children's health problems in the United States, 1981

Source: Microdata from the 1981 National Health Interview Survey, Child Health Supplement

Table 1.4 The Burden of Illness for Children under 18 Years, United States, 1981

Subject	Population	Percent Distribution	Average Annual Bed Days	Average Annual Restricted Activity Days	Average Annual Physician Visits	Hospital Days per 1,000
Children with no checklist conditions	36,686,000	58.1	3.4	7.3	2.8	132
Children with conditions in one morbidity category	17,020,000	27.0	6.0	13.7	4.7	443
Children with conditions in two morbidity categories	6,535,000	10.3	8.9	18.8	7.4	625
Children with conditions in three or more morbidity categories	2,901,000	4.6	9.6	27.7	10.8	1,476
All children	63,142,000	100.0	5.1	11.1	4.2	329

Source: Microdata from the 1981 National Health Interview Survey, Child Health Supplement.

morbidity categories; and about 5 percent, or 2.9 million children under 18 years old, had conditions in three or more illness categories. These data suggest that a substantial number of children suffer from some combination of two or more types of illness.

To determine the severity of the conditions on the checklist, data on days spent ill in bed or otherwise restricted due to acute or chronic illnesses during the two weeks before the interview were examined. Table 1.5 shows restricted activity and bed days for children with conditions in each of the 10 morbidity categories as well as for children with no reported checklist conditions. These measures were relatively high for children with acute self-limited conditions and tonsillitis—conditions that can be debilitating over short periods of time. Among chronic conditions, disability day totals were highest for children with asthma, followed by children with chronic medical and chronic specialty conditions. Children with chronic specialty conditions had few average bed days and restricted activity days. Conditions in this morbidity category are primarily physical and mental impairments including vision, hearing and speech problems, mental retardation, and orthopedic impairments. Restricted activity day totals might be expected to be higher for such conditions, but the wording of the restricted activity day question emphasizes days on which a person cut down on his or her *usual* activities (National Center for Health Statistics, 1985b). Physically or

Table 1.5 The Severity of Health Problems among Children under 18 Years, United States, 1981

Condition Group	Average Number of Restricted Activity Days per Year	Average Number of Bed Disability Days per Year
1. Acute self-limiting	24.0	14.8
2. Allergies	16.9	6.7
3. Asthma	27.7	12.7
4. Repeated ear infections	22.8	10.4
5. Tonsillitis	24.3	10.4
6. Acute, likely to recur	17.6	8.4
7. Chronic medical	19.9	8.9
8. Chronic specialty	14.8	6.1
9. Dermatologic	11.0	3.8
10. Symptoms/signs/other	18.1	9.2
11. No reported conditions	7.3	3.4

Source: Microdata from the 1981 National Health Interview Survey, Child Health Supplement.

mentally impaired children may have permanently reduced their usual activities. Fewer restricted activity days does not therefore necessarily imply better functioning for these children.

The clustering of illness described above suggests that restricted activity and bed days also might be clustered among children. Analyses show this to be the case (see Table 1.4). Both bed days and restricted activity days were reported at low levels for children without any checklist conditions but progressively increased as the number of different morbidity categories experienced by children rose. For example, children with conditions in only one morbidity category experienced almost twice as many bed days as children with no checklist conditions, while almost three times as many bed days were reported for children with conditions in three or more morbidity categories.

The use of physician services varies substantially among children in the various morbidity categories. Reported physician's visits include visits for all reasons, including checkups and other preventive services, but exclude inpatient hospitalizations. Levels of use, based on two-week recall questions weighted to reflect annual totals, were highest for children with acute self-limited conditions, followed by repeated ear infections and asthma (Table 1.6). Levels of use were lowest for children with dermatologic conditions and children with no reported checklist conditions.

Like restricted activity days, physician visits were clustered according to the number of morbidity categories experienced. For example, children with conditions in three or more morbidity categories saw physicians nearly four times as often as did children with no checklist conditions. The 4.6 percent of children in this category accounted for 16

Table 1.6 The Use of Ambulatory and Hospital Services among Children under 18 Years, United States, 1981

Condition Group	Average Number of Physician Visits per Year	Number of Hospital Discharges per 100 per Year*	Hospital Days per 1,000 per Year
1. Acute self-limiting	11.0	30.3	2,034
2. Allergies	6.6	8.1	413
3. Asthma	8.1	17.7	1,125
4. Repeated ear infections	8.9	12.3	506
5. Tonsillitis	7.3	14.9	441
6. Acute, likely to recur	6.7	14.1	1,285
7. Chronic medical	7.5	18.8	1,235
8. Chronic specialty	6.2	12.0	736
9. Dermatologic	4.2	4.8	192
10. Symptoms/signs/other	6.5	17.4	1,086
11. No reported conditions	2.8	2.9	132

Source: Microdata from the 1981 National Health Interview Survey, Child Health Supplement.

*Includes multiple admissions.

percent of all physician visits; the 15 percent of children with conditions in two or more categories accounted for 32 percent of all physician visits.

Two measures of hospital care are available from the Health Interview Survey: the number of hospital episodes per hundred and the number of hospital days per thousand. During 1981, 5.4 percent of all noninstitutionalized children had at least one hospital episode and 14 percent of hospitalized children had multiple hospital stays. Discharge rates and days spent hospitalized were highest for children with acute self-limited health conditions; children in this group experienced 10 times as many hospital discharges and 15 times as many nights hospitalized as did children with no reported checklist conditions (Table 1.6). After acute self-limited conditions, children with asthma, acute likely-to-recur conditions, and chronic medical conditions ranked as the highest users of hospital services. Children with these conditions used between 8 and 10 times the amount of inpatient hospital days as children with no reported checklist conditions. Among children with checklist conditions, the lowest rates of hospital use were found for those afflicted by dermatologic conditions.

Table 1.4 showed how hospital days varied by the number of morbidity categories experienced by children. Dramatic differences in hospital use were apparent; children with conditions in three or more morbidity categories had more than 10 times the number of hospital days as children with no checklist conditions. Stated differently, the 4.6 percent of children with conditions in three or more morbidity categories accounted for 20.6 percent of all hospital days; the 15 percent of children with conditions in two or more categories accounted for more than 40 percent of all hospital days.

Taken together, these findings indicate that health status and use of medical care services are unevenly distributed across the child population. The majority of children use few physician services and very few hospital services. A substantial minority of noninstitutionalized children suffer from multiple health problems and account for a large share of medical care services, especially those provided by hospitals.

Children at Risk

To what extent is high risk concentrated in the population? Who are the children who have more than their share of morbidity? Although the precise answers to these questions are not known, there is mounting evidence that much of the excess morbidity is concentrated in groups of children who have been exposed to risks of particular types. These types of risks include those that are sociodemographic and environmental, those that are rooted in social and physical behaviors, those that are genetic or biological, and those that are associated with prior illness experiences (Starfield, 1984).

Sociodemographic Risk

The 20–25 percent of children who are in low-income families are at increased risk of experiencing certain health problems. They are also at increased risk of experiencing complications or sequelae from these conditions. Table 1.7 indicates the magnitude of the excess risk from just some of these conditions; poor children are at increased risk of all but a few conditions. Poor children are two to three times more likely to experience many of the conditions, and two to four times as likely to have complications or sequelae from them.

Children in families with divorce, who comprise about one-third of all children, have double to triple the risk of being suspended or expelled from school or having a school behavior problem, and three to five times the likelihood of experiencing a mental health consultation (Peterson and Zill, 1986; Zill, 1988).

Perinatal Risk

Children born weighing less than 2501 grams, about 7 percent of all infants, are three times as likely to have long-term neurologic sequelae as other children, twice as likely to have one or more congenital anom-

Table 1.7 The Approximate Relative Frequency of Selected Health Problems in Low-income Children

Condition	Relative Frequency in Low-income Children
Neonatal mortality	1.5 times
Postneonatal mortality	double-triple
Child deaths	triple-quadruple
Low birthweight	double
Teenage births	triple*
Delayed immunizations	triple
Asthma	higher
Complications of appendicitis	double-triple
Diabetic ketoacidosis	double
Rheumatic fever	double-triple
Bacterial meningitis	double
Complications of bacterial meningitis	double-triple
Lead poisoning	triple

Source: Based on Starfield (1985).
*Estimated on the basis of white/black differentials.

alies, 50 percent more likely to be hospitalized in their first year of life, twice as likely to be rehospitalized if hospitalized, and, for those whose birth weight is less than 1500 grams, have 50 percent more physician visits in a year (McCormick, 1985).

Environmental Risk

Although the full nature of this risk is not known, there is information indicating the risk of at least one potent environmental agent: lead. Lead is ubiquitous in the environment (Farfel, 1985). Infants with umbilical cord blood lead levels of greater than 10 micrograms per deciliter, who comprise about 10 percent of all infants, are at twice the risk of a congenital anomaly and have an average 6–8 point deficit in IQ when tested at six months and two years of age (Bellinger et al., 1984). Almost one in ten children in the population has an elevated blood lead level, which put him or her at increased risk of impaired growth (Schwartz et al., 1986), lowered IQ, and poor classroom behavior (Needleman et al., 1984).

Behavioral Risk

Individuals who smoke are at twice the risk of cancer, 10 times the risk of lung cancer, 1.7 times the risk of coronary artery disease, and 1.5 times the risk of hospitalization than are individuals who do not smoke. Those who smoke frequently are at even greater risk (Office of Disease Prevention and Health Promotion, Office of Smoking and Health, 1985).

Smoking is also associated with a variety of poor pregnancy outcomes (U.S. Department of Health and Human Services, 1980).

Substance abuse is believed to increase greatly the risk of a variety of adverse outcomes, despite the absence of data from methodologically sound epidemiologic case-control or prospective studies. Adverse effects on the individual depend on the substance, but include fatal and nonfatal overdose, hepatitis-B infection, acquired immune deficiency syndrome, bacterial endocarditis, accidents and injuries, low birth weight and dysmorphogenesis in offspring, suicide and psychiatric problems, and interference with school achievement. Several case reports also suggest a greater than expected frequency of complications of labor and delivery. Teenage drivers accounted for 15 percent of all alcohol-related fatal crashes in the United States in 1985, but only 7 percent of the licensed drivers. In a study in California, 63 percent of 15- to 19-year-old fatally injured male drivers had elevated blood alcohol concentrations; 37 percent had elevated levels of cannabinoids (Williams, 1983–85). The extent of excess risk from substance abuse is provided by a ten-year follow-up of adolescents identified in grades 10–11 in New York State. Those who reported using illicit drugs were more likely than others to report a mental health hospitalization, being depressed, and seeing a mental health professional; the extent of increased risk was of the order of three- to fivefold (Kandel, 1985).

A History of Illness

Children who are sick—even with conditions not generally considered chronic—often continue to have health problems in the future (Starfield and Pless, 1980). Those with *general* health problems in childhood are also more likely to have them as adolescents (Table 1.8). For example, children who took regular medication when 6–11 years old were six times as likely to need medication when 12–17.

Selected problems reported by young black urban teenagers also are likely to persist to early adulthood (Starfield, 1981). Some of the reported problems (asthma, trouble hearing, hay fever or allergy, menstrual problems), were five times as likely to occur in adolescence if they initially occurred in childhood. This persistence was also found, to a lesser extent, among acute illnesses such as frequent colds, shortness of breath, stomach pains, repeated sinus trouble, sore throats, dizziness or fainting, shaking or trembling, vomiting, earaches, nosebleeds, and frequent diarrhea. The difference in risk between the group with the condition early in adolescence and the group without it was statistically significant for 23 of 33 conditions. Conversely, conditions present in the later period were frequently present earlier.

Table 1.8 The Risk of Persistence of Selected General Measures of Ill Health in Children

Taking regular medication	6.4
Hearing problems	11.1
Walking problems	19.4
Restricted activity	25.9
Frequent school absence for illness	3.6

Source: Calculated from data in Starfield and Pless (1980).

Note: Numbers are the ratio of the observed to expected prevalences of the condition in two time periods. The numerator is that proportion of children who had the problem both at childhood and adolescence. The denominator is the expected prevalence in both time periods if the two prevalences were random.

The source of information was the Health Examination Survey conducted by the National Center for Health Statistics in the early and mid-1960s. By design, a sample of households was visited in both waves of the survey so that children who were 6–11 years old in the first survey were reexamined in the second wave when they were age 12–17.

A similar persistence has been found for children who are high users of medical services. Children who fall in the upper third of the distribution of number of physician visits in early childhood have two to three times the risk of being high users later in childhood, compared to the average child.

Thus, there appears to be a group of children whose earlier problems are associated with great risk of subsequent problems. Since these earlier problems are themselves concentrated among specific groups of children, intervention and policies may be made more effective by targeting them to these groups.

It is important to note that persistence of illness is not confined to problems widely considered chronic. Targeting should therefore focus on individuals rather than on particular diagnoses.

Implications of the Concept of Risk

Table 1.9 shows how widespread even a few selected risk states are among children in the United States. If each risk state were independent of the other, most children would require extra services or interventions to reduce their likelihood of illness. On the other hand, if these risk states were associated with each other or interacted with each other, perhaps only a small minority of children would require this added attention.

Unfortunately, little is known about the degree of interaction or clustering of genetic, biological, sociodemographic, environmental, and health service factors that predispose to illness. The absence of such information leads to two possible courses of action: (1) to treat all children as potentially at risk, because of the prevalence of risk rates; or (2) to provide extra services to children in each of the risk groups

Table 1.9 Selected Risk States, United States, 1985

Risk Factor	Percentage of Children
Sociodemographic	
Poor children	20–25
Children in families with divorce	32
Perinatal	
Children born at low birthweight	7
Environmental	
Perinatal exposure to lead (cord/blood levels ≥ 10 microgms/dl)	10
Children with elevated blood lead levels	9
Behavioral	
Children using illicit drugs	5
Children who smoke	20
Children who drink heavily*	37
Use of health services	
Children with persistently high use of services	13

Sources: Johnston et al. (1985); Bellinger and Needleman (1984); Furstenberg et al. (1983); Peterson and Zill (1986); Starfield et al. (1979); and National Center for Health Statistics (1984).

*5 or more drinks in a row in 2 weeks.

separately. The policy implications of these widely discrepant approaches to health services are discussed in the next section.

Policy Implications

Five themes and their six implications for policy follow from the analyses in this chapter.

A. *Changing Health Needs and Appropriate Data Collection*

Child health needs have changed over the past several decades. In contrast, the tools used to measure and monitor child health status are essentially the same as those used fifty years ago.

Policy implication. *There is a pressing need for the development and application of new tools of measurement of child health status.*

The measurement of child health status should address at least seven domains.

1. *Longevity or projected life expectancy.* Although information to predict life expectancy for various population subgroups is rudimentary, existing life tables provide such information for major demographic categories in the population. More concerted efforts to assess risks

in other population subgroups could provide better information to make this a useful dimension in a health status profile.
2. *Activity and limitation of activity.* Instruments to assess the extent of ability and disability in children with and without chronic illnesses have been recently tested and refined (for example, Stein et al., 1985). These types of instruments, which have been developed for several child age groups, are suitable for incorporation in a more general health status measure.
3. *Comfort.* Any adequate measure of health should ascertain the presence of symptoms that are disturbing to children and may interfere with their achievement. Efforts to develop a method to categorize symptoms (Lamberts et al., 1985) offer an opportunity to incorporate this dimension into a child health status measure.
4. *Satisfaction with health.* In addition to an overall measure of the extent to which the child (or adult proxy) is satisfied with the child's state of health, this domain might also include assessment of the extent to which the demands of a medical regimen (such as the taking of medication, adherence to a prescribed regimen of activities, or requirements to keep appointments with health professionals) interfere with the child's sense of well-being.
5. *Disease rate.* This domain includes the types of measures that were the basis for the data in earlier parts of this chapter. Information obtained by various means, including health interviews and medical examinations, would be combined into categories that reflect the likelihood of persistence as well as the nature of the care required to deal with the type of conditions experienced by the child.
6. *Achievement.* In this domain are characteristics that include children's psychological and social performance. In recent years, considerable experience has been gained with measurement in this sphere (Eisen et al., 1979; Hankin and Starfield, 1986).
7. *Resilience versus vulnerability.* This domain incorporates the extent to which children are able to cope with threats to their health. Immunization status is a clear example in the biologic realm; adequate immunization is clearly associated with greatly reduced susceptibility to particular illnesses. An equally promising set of measures would tap health behaviors that predispose to good health, such as diet, exercise, and the avoidance of harmful practices such as smoking and drug misuse.

B. *Children Who Have High Burdens of Illness*

Recent data indicate that about 15 percent of children experience several types of illnesses within a year; over a six-year period, about twice this proportion will experience several types of illnesses. In any several-year period, approximately one in eight children is a persistently high user of services throughout the period.

Policy implication. *It is now possible to determine, a priori, those children who are at risk of being high users of services. Children who have been high users in the recent past, or children who have experienced several types of illnesses, are at high risk of making relatively large demands on the health care system. Therefore, facilities that undertake to provide care for a fixed negotiated fee should be compensated at higher rates for those children who require more services.*

In prepaid managed health care in which facilities contract to provide services for a defined population of children, extra compensation for needy children could take one of two forms. Capitation rates could be set at a higher level for these children. Alternatively, payment of care for these children could be on a fee-for-service basis rather than a prepayment basis.

Adverse selection can be particularly problematic for organized health systems that include large proportions of low-income children. Analyses similar to those reported in the following section, but examining for differences according to family income, indicate that children in lower-income families have greater frequencies of severe illness and greater likelihood of experiencing more types of illness (Newacheck and Starfield, 1988). These findings suggest that prospective financing based on community rating, adjusted for differences in health status between communities, would be feasible. Payment for services adjusted by need would greatly improve the incentives for health organizations to enroll low-income children.

C. The Coexistence of Physical and Psychosocial Problems

Recent data show a strong tendency for several types of health conditions to cluster in certain children. That is, children with repeated acute illnesses tend to be the children with more chronic illnesses, and children with various types of persisting illnesses tend to have persisting illnesses of other types. For example, children with psychosocial problems are at higher risk of having various types of physical problems.

Policy implication. *Psychosocial problems should not be viewed in isolation from physical problems, either in clinical settings or in the financing of services.*

More attention needs to be given to psychosocial problems in children, as they are both frequent and underrecognized (Hankin and Starfield, 1986). New and well-validated methods to screen for such problems should be judiciously applied and used to detect both the problems themselves and any related problems that may coexist.

D. Characterizing Risks of Poor Health

Although several types of factors are known to increase the risk of ill health, little is known about the extent to which various combinations of risks coexist in particular individuals or how often these combinations change over time and with new policy initiatives. As a result, we do not know whether the proportion of children at increased risk is small or large and whether it is increasing, decreasing, or staying stable. For example, low birth weight and poverty are known to be highly correlated. Are risk-taking behaviors, family disruption, and environmental exposure to toxicants equally correlated with low birth weight and poverty or with each other and are these correlations becoming stronger or weaker?

Policy implication. *The need for continued and expanded data collection and analysis is acute. Existing national surveys should be maintained and improved and state and local data collection should be encouraged and supported.*

The possibility of deterioration of health status, as occurred during the middle and late 1950s (Starfield, 1985b) and perhaps again in the early 1980s (Miller et al., 1985), suggests the need for a system of national accounting based upon periodic assessment of health status. The Child Health Supplement of the National Health Interview Survey, which provided data for some of the analyses presented in this chapter, should be repeated at regular intervals to monitor changes in child health in the population and in selected subgroups of the population. Changes in public policy that reduce access to medical services, such as cutbacks in the Medicaid program or decreased support for unemployed families, may be followed by changes in the health status of certain segments of the population. Periodic monitoring of health status, with particular attention to those who may be at this added risk, will serve to alert the public to these unintended effects.

Enhanced analyses of existing and future data should be encouraged for the purpose of providing new insights into the interaction between important risk factors. To assess the extent of impact of various risk factors, both alone and in combination, it will be necessary to provide for the collection of information on individuals over time. The capability for this longitudinal approach already exists in the form of follow-back surveys conducted by the National Center for Health Statistics. In particular, the National Natality Follow-back Survey should be maintained and expanded so that individuals can be recontacted periodically through childhood. Similar follow-up should be instituted for subsamples of the ongoing health interview surveys and health examination surveys and for special surveys such as the National Longitudinal Survey of Youth.

E. *Identifying Children at High Risk of Poor Health*

Although we now know the frequencies of most important health conditions, the frequency of some of the important states of risk, and the excess risk posed by some of the risk states, we still do not know how to identify children at high risk in their communities. The current approach to dealing with this situation is to develop interventions to deal with each health condition separately. Thus, there are programs to finance care for children with certain chronic conditions, teenagers prone to pregnancy, low-birth-weight infants, and some poor children (depending on where they live and their family circumstances). No one knows the extent to which this fragmentation of services leads to a situation in which the same children are covered by more than one program, although duplication is widely recognized as a problem.

Policy implication. *Comprehensive, coordinated, community-based services for children should be developed on a wide scale. Incentives for technology-intensive, high-cost care should be replaced with incentives for identifying children at highest risk and providing preventive interventions for reducing that risk.*

The changing burden of illness in children in general, as evident from increased rates of hospitalization associated with several types of morbidity, increased survival of infants with variety of types of minor handicaps (Shapiro et al., 1983), and increased levels of disability, argue for more attention to systems of health services based upon the identification of defined population groups who are followed over time with coordinated services. In this approach all children are viewed as potentially at risk. Such an approach can be justified by the high prevalence of the different types of risk. Even though important clusters of risks may be found in only a segment of the child population at any one time, children may move in and out of vulnerable situations over time, leaving many at risk at some point in their lives.

F. *Reducing Fragmentation*

The health care system is characterized by extraordinary fragmentation. As a result, no mechanism provides for accountability of the health services in meeting and dealing with the needs of children.

Policy implication. *Until a more coherent national health policy is feasible, federalize Medicaid, standardize eligibility requirements, and extend them to include a broader definition of medical need for children in low-income families.*

Children in low-income families are at increased risk of most health problems. Access to medical care in the form of Medicaid reduces the degree of excess risk. Whereas the proportion of children in poverty has risen over the most recent few years, Medicaid eligibility and benefits have been shrinking. Moreover, states vary enormously in the extent to which they provide Medicaid for needy families. A federalized policy would at least assure equity across the country.

G. A National Health Policy

The United States is among the very few industrialized countries to lack a national health policy for children. Instead, funding and service delivery responsibilities are spread across a number of federal, state, and local agencies. This lack of a coherent focus leads to duplication, fragmentation, and inequity.

Policy implication. *Develop a national health policy for children.*

The Western European nations, with whom we share considerable cultural heritage and many common interests, have had such policies for many years. Most Western nations rely very little on means-tested public assistance (welfare) as the means of assuring the basic necessities of living. Instead, they rely on universal income transfers, the most notable of which are child and family allowances and maternity benefits. They view families with children as targets of social policy with explicit concern for the well-being of children (Kahn and Kamerman, 1983).

In Western European nations, a separate preventive service for mothers and children has long been in existence. Every woman is entitled to prenatal care and costs are met largely from general revenues. Except in Great Britain (where the situation changed in 1974), local health authorities are responsible for well-baby, perinatal, and school health services. Preventive care is assured by law in many of the countries. In the Netherlands, for example, all Dutch children must be examined for handicapping conditions within six weeks of birth, at least four times before school entrance, several times during school attendance, and on leaving school. The data are collected and published for planning purposes. In Sweden and Denmark, local councils establish committees on children and youth which have the job of gathering information on child health and welfare. Sweden and Finland, as well as France, rely almost entirely on nurses to provide preventive care, under the supervision of physicians. In France, medical examinations are required by law at eight days, nine months, and two years, and the results are computerized and published. Sweden focuses on an examination at age four to provide remediation of identified defects well in advance of school entry (Silver, 1978).

An orderly transition to a national health policy for children in this country might start with the youngest age group (infants and preschool children). This procedure would have the advantage of focusing first on those children with the most potential to benefit from preventive interventions. Furthermore, other industrialized nations have started with the youngest ages and worked to include children at progressively older ages.

Conclusions

The problems of measuring child health and the nature and distribution of ill health in the child population have not received the attention they deserve. Both social and technological advances have increased the survival of those who heretofore would have died in infancy and early childhood from congenital and metabolic abnormalities, infections, and most other causes of death. If these survivors are compromised in their ability to ward off subsequent problems, the frequency of illness in childhood is likely to increase. Furthermore, the frequency of several risks to ill health may be increasing. The potential impact of ill health in childhood on subsequent health status and its implications for productivity of the future generation of adults have received much less attention than they deserve. Despite implications to the contrary, access to appropriate health services can improve child health and reduce disparities in health status across subgroups of children (Starfield, 1985b). If children have traditionally appeared healthy, it is largely because adult standards of health have been applied. A comprehensive perspective indicates that much more concern and remedial effort is warranted.

Appendix: The Child Health Supplement

The Child Health Supplement to the National Health Interview Survey was administered to a random sample of 41,000 households in all 50 states and the District of Columbia by Census Bureau interviewers working under contract to the National Center for Health Statistics. In each household where children were present, one child was selected at random to be the subject of an in-depth interview. In total, some 15,416 children under 18 years old were surveyed. The overall response rate exceeded 93 percent. In general, a parent (most often the mother) served as the respondent for the interviews. The questionnaire contained extensive probes on family background, prenatal care, child care, motor and social development, and a variety of other topics related to child health (National Center for Health Statistics, 1985a). Of particular importance was the inclusion of a detailed checklist of physical childhood health problems. Probes ascertained the lifetime prevalence of 59 childhood health conditions ranging from tonsillitis to cystic fibrosis but excluding minor acute illnesses, such as the cold, the "flu," and minor injuries. The large sample combined with this lengthy checklist provides an opportunity to examine children's health problems in a more comprehensive fashion than was possible from past national surveys. In addition, data from the Child Health Supplement are linked to data from the core questionnaire of the National Health Interview Survey, permitting analysis of hospital and ambulatory care use for different types of childhood conditions.

Because mental and nervous conditions are generally underreported in household interviews (National Center for Health Statistics, 1967), only limited numbers of such conditions were included on the checklist. For the purposes of describing the relationship between morbidity and use, we restricted our analysis to conditions that were present during the year before the interview. As a result, prevalence estimates presented in the remainder of this chapter refer to annual prevalence.

The conditions ascertained in the Child Health Supplement were grouped into morbidity categories based upon a method described elsewhere (Starfield et al., 1984). This categorization scheme was developed to examine the relationship between ill health and the use of services over long periods of time. The underlying rationale for the grouping was the extent to which a condition was likely to persist and whether or not it would be likely to require services other than primary care over a period of time.

As the Child Health Supplement condition list did not contain all of the separate diseases that children would experience and was particularly deficient in acute self-limited conditions, injuries, and psychosocial problems, modifications were made in the original categorization. In particular, psychosomatic conditions were subsumed in a *symptoms and signs* category, mental and developmental problems were subsumed under the *chronic specialty* category, and the *injuries* category had to be eliminated. Where certain usually acute conditions (such as hepatitis and meningitis) were reported as present more than three months, they were categorized as *likely-to-recur conditions*. Conditions reported as "other" (such as "other digestive conditions" or "other respiratory diseases") were categorized as *acute self-limited* if present three or fewer

Table 1.A Child Health Supplement Condition Groups

Group 1: Acute Self-Limiting (conditions present 3 months or less)
 1 Hepatitis
 3 Other liver trouble
 5 Other bowel trouble
 9 Digestive system disease
 15 Pneumonia
 16 Other lung, pulmonary, or respiratory condition
 30 Skin allergy
 31 Other genitourinary conditions
 33 Other skin trouble
 60 Meningitis
 63 Nephritis
 64 Urinary infection
 65 Other kidney trouble
 68 Other thyroid trouble
 77 Other heart trouble

Group 2: Allergies
 8 Allergy, respiratory
 11 Hay fever
 17 Allergy, other and multiple
 27 Eczema

Group 3: Asthma
 10 Asthma

Group 4: Repeated Ear Infections
 34 Repeated ear infections

Group 5: Tonsillitis
 12 Tonsillitis, enlarged adenoids and/or tonsils

Group 6: Acute, Likely to Recur (conditions present more than 3 months)
 1 Hepatitis
 15 Pneumonia
 30 Skin allergy
 60 Meningitis
 63 Nephritis
 64 Urinary infection

Group 7: Chronic Medical
 3 Other liver trouble*
 4 Colitis
 5 Other bowel trouble*
 7 Hernia or rupture
 9 Digestive system disease*
 13 Allergy, digestive
 14 Tuberculosis
 16 Other lung, pulmonary, or respiratory condition*
 18 Arthritis
 19 Rheumatism
 24 Ulcer, other
 31 Other genitourinary conditions*
 33 Other skin trouble*
 54 Epilepsy
 55 Convulsions (repeated)
 56 Seizures (repeated)
 57 Blackouts (repeated)
 58 Migraine
 61 Chorea
 62 St. Vitus' dance
 65 Other kidney trouble*
 66 Diabetes
 67 Goiter trouble
 68 Other thyroid trouble

 69 Cystic fibrosis
 71 Sickle cell anemia
 72 Rheumatic fever
 73 Rheumatic fever disease
 74 Congenital heart disease
 75 High blood pressure
 77 Other heart trouble*
 78 Cancer (any kind)

Group 8: Chronic Specialty
 20 Curvature of spine
 21 Trouble with flat feet
 22 Clubfoot
 23 Tendon, muscle, or cartilage disease
 26 Bone disease
 35 Deafness
 36 Trouble hearing/one ear
 37 Trouble hearing/both ears
 38 Other hearing trouble
 39 Blindness
 40 Cataracts
 41 Trouble seeing/one eye
 42 Trouble seeing/both eyes
 43 Other trouble seeing
 44 Cleft palate
 45 Harelip
 46 Stammering and stuttering
 47 Other eye trouble
 48 Other speech defect
 49 Autistic
 50 Cerebral palsy
 51 Other palsy
 52 Paralysis
 53 Mental retardation
 79 Missing finger
 80 Missing hand
 81 Missing arm
 82 Missing toe
 83 Missing foot
 84 Missing leg
 85 Permanent stiffness in back
 86 Permanent stiffness in foot
 87 Permanent stiffness in leg
 88 Permanent stiffness in fingers
 89 Permanent stiffness in hand
 90 Permanent stiffness in arm
 91 Other stiffness
 92 Deformed back
 93 Deformed foot
 94 Deformed leg
 95 Deformed fingers
 96 Deformed hand
 97 Deformed arm
 98 Other deformities

Group 9: Dermatologic
 28 Psoriasis
 29 Trouble with acne

Group 10: Symptoms/Signs/Other
 2 Yellow jaundice
 6 Ulcer of skin
 32 Skin rash
 59 Headaches
 70 Anemia
 76 Heart murmur
 99 Other, nec

*If present more than 3 months.

months or as *chronic medical* if present more than three months. Thus, the frequency distribution of morbidity types as ascertained in the Child Health Supplement would not be expected to be similar to those in the prior study (where every illness in the six-year period was known and separately categorized) but the concept underlying the categorization is the same. A list of the 10 morbidity categories used in this chapter and the Child Health Supplement conditions included in each is presented in Table 1.A.

Notes

1. To provide a proxy measure of severity, these days were summed across individuals in each diagnostic category and weighted to reflect average annual bed day and restricted activity day totals. Since the bed and restricted activity day totals reflect disability due to any acute or chronic illness (including those due to conditions not included on the checklist), their use as *absolute* measures of severity for particular morbidity categories is limited. They are, however, useful *relative* indicators of severity, assuming that bed days and restricted activity days due to conditions not included in the morbidity categories being compared were randomly distributed.

References

Annest, J., and K. Mahaffey. 1984. Blood Lead Levels for Persons Ages 6 Months–74 Years, United States, 1976–1980. *Vital and Health Statistics,* Series 11, No. 233. DHHS Publication No. 84-1683. Washington, D.C.: G.P.O.

Annest, J., K. Mahaffey, D. Cox, and J. Roberts. 1982. Blood Levels for Persons 6 Months–74 Years of Age: United States, 1976–1980. *Vital and Health Statistics.* Advance data No. 79, National Center for Health Statistics. DHHS Publication No. 82-1250. Washington, D.C.: G.P.O.

Bellinger, D., H. Needleman, A. Leviton, C. Waternaux, M. Rabinowitz, and M. Nichols. 1984. Early Sensory-Motor Development and Prenatal Exposure to Lead. *Neurobehavioral Toxicology* 6:387–402.

Eisen, M., J. Ware, C. Donald, and R. Brook. 1979. Measuring Components of Children's Health Status. *Medical Care* 17:902–921.

Farfel, M. 1985. Reducing Lead Exposure in Children. *Annual Review of Public Health* 6:333–360.

Furstenburg, F., C. Nord, J. Peterson, and N. Zill. 1983. The Life Course of Children with Divorce. *American Social Review* 48:656–668.

Gortmaker, S., and W. Sappenfield. 1984. Chronic Childhood Disorders: Prevalence and Impact. *Pediatric Clinics of North America* 31:3–17.

Hankin, J., and B. Starfield. 1986. Epidemiologic Perspectives on Psychosocial Problems in Children. In N. Krasnegor, J. Arasteh, and M. Cataldo (eds.), *Child Health Behavior,* pp. 70–93. New York: John Wiley and Sons.

Johnston, L., P. O'Malley, and J. Bachman. 1985. *Use of Licit and Illicit Drugs by America's High School Students, 1975–1984,* p. 46. National Institute of Drug Abuse. DHHS Publication No. (ADM) 85-1394. Rockville, Md.

Kahn, A., and S. Kamerman. 1983. Income Maintenance, Wages and Family Income. *Public Welfare* 41(4):23–30.

Kandel, D., D. Murphy, and D. Karus. 1985. Cocaine Use in Young Adulthood: Patterns of Use and Psychosocial Correlates. In N. Kozel and E. Adams (eds.), *Cocaine Use in America: Epidemiologic and Clinical Perspectives.* NIDA Research Monograph 51, DHHS, Rockville, Md.

Lamberts, H., S. Meads, and M. Wood. 1984. Classification of Reasons Why Persons Seek Primary Care: Pilot Study of a New System. *Public Health Reports* 99:597–605.

McCormick, M. 1985. The Contribution of Low Birth Weight to Infant Mortality and Childhood Morbidity. *New England Journal of Medicine* 312:82–90.

Mahaffey, K., J. Annest, J. Roberts, and R. Murphy. 1982. National Estimates of Blood Lead Levels: United States, 1976–1980: Association with Selected Demographic and Socioeconomic Factors. *New England Journal of Medicine* 307:573–579.

Miller, C.A., E. Coulter, A. Fine, S. Adams-Taylor, and L. Schorr. 1985. 1984 Update on the World Economic Crisis and Children: A United States Case Study. *International Journal of Health Services* 15:431–450.

National Center for Health Statistics. 1967. Interview Data on Chronic Conditions Compared with Information Derived from Medical Records, Series 2, No. 23. DHHS Publication No. 1000. Washington, D.C.: G.P.O.

———. 1982. Current Estimates from the Health Interview Survey: United States, 1981. *Vital and Health Statistics,* Series 10, No. 141. DHEW Publication No. (PHS) 82-1569. Hyattsville, Md.

———. Utilization of Short-Stay Hospitals, United States. *Vital and Health Statistics.* Hyattsville, Md.

1971: DHEW (HRA) Publication No. 75-1767, 1974 Series 13, No. 16.
1975: DHEW (PHS) Publication No. 78-1786, 1978 Series 13, No. 35.
1980: DHHS (PHS) Publication No. 83-1735, 1983 Series 13, No. 74.
1984: DHHS (PHS) Publication No. 86-1745, 1986 Series 13, No. 84.

National Center for Health Statistics. 1985a. National Health Interview Survey Child Health Supplement for 1981: Public Use Tape Record (Outline of items and codes). Hyattsville, Md.

———. 1985b. Persons Injured and Disability Days Due to Injuries: United States, 1980–1981. *Vital and Health Statistics,* Series 10, No. 149. DHHS Publication No. 85-1577. Washington, D.C.: G.P.O.

———. 1986, September 25. 1985 Summary, National Hospital Discharge Survey. Advance Data from *Vital and Health Statistics* No. 127. DHHS Publication No. 86-1250. Hyattsville, Md.: Public Health Service.

Needleman, H., and D. Bellinger. 1984. The Developmental Consequences of Childhood Exposure to Lead. *Advances in Clinical and Child Psychology* 7:195–220.

Newacheck, P., P. Budetti, and P. McManus. 1984. Trends in Childhood Disability. *American Journal of Public Health* 74:232–236.

Newacheck, P., N. Halfon, and P. Budetti. 1986. Prevalence of Activity Limiting Chronic Conditions among Children Based on Household Interviews. *Journal of Chronic Disease* 39(2):63–71.

Newacheck, P., and B. Starfield. 1988. Morbidity and Use of Ambulatory Care Services among Poor and Nonpoor Children. *American Journal of Public Health* 78:927–933.

Office of Disease Prevention and Health Promotion and Office on Smoking and Health (ODPHP/OSH). 1985. *A Decision Maker's Guide to Reducing Smoking at the Worksite.* Washington, D.C.: Washington Business Group on Health.

Peterson, J., and N. Zill. 1986. Marital Disruption, Parent-Child Relationships and Behavioral Problems in Children. *Journal of Marriage and Family* 48:295–307.

Schwartz, J., C. Angle, and H. Pitcher. 1986. Relationship between Childhood Blood Lead Levels and Stature. *Pediatrics* 77:281–288.

Shapiro, S., M. McCormick, B. Starfield, and B. Crawley. 1983. Changes in Infant Morbidity Associated with Decreases in Neonatal Mortality. *Pediatrics* 72:408–415.

Silver, G.A. 1978. *Child Health: America's Future.* Germantown, Md.: Aspen Publications.

Starfield, B. 1985a. Giant Steps and Baby Steps: Toward Child Health. *American Journal of Public Health* 75:599–604.

———. 1985b. *Effectiveness of Medical Care: Validating Clinical Wisdom.* Baltimore: Johns Hopkins University Press.

Starfield, B., and P. Budetti. 1985. Child Health Status and Risk Factors. *Health Services Research* 19(pt. II):817–886.

Starfield, B., J. Hankin, D. Steinwachs, S. Horn, P. Benson, H. Katz, and A. Gabriel. 1985. Utilization and Morbidity: Random or Tandem? *Pediatrics* 75(2):241–247.

Starfield, B., B. van den Berg, D. Steinwachs, H. Katz, and S. Horn. 1984. Morbidity in Childhood: A Longitudinal View. *New England Journal of Medicine* 310:824–829.

Stein, R.E.K., and D.J. Jessop. 1985. Further Development of a Functional Status Measure for Chronically Ill Children. Final Report to the William T. Grant Foundation, 1985.

U.S. Department of Health and Human Services. 1980. *The Health Consequences of Smoking for Women: The Surgeon General's Report.* Washington, D.C.: DHHS, Public Health Service.

Waller, J. 1986. State Liquor Laws as Enablers for Impaired Drinking and Other Impaired Behaviors. *American Journal of Public Health* 76:787–792.

Williams, A. 1983–85. Fatal Motor Crashes Involving Teenagers. *Pediatrician* 12:37–40.

Wynn, M., and A. Wynn. 1979. Some Developments in Child Health Care in Europe. *Royal Society of Health Journal* 99(6):259–264.

Zill, M. 1988. Behaviors, Achievements and Health Problems among Children in Stepfamilies. Findings from a National Survey of Child Health, in E. Mavis Hetherington and J. Arasteh (eds.), *The Impact of Divorce, Single-Parenting and Step-Parenting in Children.* Hillside, N.J.: Earlbaum.

2

Health Care for Children with Special Needs

Ann B. Taylor, Ed.D., Susan G. Epstein, M.S.W., and Allen C. Crocker, M.D.

This chapter examines the health care needs of a special population of children, those with chronic illness or disabling conditions, and the capacity of current health care financing and delivery systems to meet those needs. In our assessment, the present system fails to support adequately family involvement in the planning for care, and inadequately meets the health-related needs of these children and their families. In addition, innovative organizational and financing mechanisms in American health care, though beneficial to other groups, may exacerbate problems faced by children with costly specialized needs.

Who Are These Children?

For present purposes, we define "chronic illness" as any illness of extended duration or with effects of extended duration, and "disabling condition (or disability)" as any condition that interferes significantly with normal functioning and development. This chapter focuses on children with either chronic illness or disability or both. They have in common a persistent collection of health and developmental problems which have serious personal implications for the child and the family. It is a diverse population with varied needs. Problems are characterized by early onset, long duration of impairment, and serious impositions on health and functioning. Most of the disorders are now not fatal within the childhood years; many are only partially remediable.

A review of typical diagnoses for such children reveals that some are heterogeneous symptom complexes (such as scoliosis or hearing impairment), while others are discrete disorders (Down syndrome, juvenile rheumatoid arthritis). The biomedical origins cover the full range of human exceptionality, including hereditary conditions, chromosomal aberrations, congenital anomaly syndromes, complications of pregnancy and childbirth, early injury, serious infections, malignancy, and hypersensitivity states.

In recent years, mortality during childhood has been dramatically reduced for many anomalies and chronic illnesses. It is difficult, however, to make precise statements about the size of this group of children.

There are no solid national prevalence figures, because there are no broadly based registrations of children with chronic conditions. Although some children with disabling conditions such as mental retardation and cerebral palsy are reported by public schools, this would not usually include the majority of children with chronic illnesses who may not require specialized educational services. Birth records provide one source of information for estimating the incidence of congenital anomalies, but this source will fail to report diagnoses of chronic conditions that are identified after the perinatal period.

Recent studies suggest a range of estimated prevalence. Kiernan and Bruininks (1986) estimated the prevalence of developmental disabilities at 10/1000 persons with significant mental retardation, 7.5 with epilepsy, 3.5 with cerebral palsy, and 0.5 with autism. The Vanderbilt study concluded that 10 percent of children have chronic medical conditions, with 10 percent of those problems (or 1 percent of the childhood population) representing severe affliction (Hobbs, Perrin and Ireys, 1985). Current experience in school districts in this country shows that between 8 and 16 percent of children require individual educational plans and special education assistance, but many of these are for relatively mild language or learning disorders requiring no specialized health care services.

Based on these estimates, we conclude that about 5 percent of all children have nontrivial special health needs, with 1–2 percent having severe impairments that can be expected to create special burdens for the child and family (Gortmaker, 1985; Kiernan and Bruinincks, 1986; Pueschel et al., 1987). The degree of this burden depends on the intrusiveness of the disorder, the resources and accommodation of the family, and the abundance and flexibility of local services.

What Are the Needs of Families and What Is Family-Centered Care?

The role of the family as care-giver assumes new dimensions when it involves attention to the needs of a chronically ill child or one with a disability. In recent years, there has been increased recognition and respect for the family as a significant participant in the complex process of accessing, coordinating, and actually providing specialized care. It is our contention that health care delivery and financing systems should be reshaped to take into account these critical roles that families play.

Family-centered care was defined by the Association for the Care of Children's Health (1987) as:

> a philosophy of care that recognizes and respects the pivotal role of the family in the lives of children with special health needs. It is a philosophy

that strives to support families in their natural care-giving roles by building upon their unique strengths as individuals and families. It is a philosophy that promotes normal patterns of living at home and in the community. It is a philosophy that views parents and professionals as equals in a partnership committed to excellence at all levels of health care. (P. 1)

The Family as Care-Giver

Care-giving includes several critical tasks in the life of a family: physical maintenance (the provision of food, clothing, housing, and health care); providing emotional and psychological support; assuring access to education; providing social and recreational opportunities; and providing a transition to adulthood. Each of these tasks becomes much more complex and stressful when the child who is being cared for has a chronic illness or disability. There are also major implications for other children in the family as well as for the careers and personal lives of the adults.

In achieving what is regarded as simple *physical maintenance,* children with chronic illness or disabling conditions may require special diets, adaptive equipment, home adaptations, and access to specialized health care available only in major medical centers. To be geographically close to necessary providers, parents may have to limit their career opportunities. To pay for the care as well as the other physical needs of children, parents may choose to stay with a job that offers good health insurance but is not otherwise preferred.

It has been estimated that parents pay out of pocket for one-third of all the expenditures of health care for children (Weeks, 1985). In one survey of parents of children with hemophilia, one-third of the mothers worked to meet expenses, one-fifth of the fathers had a second job, and 11 percent of the fathers reported that the child's illness influenced their choice of a job (Hilgartner, Aledort and Giardina, 1985). These financial burdens often lead to significant stress on families (Turk, 1964; Salk, Hilgartner and Cranich, 1972; Vance et al., 1980; Burr, 1985).

The *provision of emotional and psychological support* to children is also affected by a chronic illness or disability. The ability of a family to provide this support to a child is determined to a great extent by the level of stress within the family and the family's ability to deal with that stress. The reactions a family may have to a child with a disability or chronic illness have been addressed by a number of researchers (Talbot and Howell, 1971) and chronicled by parents as well (Greenfeld, 1978; Featherstone, 1980; Pieper, undated). These reactions are complex and change over time but are important determinants of the well-being of both the child and family members.

Magrab (1985) identified psychosocial issues that are prevalent at different stages of a child's life and the impact chronic illness may have on these developmental tasks. These include the importance of parent/child bonding, developing autonomy, emergence of self-concept, need for social interaction with peers and adults, development of gender identification, and personality definition. Children's concepts of their own illness, reactions to hospitalizations, and perception of death all have an impact on these critical aspects of psychosocial development. For example, repeated hospitalization interferes with the bonding process in infancy as well as with the primary need for young children to have their parent close. Repeated separations can cause anxiety in the child and arouse fears of abandonment.

Facilitating the development of family relationships is a critical component of care-giving. Various studies have indicated that brothers and sisters of children with chronic illness are more at risk for emotional and behavior problems (Lavigne and Ryan, 1979). Increased responsibility for care and treatment within the home by family members implies that additional attention and support be provided to the needs of brothers and sisters as well (Crocker, 1983).

Assuring access to education has been greatly supported in the last ten years by the passage in 1977 of Public Law 94-142, the federal law that mandates that public schools provide a free and appropriate education for all children regardless of disability. Thus, obtaining a public education has become an entitlement in this country for all children regardless of special needs. This right was reaffirmed in 1987 with the reauthorization and expansion of the law, now referred to as Public Law 99-457.

While children with disabilities have the protection of this federal mandate, many chronically ill children (e.g., those with diabetes or juvenile rheumatoid arthritis) are not considered eligible for special education services, and therefore do not receive the necessary support services that they may require in the school setting. These children may be offered inferior home-based educational programs when schools are reluctant to assume responsibility for even routine medical procedures such as finger pricks.

Even when children do receive special education services under these federal mandates, it is still necessary for families to monitor whether the education is appropriate, whether it is being delivered in the least restrictive setting, and whether all the support services that the child requires are being provided. These health and related support services are often complex and may require considerable expenditure of local education dollars. Parental advocacy increases the likelihood of full implementation of promised services. However, educational and related services that may be delivered in the school must also be coordinated with ongoing health care in the home and community. Teachers need accurate information concerning the child's health status and/or limitations to interact effectively and sensitively with the child and his or her family and to apply appropriate expectations and performance standards. School is the child's primary environment for acquiring new skills and developing friendships. Therefore, coordination of health and educational services, and information and support to the school, become a major management task for parents.

Social and recreational opportunities are essential components of a child's life. For most children, these opportunities occur naturally in the course of school and play. Additional opportunities are often available through summer camps, organized groups such as Girl or Boy Scouts, and sports. If a chronically ill child or a child with a disability is to take advantage of these activities, this may require considerable effort on the part of the family as well as the recreation program staff. Often camps or other organized groups are reluctant to accept a child who has a disability or illness because of perceived liability issues. In addition, they may not feel competent or secure in working with a child who has specialized health care needs. Other children or parents may not understand a child's limitations and may be reluctant to include the child in social and recreational activities. The result is that children with special health needs often have limited recreational opportunities and are at risk for missing many of the normal socialization experiences available to other children.

The *transition to adulthood* is challenging for normal children. Adolescence is a time when young people are attempting to establish independence from their families, developing a separate definition of self, and consequently it is often a time of increased family stress. When adolescents also have a chronic illness or disability, this process of increasing autonomy becomes much more complex. The young person may have severe limitations on his or her ability to perform personal care functions and resent having to depend on family assistance in these areas. Occasionally, the need for independence and autonomy is demonstrated by noncompliance with medication or other therapeutic requirements. In addition to these areas of possible conflict, there may be considerable concern and anxiety on the part of parents regarding future care of their child, in terms of both continued eligibility for health insurance and the young adult's ability to support himself or herself financially and live independently.

The Family as Full Partner in the Health Care System

Despite the roles and responsibilities that families perform as caregivers, the health and medical system often regards the family in a patronizing and paternalistic manner (Weil, 1986). While parents may be willing to accept this attitude when an acute medical crisis requires total dependency on professional care-takers, it is much more difficult to tolerate a subservient role on an ongoing basis. This is particularly difficult when a child's chronic condition requires the active intervention and monitoring by family members who possess unique knowledge and understanding to ensure continuity of care.

The current trend toward home care for children who until recently would have been confined to hospitals or other institutional settings illustrates the need for recognizing the family as both the provider and the consumer of health care services.

Since it is the family who must carry additional responsibilities for protecting the rights and interests of the child, it is critical that family members be involved as equal partners in the health care team that defines the needs for service and designs the solutions to meet those needs in all settings.

How Do Families and Providers Define the Needs?

To increase the understanding of how parents perceive their needs, Massachusetts conducted a statewide survey of parents of children with a wide range of chronic illnesses or disabling conditions. Respondents ($N=910$) were asked to rank a checklist of twenty-six services in terms of importance (Project SERVE, 1985). The findings suggest that, in addition to condition-specific needs, generic services are consistently viewed as important by families. The cumulative rating of services as reported by families across sixteen diagnostic groups (Table 2.1) demonstrates a strongly expressed need for parental education on rights and entitlements (74 percent rated as "very important") as well as help in getting needed services (72 percent rated as "very important"). These were the two most consistently highly ranked services for the entire sample.

These findings were confirmed by interview data from providers of specialty care who declared a surprising degree of agreement that the greatest unmet need for this group of children is the provision of support services to families. Support services were defined as including case management, service coordination, and advocacy services as well as counseling, parental support groups, support groups for brothers and sisters, a hotline for information and referrals, specialized equipment, and housing adaptation.

These services are critical components in delivering family-centered care. However, since family support services are frequently viewed as

Table 2.1 The Importance of Services for Family and Child

Child's Condition	Parent Education on Rights and Entitlements	Help in Getting Needed Services	P.T.	Financial Help	Speech Therapy	Information on Community Resources	Early Intervention Services	Social/Recreational Opportunities	O.T.	Parent Support Groups
Asthma (N = 49)	88%	74%	73%	81%	55%	55%	56%	61%	57%	49%
Autism (N = 43)	79	77	35	61	91	73	68	74	50	67
Cerebral palsy (N = 123)	84	78	91	65	82	62	60	60	83	38
Cleft lip/palate (N = 59)	71	59	39	26	86	52	68	36	35	55
Congenital heart disease (N = 112)	69	63	49	56	52	54	57	49	42	56
Cystic fibrosis (N = 33)	74	73	71	88	6	52	36	55	6	41
Down syndrome (N = 93)	81	76	73	54	94	75	87	64	72	54
Hemophilia (N = 38)	77	56	50	67	22	42	19	52	25	52
Juvenile rheumatoid arthritis (N = 33)	61	43	52	50	14	35	30	41	36	38
Mental retardation (N = 182)	82	83	79	62	90	72	64	60	77	48
Neurofibromatosis (N = 39)	65	66	35	50	43	62	28	55	36	52
Scoliosis (N = 99)	73	86	77	70	60	69	48	65	65	51
Seizure disorder (N = 151)	82	84	80	76	75	66	67	52	74	45
Severe hearing impairment (N = 47)	92	82	62	72	90	70	74	65	50	53
Severe visual impairment (N = 74)	89	87	80	78	83	70	69	60	74	48
Spina bifida (N = 108)	82	83	84	75	45	71	57	68	68	58

Note: Figures indicate the percentage of parents in each diagnostic group who ranked each service as "very important."

nonreimbursable by health insurance, they are not likely to be provided in sufficient quantity to meet the demand or to be available at all in most medical settings. Yet, many families report that they prefer to have such support services available through the medical setting because they lack the time and energy to seek them elsewhere.

These parent survey data (Project SERVE, 1985) support previous studies that documented the financial stress on families who are caring for children with chronic illness or disability. Specifically, parents reported significant concern regarding the future stability of health insurance coverage for their children, as well as some estimates of out-of-pocket expenditures. Despite the sample's being basically well insured (96 percent reported some kind of public or private insurance), less than half (48 percent) reported that they were confident that their child had or would have in the future adequate health insurance. Parents of children with chronic illness (e.g., cystic fibrosis, asthma, etc.) were notably less confident (29–30 percent) than parents of children with a physical disability (e.g., hearing impairment, 55 percent; visual impairment, 58 percent). In addition to these concerns about insurance, 89 percent of the parents reported significant out-of-pocket expenses during the previous year because of their child's medical condition (Table 2.2).

The Current Financing System and Its Impact on Families with Children with Special Health Care Needs

Given the characteristic service needs of the population of children and families with whom we are concerned, how well does the current health care system perform in providing financial assistance to meet these needs? Traditional insurance was not meant to be a guarantee that the individual would receive the necessary, most appropriate, and highest-quality health care, only that the family or individual would not be overwhelmed by the financial consequences of illness or accident. Therefore, it is not surprising that there are real limitations in the degree to

Table 2.2 Significant Out-of-Pocket Expenses as Reported by Families, (N = 910)

Type of Expense	Percentage Reporting
Travel	65%
Parking	52
Drugs and medication	50
Bills after insurance	40
Physical changes in house	39
Lost wages	25
Special equipment	23
Babysitters for other children	22

which the existing health-financing arrangements meet the costly and specialized health care needs of chronically ill and disabled children. We review here these limitations in private and public health financing programs, including managed-care arrangements in prepaid health plans.

Problems in Obtaining Health Insurance

A significant number of American families are unable to obtain affordable health insurance. The national figure of uninsured persons is estimated to be 33 million and increasing as the economy shifts from industry to service components. While it is not known how many of these uninsured are children with a chronic illness or disabling condition, Butler et al. (1985) estimated that 10.3 percent of all children with functional disabilities have no insurance. This percentage jumps to 19.5 percent among low-income children.

Even families who could normally afford to purchase health insurance outside of employer-sponsored programs face significant problems if caring for a chronically ill child. Such children are expensive to serve and therefore are not viewed as desirable risks by private insurance plans. Butler et al. (1985) estimated that in 1980, total expenditures for physician visits and hospitalizations for children with activity limitations were in excess of $1.7 billion. Average annual hospitalization costs for this population were estimated at $511, compared to a cost of $48 for an average child. Physician visits for this population averaged $237, as compared to $98 for those with no functional limitation. These differences were even more dramatic when data for children with severe problems were examined: this group had average physician costs of $330 per child and hospitalization costs of $758 per child.

While children with a disability or chronic illness whose families may be eligible for group membership in a private insurance plan or HMO cannot be denied coverage simply because they present a high risk for costly care, they could confront a denial of benefits due to preexisting conditions if applying for coverage outside of a group.

Private nongroup health insurance policies may exclude individual family members with chronic or disabling conditions or exclude coverage of those preexisting conditions for an extended period of time. Although in Massachusetts, Blue Cross/Blue Shield, by law, cannot deny membership on the basis of health status, it can restrict benefits for the treatment of a chronic illness or for any anticipated complications of the illness for up to three years from the date of enrollment. Full and immediate coverage of a child with a disability by a nongroup policy is generally restricted to families who received continuous coverage under a previous group plan or purchased the nongroup policy before the child's disabling condition was discovered.

In recent public hearings in Massachusetts, one family testified about the hardships involved in not being able to purchase health insurance that would cover their disabled child. This was a middle-class family with two working parents. They did not, however, have access to a group health plan and their child was excluded from their family's nongroup policy. They described bills of $15,000 for brief hospitalizations and their dealings with collection agencies when they fell behind on the negotiated payment schedules. The only way they found to finance care was to utilize the major urban hospital that provided free care, even though it was located a considerable distance from their home. They told of driving six hours to reach this city hospital when their child broke his arm while on a family trip because they could not incur any additional medical bills.

Because of the significant advantages of having employer-sponsored group membership in an insurance plan, families do everything they can to retain their health insurance benefits once they have been secured. This has a major impact on the employment mobility of families, since a family may become ineligible for group insurance if they change their employment status.

The Limitations of Private Health Insurance

The limitations of private insurance in meeting the health care needs of the general population are discussed Chapter 5. The special problems for this group of children include exclusions for preexisting conditions, mandatory waiting periods before coverage may take effect, high deductibles and copayments, lifetime ceilings, and annual limits on specific benefits. Even when private health insurance is obtained, families with children with special health needs must face limited coverage for medication, appliances, and health-related services such as physical therapy, occupational therapy, and speech therapy. An analysis of existing private insurance programs demonstrates that the breadth and depth of coverage necessary to meet the specialized needs of these children and their families are not readily available (Project SERVE, 1985).

For families with private health insurance, out-of-pocket expenses can still remain a major financial burden, because cost-sharing requirements that are reasonable for most enrollees become excessive for chronically ill children. Twenty percent copayments on inpatient bills or outpatient services such as adaptive equipment or appliances can quickly reach very costly levels. In data reported by Butler et al. (1985) on payment for health care for children with myelomeningocele in Oregon during 1971–74, families paid for 10.7 percent of inpatient costs, 32.1 percent of outpatient costs, and 56.7 percent of social and related costs. Data collected from families by Project SERVE[1] in Massachusetts showed that 87 percent of the families sampled had significant out-of-pocket expenses for such things as drugs and medication, bills after insurance payments, physician charges, lost wages, special equipment, travel, and parking.

This problem is growing worse. Recent health insurance data show the trend toward higher cost-sharing requirements for individual beneficiaries, with increasing front-end deductibles. Only 50 percent of group-insured individuals were entitled to full hospital coverage in 1986, as compared with 87 percent in 1980 (Hewitt Associates, 1985). These are serious trends for families with children with special health care needs.

Families with third-party coverage remain under enormous pressure to manage their limited benefits by monitoring utilization in relation to lifetime ceilings, as well as annual limits on specific benefit categories. While limitations on annual and lifetime benefits may seem reasonable and manageable for families with healthy children, they may be overwhelming to a family with a chronically ill or disabled child. Twelve months of physical therapy is more than an adequate lifetime allotment in the case of a leg fracture, but totally inadequate for a child with a chronic condition such as cerebral palsy. Nonreimbursable supplies such as syringes, special diets, or disposable diapers for an older child may cost a family hundreds of dollars each month. A lifetime benefit ceiling of $250,000 may be reached in just a few years when a child requires frequent hospitalizations. A child in Massachusetts with cystic fibrosis, for example, incurred hospitalization costs of $83,000 in one calendar year for four separate admissions totaling 193 days (Nickerson, 1985).

Ventilator-dependent children present a dramatic example of costly inpatient care. Many of these children could live at home in a more normalized setting at reduced cost. However, before this is possible, families must work through a maze of bureaucratic procedures as well as negotiate the financing of all aspects of home care. Even after home care benefits are achieved, a family must continue to monitor the utilization of benefits very closely. For example, one family in Massachusetts described how they keep detailed books on their hospital costs to try to maximize the use of their private health insurance. This family confronted a terrible dilemma when hurricane Gloria hit in 1984. Their child was dependent on a ventilator and the hurricane threatened the very real possibility of a power failure for a period of days, while their backup generator would be good for only a few hours. Should they hospitalize their child even though she was not ill and use up some of those valuable hospital days or should they take a chance on losing power? Families are confronting such health care financing dilemmas all the time as they negotiate a system that has not been designed or adapted to meet the needs of children with chronic illnesses or disabilities.

The lack of standardization of private medical benefit packages can also be problematic. Written materials describing benefits are often vague and/or difficult to understand, and a variety of benefit coverage decisions are made on a case-by-case basis after the service has been delivered and the insurer has been presented with a bill. Furthermore, insurers are reluctant to establish precedent by publicizing the results of individual coverage decisions. Thus, it is difficult for subscribers to know in advance precisely what benefits will be available for paying for their child's medical expenses (Project SERVE, 1985).

Is managed care a solution? Health maintenance organizations (HMOs), with their emphasis on prevention and incentives to avoid costly inpatient care, may seem ideally suited for families of children with chronic illness or disability. These children require close monitoring and sustained preventive services to avert or ameliorate complications associated with their chronic conditions and often incur high ambulatory as well as inpatient costs for care. HMOs, however, operate with a financial incentive to exclude such families, since they must provide this medical care within a fixed budget.

Should an HMO enroll a family with a child with a chronic condition, it would presumably seek to provide appropriate preventive services and to avert unnecessary hospitalizations. A four-year study of Medicaid beneficiaries voluntarily enrolled in a Washington, D.C., HMO supports this presumption (Fuller, Patera and Koziol, 1977). While physician encounter and drug prescription rates for nondisabled Medicaid enrollees were steadily and significantly lower 22 months after HMO enrollment than during the same period before, rates for Medicaid enrollees with disabilities remained stable or rose. At the same time, hospital admissions and total hospital days declined more for the group with disabilities than for the nondisabled. Furthermore, more than 90 percent of persons with disabilities found care in the HMO equal to or better than the care they had received in the fee-for-service sector. Receiving medical care from an HMO seems an option that should be available to families who have children with disabilities, an option with the potential to support family-centered care.

But HMO enrollment carries disadvantages for this group of children. Traditional fee-for-service insurance plans offer complete freedom of choice in selecting providers, while HMOs restrict the choice to a panel of physicians and a limited number of hospitals. This can be a critical limitation for the child with a chronic condition. Families may have established relationships with medical specialists in tertiary-care centers who do not belong to an HMO—therefore, to maintain this relationship or feel free to access other highly trained specialists by choice, the families must retain a fee-for-service plan. In addition, participants in HMOs report that many plans have limited access to the highly necessary specialists with particular pediatric training and expertise. It is not clear whether this is a function of the size of a particular HMO or whether it is just that it has been determined not to be cost-effective to provide certain types of services.

An evaluation of a pilot program in Wisconsin, which mandated that AFDC Medicaid recipients enroll in HMOs in two counties, raised questions about the availability of needed specialized services within HMO assignments. In addition, families reported a concern regarding the continuity of care when previous ties to pediatric specialists were disrupted (Brazner and Gaylord, 1986). In other analyses of the desirability of HMOs as a potential solution to providing comprehensive health care to specialized populations, questions have been raised as to whether the proper financial incentives exist in the current system to assure both enrollment and appropriate service delivery (Schlesinger, 1986).

Though HMOs generally provide fuller outpatient coverage than conventional fee-for-service insurance plans, HMOs can and do exclude from nongroup policies chronically ill family members or those with disabilities. In addition, since there are no incentives for HMOs to recruit this population, they often restrict the amount of support and related services they provide (i.e., one large HMO in Massachusetts will not pay for orthopedic braces, a significant expense if a child requires adaptive appliances on a continuing basis).

The current pressures for cost containment have encouraged many insurance companies and HMOs to institute a case-management function, which attempts to individualize benefits planning for a subset of very costly patients. Such patients may be capable of leaving a high-cost inpatient bed if their benefits could follow them to purchase alternative care. Application of such an individualized case-management service may result in significant savings to the insurer. Aetna Insurance Company reportedly saved $36 million in 1985 by financing home care for 800 patients (American Academy of Pediatrics, 1986). These are clear incentives for managed care—incentives that may work in favor of chronically ill children if they increase the comprehensiveness and coordination of care or encourage innovative, more normalizing solutions for children—or may work to their disadvantage if pressure for cost savings leads to inadequate provision of services.

In summary, the current private mechanisms for financing health care fail to protect families with children who have a disability or chronic illness from significant and potentially catastrophic costs of care. In addition, these financing mechanisms are not designed to support family-centered care. As a result, these families absorb a heavy financial and emotional burden in trying to secure the comprehensive and coordinated services their children require. Prepaid care in HMOs may offer a means of addressing some of these limitations, but only if a comprehensive range of specialty services is available.

Medicaid

Medicaid is a potential financing source for medical care for children with disabilities whose families cannot afford or obtain adequate benefits under a private insurance plan, *if* they meet Medicaid financial eligibility standards. The inequities resulting from difficulties in "spending down" to Medicaid eligibility and interstate variations in eligibility standards are discussed in Chapter 6. For those who qualify, Medicaid has the potential to provide comprehensive care, including extended benefit coverage for home care, transportation, and mental health services. But here, too, interstate variations in coverage make Medicaid an unreliable safety net, since many of the services required by disabled children are provided only at state option and are not covered in many states. For example, as of 1983, less than half the state Medicaid programs paid for physical therapy, prescription drugs, or personal care services for families who "spend down" (i.e., are not on welfare) to Medicaid eligibility (U.S. Department of Health and Human Services, 1986).

State Programs for Children with Special Health Care Needs: The Public Health Role

State-sponsored Programs for Children with Special Health Care Needs (formerly known as Crippled Children's Services programs) are funded under Title V of the Social Security Act of 1935. This act was amended in 1981 to create the Title V Maternal and Child Health Services Block Grant, which consolidated several federal programs and provided states with greater flexibility in meeting the goals of Title V.

Historically, the state-operated programs have provided another source of assistance for families seeking health care for children with some chronic illnesses or disabling conditions. These programs typically provide or may purchase direct medical services for some specific groups of children. Eligibility is generally defined by condition, although in some states income is also a determining factor (Ireys, 1980). Orthopedic diagnoses are prominently covered, as the programs were initiated in the 1930s, times of significant prevalence of bone infections, poliomyelitis, and handicapping anomalies.

States have had considerable flexibility in establishing their programs and there is great variation in the numbers served, eligibility requirements, conditions treated, and comprehensiveness of services provided. Another important characteristic of the state programs is that they are small in relation to the larger system of health care. Ireys estimated in 1979 that the state programs served about 700,000 children nationwide—about 8/10 of 1 percent of the children under twenty-one (Ireys, 1980). This is less than most estimates of the number of children with the most severe disabling conditions and far short of the 5 percent with some chronic condition.

Conclusions and Policy Recommendations

The characteristic health care needs of this population are broader, deeper, and more costly than those of other children. We are witnessing and can continue to expect major changes and reforms that will govern how health care in America is both organized and financed. It is critical that this group of children benefit from effective advocacy so that their special needs in the health care market are not overlooked in the continuing development of health policy in our country.

In addition to children with chronic illness or disability who are described earlier in this chapter, a new group of children with special needs is emerging. As the AIDS epidemic is forcing a reexamination of the provision and financing of health care for adults, the growing numbers of children with HIV infection will bring additional pressure on the health care system. While these children and their families have many of the same needs as children and families who have other chronic illnesses, the needs are complicated by other concerns. These include the fear of infection surrounding the disease, the fact that many are infants whose parents are dead or dying, and the resulting need to provide other social services beyond health care, such as residential services or foster care. The current challenge to our health and social service systems to finance and care for children with HIV infection or AIDS provides a dramatic illustration of the shortcomings of these systems in serving a broad range of children with special health needs.

Good-quality health care for children with chronic or disabling conditions must be family centered and characterized by: (1) adequate access to appropriate, high-quality specialty care, (2) coordination of primary care with specialty care, (3) extensive coordination and integration of multiple services and entitlements, (4) high degree of responsiveness to family needs, (5) support for the role of parent as caregiver and partner in the delivery of health care, and (6) respect for the financial integrity of the family. This chapter describes a health care system that provides inadequate safeguards for families with children who have specialized needs and falls far short of these six criteria.

The six characteristics of high-quality health care for this population of children imply a guaranteed and universal access to primary health care for all children, as well as access to specialized health care for children with disabilities or chronic illnesses. To achieve such substantial goals, a diverse and effective advocacy effort will be required. It will be necessary to support and encourage the development of a broad coalition of parent-based advocacy groups that can cut across diagnostic categories and collaborate in seeking the necessary reforms. In addition, states must build a public capacity to monitor the health care system's ability to deliver high-quality care that meets the needs of children and families.

Toward these ends, we recommend the following for both the private and the public roles in the health care system on behalf of children with chronic illness or disabling conditions and their families. The proposed changes seek to redesign the system so that it is accessible regardless of employment status, income, family structure, or special health care needs. Each of the recommendations builds upon the existing public/private patchwork of health care financing that currently exists in this country. It is tempting to make one sweeping recommendation to establish a one-tiered publicly financed system of care that would guarantee equal access for all. We have forgone this temptation in the interest of political realism in the short term. It is our opinion that the achievement of each of these recommendations would make incremental progress toward the goal of equal access to quality health care for all. These reforms thus are steps that will protect the needs of this group of children and their families while assisting in the attainment of more comprehensive reform.

The recommendations fall into three categories: (1) expansion of the existing health insurance system, both public and private; (2) expanded benefits for children with special health care needs; and (3) new and expanded roles for public health agencies which increase their responsibilities for quality assurance, advocacy, and family support.

The Expansion of Access to Basic Health Insurance

Current national surveys document that approximately 33 million people in this country are uninsured, of whom approximately one-third, more than 10 million, are children. An initial priority must be to decrease the percentage of uninsured children. Initiatives should increase access to private insurance, publicly sponsored programs that make insurance available to the uninsured, and expanded state and federal Medicaid programs.

1. Improve incentives for expanding access to employer-based insurance. A variety of mechanisms could provide incentives to both employers and employees to participate in expanded family benefits through the workplace. Examples include: (a) state mandate for employers to provide basic health insurance or contribute to a state-sponsored insurance program such as the recently enacted Massachusetts legislation; (b) tax incentives for both employers and employees which reward participation in family coverage extending to adult dependents; (c) state-sponsored insurance programs for small employers (i.e., multiple employer trusts); and (d) state legislation that eliminates the waiting period for preexisting conditions for all group and nongroup policies.

2. Develop state programs that guarantee access to adequate health insurance. State governments have the ability to establish programs that could assure access to nongroup options for uninsured individuals and their families. State programs could be operated independently or utilize vouchers that could purchase private insurance products. Publicly established systems could be financed by a tax on employers not providing insurance, a surcharge on unemployment insurance, general tax revenues, or through sliding fees for families and individuals who participate. General coverage for uninsured children with special health care needs would be incorporated into a program for all uninsured children and adults. A supplemental benefits package could be designed for special needs groups. State-sponsored programs should result in a substantial, if not total, reduction in the number of uninsured families in the general population. More than a dozen states currently operate programs to insure so-called high-risk individuals. Several states, including Massachusetts and Wisconsin, recently established programs to offer insurance explicitly for the disabled.

3. Expand eligibility for Medicaid. Another strategy for increasing the percentage of the general population which is covered by some type of health insurance is for states to take full advantage of the existing options in the Medicaid program. Alternatively, federal regulations could be revised to require broadened eligibility criteria. A reasonable goal would be to have a Medicaid program that covers families under 150 percent of federal poverty standards without regard to family structure.

In addition, the "Medically Needy Options" should be comparably broadened to cover an expanded proportion of the population of children with chronic conditions. The current limitation on the Medically Needy Program is 133 1/3 percent of the state-established Medicaid eligibility standard. If increased to 200 percent, an expanded Medically Needy Program would extend coverage to an additional group of children with special health care needs who are still within the low-income population.

The Expansion of Benefits Available to Children with Special Health Care Needs

Both the kinds and the amount of benefits available to children and families must be expanded if the insurance system is to provide adequately for the health care of these children and to protect families from an overwhelming financial burden. Benefits should be broadened to include: expanded home care, provision of related medical services that are delivered outside of hospital settings, provision of adaptive equipment, coverage for medications, dependent coverage beyond age 18, and caps on the amount of copayments and deductibles based on income.

The provision of these benefits to the population needing them could be provided by: (1) the inclusion of a supplemental benefits package for eligible families in the state-sponsored program described above, or (2) the creation of a Medicaid buy-in program.

1. Develop a state-sponsored benefits package. Access to an expanded benefits package could be included as part of a larger program that provides health insurance to the general population of the uninsured. Access to these supplemental benefits would be available to families who could document health care needs that are not covered by their existing insurance. An extended benefits package should include services such as home health care; nutritional counseling and supplements; adaptive equipment and adaptive clothing; medications; specialized orthodontia; hospice care; long-term occupational therapy, physical therapy, speech, language, and hearing services; genetic services; specialized transportation; and preventive mental health services. Premiums should be based on income.

2. Establish a Medicaid buy-in program for eligible families. An alternative strategy would be to amend the federal Medicaid regulations to give states the option of establishing a program that would allow families with children who have a chronic illness or disability and whose private insurance is inadequate to purchase supplementary benefits through Medicaid at an income-adjusted monthly premium. Benefits available through this program should be the same as those for the state-sponsored program described above. The cost of this program, however, would be shared by the federal and state governments, as well as families themselves.

The Expansion of Roles for Public Agencies

State Programs for Children with Special Health Care Needs under Title V have traditionally provided direct clinical services to a small proportion of the childhood population (Ireys, 1980). This model of providing medical services was encouraged by the original legislation (Title V of the Social Security Act of 1935) and has not been substantially changed in intervening years.

A reexamination of the roles that the state programs play across the nation appears timely to question whether the direct provision of medical services to a narrowly defined population is the most efficacious and equitable use of these public funds (see also Chapter 12).

Since 1935, access to medical care has changed dramatically. Far greater numbers of physicians and specialty clinics are available to children nationwide. The proportion of the population which has some type of health insurance has greatly increased and the federal government has established the Medicaid program to improve access for the poor. While there remain problems with this system, both increasing medical costs and greater numbers of provider resources cause states to question their role as direct providers of specialty care through Title V programs. Though some argue for a continuing service delivery role for state Title V programs (see Chapter 12) to "fill the gaps," increased attention must be paid to the critical roles that state agencies can play in providing quality assurance, family support services, and advocacy functions.

1. Expand state Title V quality-assurance activities for children with special health care needs. State Title V Programs for Children with Special Health Care Needs should increase their standard setting, monitoring, and regulatory activities to build a quality-assurance capacity for children needing specialized health care.

State personnel can bring their experience and expertise developed as a result of a long history as providers of direct care to this population to a new task of developing quality-assurance programs. Standards that define the minimal set of services and personnel required to provide quality care in public or private settings should be developed. State Title V programs could then apply such standards in certifying specialty teams within managed-care systems as well as fee-for-service systems. Standards could also be used to educate consumers and providers regarding necessary components of quality care.

The successful development of these functions within state Title V programs requires the establishment of several critical partnerships. Negotiations with payers of care such as Medicaid, Blue Cross/Blue Shield, or commercial insurers would be necessary if these standards of care were to be adopted by providers. If major payers were convinced that the use of these standards would be to their benefit (i.e., cost effective), then it would be possible to develop a certification process for providers which would be a requirement for their services to be reimbursable. This type of role would improve care for all children receiving services in the participating institutions, regardless of diagnoses or eligibility for Title V services.

State Title V programs that establish agreements with state Medicaid agencies could assist in managing complex cases to determine whether care currently paid for with Medicaid dollars is the most appropriate and/or cost effective.

A formalized collaboration between state Title V programs and Medicaid which endorsed such a standard-setting role would facilitate similar collaborations between the Programs for Children with Special Health Care Needs and private payers such as Blue Cross/Blue Shield. These collaborative agreements would result in state Title V programs influencing the quality of the care that is purchased through larger sums of private health care dollars for children with special health needs. Such quality-assurance measures would also serve to protect children from current system incentives for the underutilization of costly services.

2. *Expand state programs that provide family support and advocacy.* Another potential role for state Programs for Children with Special Health Care Needs includes the provision of support services for families.

These services are less available in the private sector, are not typically reimbursed by private insurers, and therefore constitute a gap where public dollars could have a substantial impact. They include such services as respite care, case management, financial counseling, advocacy with both the public and private health care system, and financial support for parent networks and self-help groups. These services are the ones often identified by families as being the most important and the most difficult to obtain (Project SERVE, 1985). It is by providing these kinds of services that state public programs may have the greatest and most broad-based effect in facilitating family-centered, community-based care for children with special health care needs. While many state programs provide some of these services to the population they currently serve, we envision greatly expanded programs with a much more visible role as an agency that provides support services for families. Eligibility for these kinds of support programs need not be restricted in terms of disabilities, and thus the population served could be broadened to include families with children with chronic illnesses and medical disabilities who may have been previously excluded from direct medical care under state Title V programs.

Providing services such as case management and financial counseling also provides the state agency with insight into the kinds of problems families encounter as they attempt to access and coordinate services for their children. This knowledge can enable the state program to act as a much more effective advocate with other state agencies, private providers, and the state legislatures.

Notes

1. Project SERVE was a collaborative project involving the Massachusetts Department of Public Health, the Harvard School of Public Health, and the Developmental Evaluation Clinic at The Children's Hospital. The principal investigators were Allen Crocker, M.D., Gerald Tuttle, Ph.D., and Deborah Klein Walker, Ed.D. Other members of the group included Jane Gardner, R.N., Sc.D., Ann Murphy, M.S.W., Serena Mailloux, M.D., Susan Epstein, M.S.W., Ann Taylor, Ed.D., and Alexa Halberg. Penny Feldman, Ph.D., and Betsy Anderson provided consultant services.

References

American Academy of Pediatrics. 1986. Government Activities Report. April. Washington, D.C.

Association for the Care of Children's Health. 1987. *Family Centered Care: What Does It Mean?* Washington, D.C.

Brazner, K., and C.L. Gaylord. 1986. *Medicaid, HMOs and Maternal and Child Health. An Assessment of Wisconsin's Mandatory HMO Enrollment Program for AFDC Families.* Madison, Wis.: Center for Public Representation.

Blenden, R.J. 1986. Health Policy Choices for the 1990s. *Issues in Science and Technology* 2(4):65–73.

Butler, J.A., P. Budetti, M.A. McManus, S. Stenmark, and P.W. Newacheck. 1985. Health Care Expenditures for Children with Chronic Illnesses. In N. Hobbs and J.M. Perrin (eds.), *Issues in the Care of Children with Chronic Illness*, pp. 827–863. San Francisco: Jossey-Bass.

Burr, C.K. 1985. Impact on the Family of a Chronically Ill Child. In N. Hobbs and J.M. Perrin (eds.), *Issues in the Care of Children with Chronic Illness*, pp. 24–40. San Francisco: Jossey-Bass.

Crocker, A.C. 1983. Sisters and Brothers. In J.A. Mulick and S.M. Pueschel (eds.), *Parent-Professional Partnerships in Developmental Disability Services.* Cambridge, Mass.: Ware Press.

Executive Office of Human Services, Commonwealth of Massachusetts. 1986. *Hospital Reimbursement and Access to Care: Chapter 372 and Beyond.* Publication #14-423-243-300-4-86-C.R.

Featherstone, H. 1980. *A Difference in the Family.* New York: Penguin Books.

Force, J. 1986. Supplemental Security Income Benefit for Children with Chronic Impairment. In E.M. Eklund (ed.), *Developmental Handicaps IV.* Silver Spring, Md.: American Association of University Affiliated Programs for Persons with Developmental Disabilities.

Fuller, N.A., M.W. Patera, and K. Koziol. 1977. Medical Utilization of Services in a Prepaid Group Practice Health Plan. *Medical Care* 15:705–737.

Gortmaker, S.L. 1985. Demography of Chronic Childhood Diseases. In H. Hobbs and J.M. Perrin (eds.), *Issues in the Care of Children With Chronic Illness*, pp. 135–154. San Francisco: Jossey-Bass.

Greenfeld, J. 1979. *A Place for Noah*. New York: Pocket Books.

Hewitt Associates. 1985. *Salaried Employee Benefits Provided by Major U.S. Employers: A Comparison Study, 1979 through 1984*. Lincolnshire, Ill.

Hilgartner, M.W., L. Aledort, and P. Giardina. 1985. Thalassemia and Hemophilia. In N. Hobbs and J.M. Perrin (eds.), *Issues in the Care of Children with Chronic Illness*, pp. 299–323. San Francisco: Jossey-Bass.

Hobbs, N., J.M. Perrin, and H.T. Ireys. 1985. *Chronically Ill Children and Their Families*. San Francisco: Jossey-Bass.

Ireys, H. 1980. *The Crippled Children's Service: A Comparative Analysis of Four State Programs*. Nashville: Center for the Study of Families and Children.

Kiernan, W.E., and R.H. Bruininks. 1986. Demographic Characteristics. In W.E. Kiernan and J.A. Stark (eds.), *Pathways to Employment for Adults with Developmental Disabilities*. Baltimore: Paul H. Brookes.

Kovar, M.G., and D. Meny. 1981. *Better Health for Our Children: A National Strategy*. Vol. 3., *A Statistical Profile*. Washington, D.C.: G.P.O.

Lavigne, J.V., and M. Ryan. 1979. Psychologic Adjustment of Siblings of Children with Chronic Illness. *Pediatrics* 63:616–627.

Magrab, P.R. 1985. Psychosocial Development of Chronically Ill Children. In H. Hobbs and J.M. Perrin (eds.), *Issues in the Care of Children with Chronic Illness*, pp. 698–715. San Francisco: Jossey-Bass.

Nickerson, H. 1985, February 1. *Hospitalization Payments Made by SHC in 1984*. Unpublished department memo, Massachusetts Department of Public Health, Boston.

Pieper, E. Undated. *Sticks and Stones: The Story of Loving a Child*. Syracuse, N.Y.: Human Policy Press.

Project SERVE, Massachusetts Health Research Institute, Inc. 1985. *New Directions: Serving Children with Special Health Care Needs in Massachusetts*. Unpublished report to the Massachusetts Department of Public Health, Boston.

Pueschel, S.M., C. Tingey, J.E. Fynders, A.C. Crocker, and D.M. Crutcher (eds.). 1987. *New Perspectives on Down Syndrome*. Baltimore: Paul H. Brookes.

Salk, L., M. Hilgartner, and B. Cranich. 1972. The Psychosocial Impact of Hemophilia on the Patient and His Family. *Social Science and Medicine* 6:491–505.

Schlesinger, M. 1986. On the Limits of Expanding Health Care Reform: Chronic Care in Prepaid Settings. *Milbank Memorial Fund Quarterly* 64(2):189–215.

Talbot, N.B., and M.C. Howell. 1971. Social and Behavioral Causes and Consequences of Disease Among Children. In N.B. Talbot, J. Kagan, and L. Eisenberg (eds.), *Behavioral Science in Pediatric Medicine*. Philadelphia: W.B. Saunders.

Title V of the Social Security Act of 1935. *Statutes at Large*. Chapter 531, XL (IX), Part 1, 531.

Turk, J. 1964. Impact of Cystic Fibrosis on Family Functioning. *Pediatrics* 34:67–71.

U.S. Department of Health and Human Services. 1986. *Medicare and Medicaid Data Book, 1984*. Washington, D.C.: G.P.O.

Vance, J.C., et al. 1980. Effects of Nephrotic Syndrome on the Family: A Controlled Study. *Pediatrics* 65:948–955.

Weeks, K.H. 1985. Private Health Insurance and Chronically Ill Children. In H. Hobbs and J.M. Perrin (eds.), *Issues in the Care of Children with Chronic Illness*, pp. 880–911. San Francisco: Jossey-Bass.

Weil, W.B. 1986. Review of Neglect of Chronically Ill Children. *American Journal of Diseases of Children* 140:628.

3

Legal Issues in Children's Health Care

Gary Melton, Ph.D., Ira M. Schwartz, M.S.W., and Michael D. Resnick, Ph.D.

The health care system in the United States is undergoing major and fundamental changes. At the same time, some legal concepts and issues regarding children are emerging that are likely both to influence and to be influenced by these changes. This chapter explores some of the more important of these legal issues and their implications for children's health care policy.

The General Legal Framework

There are two primary and sometimes mutually exclusive perspectives about children among child advocates (Mnookin, 1978; Rogers and Wrightsman, 1978; Melton, 1983a). One group, colloquially described as "kiddie libbers," argues for the recognition of rights to liberty and privacy for children. The other, historically known as the "child savers," seeks to establish special entitlements for children to protect their welfare. The case for both groups is made harder by the fact that, for most purposes, the law treats all "infants" (in most jurisdictions those under the age of 18) the same. Therefore, the kiddie libber must develop a legal theory that embraces young children, and the child saver must consider whether 17-year-olds are really in need of protection.

The Promotion of Self-Determination

Child liberationists assume children to be persons who are more like adults than not. Typically, this assumption is both empirical and normative. That is, child liberationists perceive children and particularly adolescents as capable of competent decision making but oppressed by dependency that is legally and socially imposed. Regardless, they believe that the differences between children and adults generally are not morally meaningful. Even if children don't possess sufficient capacity for practical reasoning and *a fortiori* full membership in the moral community, the child liberationists feel that children's *potential* for moral citizenship—their humanity—makes them deserving of respect as persons (Worsfold, 1974; Brown, 1982). From such a perspective, children are entitled to respect for autonomy and privacy and to an equitable share of social resources (Rawls, 1971).

The child liberationist perspective is of relatively recent origin. Special legal requirements for children—juvenile courts, compulsory education, child labor laws—from which to be "liberated" did not occur until about the turn of the century. Controversies about whether those changes had served more to oppress or harm than to liberate or protect children did not become widespread until the social movements of the 1960s raised questions about the status of various politically powerless groups.

In a landmark decision in 1967 (In re Gault), the U.S. Supreme Court announced for the first time that "neither the Fourteenth Amendment nor the Bill of Rights is for adults alone" (p. 13). Having recognized that children are "persons" for purposes of constitutional analysis, the Court enlivened the question of when states may infringe upon children's liberty and privacy in ways that would be unconstitutional if applied to adults. Since *Gault,* the Court has had occasion to consider this general question in a broad array of contexts, including whether schoolchildren may be punished for expressing unconventional political beliefs (no) or making a speech containing sexual innuendo (yes); whether they may be required to engage in meditation or prayer (no); whether school officials may suspend a pupil without a hearing (no, but all that is required is a conversation) or search her purse without a warrant (yes); whether they may censor the school newspaper (yes) or remove politically controversial books from the school library (no); whether respondents in delinquency proceedings are entitled to release pending a hearing (no), a stringent standard of proof (yes), and a trial by jury (no); whether states may bar sales to youth of marginally obscene materials that are not forbidden for adults (yes); even whether municipalities may limit children's access to video game parlors (remanded without a decision on the merits).

The Supreme Court's decisions about minors' privacy in health-related matters illustrate the ambivalence with which it has approached children's issues generally. Since 1976, the Court has decided nine cases about the limits of minors' self-determination in decisions related to abortion,[1] contraception (*Carey v. Population Services International,* 1977), and psychiatric treatment (*Parham v. J.R.,* 1979; see Melton, 1984; Perry and Melton, 1984). In this line of cases, the Court consistently recognized minors' right to make decisions in matters involving control of body or mind. However, the Court also consistently gave substantially more attention to the reasons why this right may be properly limited for minors than to the reasons why such a right should be recognized. Contrary to empirical evidence, as we shall see, the Court typically assumed most minors, including adolescents, to be incapable of making reasoned judgments about their health care and extremely vulnerable to "grave" and "lasting" consequences of ill-informed decisions, especially those about abortion. At the same time, the Court curiously ignored harm that might result from intrusion upon the minor's privacy. For example, to "protect" pregnant minors, states may require them to secure an attorney and go to court to present their rationale for an abortion. This legal procedure creates stress, embarrassment, and delay in securing an abortion, and therefore increases the medical and psychological risks (Melton, 1987b).

The Promotion of Child Welfare

The child-saving movement commonly supports increased *state* control to protect children from bad decisions. Perhaps because child-saving advocates would not give power to youth themselves, many of their arguments, initially appear less controversial than those favored by kiddie libbers. The entitlements commonly espoused by child savers, however, often are costly, and the amount that is reasonable for government to invest as well as the level of government that should bear such a responsibility may be highly controversial. Child saving also becomes controversial when it begins to intrude on parental autonomy (e.g., when parental religious beliefs conflict with a treatment regimen the state would impose on a child).[2]

Child savers generally assume that children are vulnerable, dependent, and in need of special protection by their parents and/or the state.[3] Whether because of a moral obligation to assist dependent persons or a utilitarian desire to facilitate the healthy development of citizens and diminish future economic and social burdens, child savers advocate special positive rights (entitlements). The United Nations Declaration of the Rights of the Child (1959) reflected this view. It recognized a cornucopia of special rights for children including: a name and nationality, social security, special education when needed, adequate nutrition, housing, and recreation, "an atmosphere of affection and of moral and material security," priority for disaster relief, and freedom from harmful labor.

Regardless of whether these rights are "natural" moral endowments, it is clear that they are not fundamental legal rights. The U.S. Constitution places no burden on states to provide social welfare services, including education (*San Antonio Independent School District v. Rodriguez,* 1973) and health care (*Harris v. McRae,* 1980; *Maher v. Roe,* 1977). There are two important exceptions to this general rule.

First, if a state wholly assumes the care of persons (as in an institution or foster care), the state also has a duty to provide them all the basic necessities of life (including adequate health care), safety, freedom from undue bodily restraint, and reasonable training to ensure safety and freedom from undue bodily restraint (*Youngberg v. Romeo*, 1982,). The *Youngberg* standard may include a broader duty to protect from harm, including regression (i.e., loss of skills already developed; see *Youngberg v. Romeo*, 1982, Blackmun, J., concurring) or lack of development of an individual's capacities (*New York State Association for Retarded Children v. Carey*, 1975).

Second, if a state chooses to provide services, it must exercise due process in denying or terminating services, and it must distribute the services equitably. Thus, although the Constitution does not provide a right to education, it does guarantee equality of access to public education, regardless of race (*Brown v. Board of Education*, 1954) or disability (*Pennsylvania Association for Retarded Children (PARC) v. Pennsylvania*, 1971, 1972).

At the same time, the constitutional mandate for equal protection generally does not preclude discrimination in favor of children. Age is not a suspect classification (*Felix v. Milliken*, 1978; *Massachusetts Board of Retirement v. Murgia*, 1976). Therefore, states need establish only a rational basis for age-based discrimination. In view of the states' historic interest in the healthy socialization of children and the developmental aspects of health needs, legislatures generally would have little difficulty justifying special entitlements to children for health care.

The lack of a constitutional requirement for provision of health services also obviously does not bar their provision. However, it is important to note that the Supreme Court in recent years has tended to read entitlement legislation narrowly (*Board of Education v. Rowley*, 1982; *Halderman v. Pennhurst State School and Hospital*, 1981.) Without an express, unequivocal expression of congressional intent, the Court is unlikely to permit "strings" to be placed on federal grants to state or local agencies.

Access to Health Care for Older Minors

Reform in Consent Laws

Neither child advocacy movement has come close to achieving its agenda, though not necessarily because the views conflict with one another. For the most part, the goals of the two movements have overlapped little. Child liberationists focus on increasing children's autonomy in decision making, but child savers are more concerned with enacting entitlement legislation. Put somewhat differently, child liberationists tend to be concerned with procedure and control, child savers with appropriations.

However, there are some issues on which the two schools of thought come together. For example, because information is critical to decision making in pursuit of one's interests, kiddie libbers, like child savers, are likely to support universal *opportunity* for education, even if they part company about whether children should be able to refuse education. Similarly, both schools are likely to advocate permitting children to consent independently to physical or mental health care. Kiddie libbers wish simply to increase the recognition of children's privacy. Child savers want to ensure that children have access to necessary health care they would not receive without the right to consent independently, whether because of parental neglect or children's discomfort in informing their parents about a particular problem.

The prevailing legal doctrine is that minors are per se incompetent to consent to health care. However, this doctrine has eroded because of a patchwork of constitutional, common-law, and statutory developments. In constitutional law, the adolescent abortion cases have established that mature minors have a right to consent to an abortion without parental assent or knowledge, although the state may compel them to prove their maturity to a judge. Access to contraceptives also is constitutionally guaranteed, but it remains unclear whether the constitutional right to privacy can be applied to adolescents' decisions about health care matters unrelated to reproduction.[4]

In the common law of torts, a rule regarding mature minors developed from practical considerations more than principled reasons (see Wadlington, 1973, 1983). Before the age of majority was lowered from 21, a few cases reached the courts in which physicians were sued for "technical batteries" in which they had acted on the consent of clearly competent older adolescents. Holding physicians liable for treating patients who consent seemed to be a travesty of justice. Therefore, a de facto common-law rule developed, in which physicians would not be liable for the treatment of older minors (aged 16 or older) that was beneficial to the minors and for which he or she had given informed consent.[5] A few states have adopted the mature minor rule in their statutory frameworks, but in most jurisdictions the law remains unclear and seldom tested in litigation.

To reduce the ambiguity about whether mature minors' consent is legally acceptable, some legislatures have adopted statutes expressly recognizing minors' consent to some forms of health care. These statutes form a patchwork that typically results from pragmatic responses to particular problems and not an overarching policy about either protection of children or respect for their privacy and autonomy. In all states, minors may consent independently to evaluation and treatment for some conditions (e.g., venereal disease) that may endanger the public health. Minors' consent often also is recognized for the treatment of conditions for which they might not seek help without a guarantee of privacy (e.g., pregnancy, drug dependency, mental disorder). Moreover, emancipated minors may be considered adults for purposes of consent. The standards for emancipation vary across jurisdictions, but they often include marriage, parenthood, military service, and independence of finances and domicile.

Even where such statutes are in place, however, ambiguity remains about the status of minors in the health care system. For example, does the power of consent imply a right to refuse treatment if parents bring the child to a clinic? Does a minor who consents independently to health care also control the confidentiality of information in the medical records? Are parents financially liable for treatment to which their child has consented independently?

In adopting statutes that grant minors power of consent, legislatures often have ignored these questions. When they have addressed the issues, they often have done so inconsistently. For example, Nebraska law permits minors to consent independently to counseling for substance abuse after an attempt has been made to involve the parents. No parallel provisions exist for other mental health treatment. Nebraska law also permits minors to seek treatment for venereal disease independently and confidentially. However, the same statute makes parents financially liable for the treatment. How parents are to be billed while the minor's confidentiality is protected is unclear.

These issues are likely to assume increasing importance in the future because of recent research findings that challenge historic presumptions of incompetency in adolescence and, to a lesser extent, middle childhood (see, generally, Melton, Koocher and Saks, 1983). The findings show that, on average, adolescents are indistinguishable from adults in their ability to express a preference about treatment, understand and weigh the risks and benefits of treatment alternatives, and ultimately choose particular "reasonable" treatments. Interestingly, even elementary-school children are like adults in their ability to express a preference and make reasonable choices, even though the process of their decision making is less thorough. Moreover, both laboratory and field studies suggest that decision making itself has positive effects, including increased treatment compliance. Taken together, these findings indicate that there is no factual basis for depriving adolescents of the power of consent to treatment. Insofar as concern with children's competence is on protecting them from harm resulting from bad decisions, research indicates that giving even elementary-school children power of consent would be feasible, at least in regard to "routine" medical decisions (see Lewis, 1983; Lewis and Lewis, 1983).

If providers take changes in the law seriously, then it implies changes in the marketing of services, the process of giving children information about their condition and treatment, policies about confidentiality, and, given the indigence of most minors as individuals, the financing of services. Even without changes in the law, providers' ethical duty, given the competence of many minors, may be to involve them at least in shared decision making (Division of Child, Youth, and Family Services, 1982; Weithorn, 1983).

Some state legislatures already have acted to increase minors' legal authority to make treatment decisions. If health care providers take such statutory changes seriously, the implications for the organization and financing of pediatric health care (particularly adolescent health care) are profound. However, most providers have been slow to respond to such legal changes. For example, an evaluation of Virginia's law of permitting minors to consent to psychotherapy with parental permission showed no effect on the frequency (more precisely, the infrequency) of minors' seeking treatment independently (Melton, 1981). Sixty percent of the community mental health clinics in the state were unaware of the law almost a year after its passage. Of the remaining clinics, only one had made any effort to inform youth in its catchment area about the availability of services without parental involvement. The effect of the law was merely to free clinics from possible liability for services that they already were offering the few adolescents who sought treatment independently.

There is reason to believe that movement toward the extension of adolescents' rights will be reasonably well received by many health care providers. For example, surveys of physician attitudes and behavior suggest, on the whole, that physicians show favorable attitudes toward confidentiality of treatment for youth (Resnick, 1986a). For example, in a study of community-based pediatricians, family and general practitioners in the Upper Midwest area (Minnesota, Wisconsin, Iowa, North Dakota, South Dakota), 75 percent of respondents expressed favorable attitudes toward the confidential provision of services to adolescents. The majority of physicians also indicated a desire to retain authority for decision making about parental notification. Practitioners' judgments about whether confidentiality was in the best interest of the minor patient were based upon such factors as familiarity with the patient and his or her family, the nature of the condition (including severity, and risk of treatment), anticipated consequences (physical, social, psychological) of not extending confidentiality of care, and the adolescent's ability to pay (Resnick, 1981). In other words, clinicians tend to support discretionary decision making based on the practical consequences of (not) protecting confidentiality.

However, given the fact that adolescents are not particularly knowledgeable about laws that either promote or inhibit autonomy in the use of health services (Resnick, Blum and Hedin, 1981; Blum, Resnick and Stark, 1987), laws that expand adolescents' rights must be accompanied by new and more effective approaches toward provider and patient education. At the very least, county medical societies, medical schools, public and private schools for adolescents, social service agencies, public interest groups, health care reform organizations, and child advocates should play an active role in informing their respective constituencies of youths' right to obtain services without parental knowledge.

Health Care Financing Dilemmas

Most adolescents are covered by their parents' insurance policy, issued through employers (Resnick, 1986b). Most adolescents who are Medicaid recipients do not have a separate coverage. The net result is that laws that expand adolescent rights to confidential utilization are countermanded by standard private and public insurance procedures that document the utilization of covered members for the holder of the policy. This disclosure may be obviated to some degree if insurers maintain separate records for each client and simply report overall expenditures without specifying the exact nature of the treatment. Such procedures partially protect adolescent confidentiality, but can be vitiated by demands of accountability by parents or guardians, or employers concerned with limiting health care expenditures.

Some possible alternatives to current practices might alleviate these dilemmas. For example, entitlement legislation could be enacted to underwrite services to children and youth and thus preclude automatic disclosure to parents. Also, sliding fee scales among providers might increase the ability of adolescents to meet their own medical expenses. However, reduced billing and payment may not be a viable option in the case of chronic illness or expensive treatment.

Trends in the Health Care System

The changing organization of health services in the United States may limit adolescents' ability to exercise their rights to give consent for and utilize services. For example, the growing corporatization of health services will likely be accompanied by diminished autonomy and authority for individual health professionals (Starr, 1982; Tarlov, 1983).

This loss of discretion may inhibit appropriate determination of autonomy and confidentiality for younger patients. As already noted, physicians emphasize the importance of retaining their autonomy and discretionary power in medical decision making, including the confidential treatment of youth (Crane, 1975; Resnick, 1981; Blum, 1982). As larger numbers of physicians practice in organized settings, autonomy may be increasingly circumscribed by employee-employer relationships between clinician and their corporate managers (Tarlov, 1983). Organizational policies on confidentiality and treatment of adolescents may predominate in the future over the loose individual provider discretion that now exists among professional providers. Such structural factors may be more powerful in shaping de facto policies than statutes permitting confidentiality of care.

Some observers do maintain that adolescents' rights to health care services may increase as the health care system becomes more competitive, as providers more aggressively develop and market an array of new services (Rodman, Lewis and Griffith, 1984). Such market expansion will create greater independent access to services, though, only if adolescents are able to pay for care independently or if they are provided public funds for such services. Neither financing strategy is likely to be a viable political option in the foreseeable future.

To maximize adolescents' access to services, not only the financing but also the organization of services must change, so that they are both psychologically and geographically approachable by adolescents. Public and privately supported school-based health services have provided a particularly accessible vehicle for the delivery of health services on a confidential basis to school-aged youth in some communities. Such services can provide an entry point for comprehensive assessment, treatment, and/or referral, and work effectively to meet unmet health needs (Gephart, Egan and Hutchins, 1984; Resnick and Bearinger, 1986). The decision whether the parents are notified of their child's use of the services is usually left in the hands of the patient. Although school-based clinics commonly seek parents' permission for students' use of services, the consent often is no more than blanket permission at the beginning of the school year to cover all subsequent utilization. This procedure preserves a modicum of parental control, but it is less than fully informed and of dubious legal validity.

Although school-based health services are a potential vehicle for giving older youth independent access to health care services, such programs may be constrained by contrary legal developments. For example, revisions in health law to permit greater autonomy and privacy for youth may conflict with state and federal statutes in the area of education. Health care reforms may not apply to school-based health services because of statutes and regulations protecting family privacy and establishing parents' rights to obtain information in school records and consent to special services for their children (e.g., Family Educational and Privacy Rights Act of 1974; Hatch Amendment of 1978; Department of Education, 1984).

The New Paternalism

The trend toward increased recognition of adolescents' autonomy promises to collide squarely with an independent trend toward increased governmental involvement in regulating unhealthy behavior—the "new paternalism" (see Bonnie, 1985, for a comprehensive review). With the reconceptualization even of interpersonal violence as a public health problem, adolescents are apt to be the target of attempts to exercise greater legal control over behavior in the name of public health.

The focus on youth is based on several assumptions that remarkably parallel assumptions made at the turn of the century that led to a separate juvenile court. First, the state has a special interest in the health and socialization of children and youth, the voters and workers of the future. Efforts to require child restraints in cars, rather than restraints for all passengers, could be justified on such grounds. Second, it is assumed that behavior in youth is especially malleable, and, third, that reform of adolescent behavior will prevent unhealthy adult behavior. Finally, it is assumed that, without special legal structures, a disproportionate number of youths will engage in unhealthy behavior.

There is some truth in these assumptions. Adolescents and young adults (the latter group is typically not singled out for special legal sanctions) are at higher risk than people from other age groups for injury and death from traffic accidents and interpersonal violence. Patterns of habitual risk-taking (e.g., cigarette smoking and drug abuse) commonly are established in adolescence. Adolescents' unhealthy behavior is usually responsive to legally induced economic pressures (see Lewitt, Coate and Grossman, 1981; Harris, 1982).

However, age-based regulation of unhealthy behavior is sometimes ineffective or even counterproductive. For example, motorcycle helmet laws aimed solely at riders under 18 have had no effect in lessening the rates of injury or death (Williams, Ginsburg and Burchman, 1977). Bonnie (1985) suggested two possible explanations. First, because it is difficult for police to identify riders under 18, they may not enforce such limited prohibitions. Second, the selective imposition upon adolescents' liberty may increase their reactance and, therefore, any tendency to eschew helmets as a form of protest behavior.

Indeed, for some forms of unhealthy behavior, age-based prohibitions may be inherently unsuccessful. If high rates of risky behavior are the product of inexperience, raising the minimum age for drinking, driving, and so forth simply postpones the modal age of injury. Thus, although lowering the drinking age may have decreased alcohol-related accidents among teenagers overall (see, generally, Wechsler, 1980), raising the drinking age may increase the accident rate during the threshold year, regardless of the age at which it is set (males, 1986; but see Williams, 1986).

The new paternalism may collide not only with adolescents' autonomy but also with family privacy, parental autonomy, and parental privacy (Robertson, 1983; Melton, 1987b). For example, the desire to prevent prenatal injuries may result in the application of occupational safety laws to bar women of childbearing age from toxic workplaces (see, e.g., *Hayes v. Shelby Memorial Hospital,* 1984). It also may result in selective public health regulation or child-protective jurisdiction to prevent women from smoking, drinking, or ingesting illicit drugs during pregnancy (see, e.g., *In re Baby X,* 1980).

Policy Considerations

The primary message of this chapter is twofold. Child health policy, like policies governing other child child service systems (Gilgun, Schwartz, Melton and Eisikovits, in press), is inconsistent and largely unplanned. Second, if a more coherent child health policy is to emerge, it must take into account developments in the law affecting children and families. That body of law itself is largely incoherent and on a collision course with itself. As one of us summarized elsewhere:

> [W]e currently are confronted with unprecedented child self-determination, family privacy, state intervention to protect children (especially in regard to their health), and state intervention to disrupt families and constrain child autonomy! Each of the major schools of thought about children's rights seem[s] to have identified issues in which it can pursue its agenda with little controversy. On the other hand, the ultimate incompatibility of such perspectives can not be avoided. If, for example, a school district relies on the new paternalism to provide the ideological foundation for establishment of school health clinics, it eventually will be confronted with the question of who may give (and refuse) consent to the clinic's services. It also eventually will have to decide whether to seek state authority to coerce receipt of services, to require parental involvement, or to enforce confidentiality against parents (Melton, 1987a, p. 86).

Such questions obviously are not merely academic. To continue with the example of school health clinics, such programs fit well with the ecology of childhood and adolescence. Nonetheless, simply identifying such a program model as sensible (in terms of enhancement of health) obviously does not implement it, as groups proposing such programs often have experienced when they become involved in ideological crossfire, all among purported child advocates. Neither is such thoughtfulness in adoption of a program model necessarily accompanied by a legal structure that facilitates the financing of the new program. Neither does it result in a policy about the limits on access to services or personal and family privacy. Neither does it yield clarity about the relationships among the various child service agencies charged with providing essentially the same services to essentially the same population under varying auspices, streams of funding, and degrees of coercion.

At the same time, it is useful to think of such issues at the level of concrete policy decisions. For example, the debate over the symbolic distribution of authority among child, family, and state in allocating responsibility for decision making about mental health treatment has often resulted in obfuscation of the actual policy dilemmas. As a practical matter, several facts dominate child mental health policy: (a) the prospective inmates of various residential treatment programs, regardless of service system, typically are conduct-disordered adolescents from dysfunctional families, (b) closing the door to one system (e.g., mental health) is apt to lead troubling youth through another door (e.g., juvenile justice), and (c) an underlying undebated assumption in law and policy is that youth cannot be left totally on their own. In such a context, the critical policy question is not how to allocate responsibility but instead how to design procedures that ensure that troubling youth across systems are placed in relatively unintrusive settings and that provide means to prevent out-of-home placement altogether (Melton and Spaulding, in press).

In that regard, the interests of the various parties are compatible, even though they are contrary to current de facto policy. Because high-intensity, middle-restrictiveness services (e.g., intensive home-based services) have the best outcome for conduct-disordered youth and their families (Melton and Hargrove, in press) and because they are less expensive than residential programs, the state's interests are served by such a policy.

Even when some ultimate reconciliation of diverse perspectives and ostensibly conflicting interests can be reached, though, the development of sound policy can be hampered by avoidance of the hard policy questions. For too long, child policy has proceeded in essentially unplanned fashion, with the result that financing mechanisms drawn from adult services are unquestionably applied to children's services and that pernicious de facto policies become the order of the day (e.g., reliance on institutionalization as a primary means of service delivery). Too often, well-conceptualized plans have been derailed by a failure to consider relevant legal doctrines, structures, and ambiguities. As the movement for full recognition of the personhood of children and youth grows (and countermovements are heard), health planners must consider the implications of such movements for their work.

Notes

1. In the following cases, the Court considered whether minors' privacy in abortion decisions may be limited in ways that would be unconstitutional if applied to adult women: *Bellotti v. Baird I* (1976); *Bellotti v. Baird II* (1979); *City of Akron v. Akron Center for Reproductive Health* (1983); *H.L. v. Matheson* (1981); *Planned Parenthood of Central Missouri v. Danforth* (1976); *Planned Parenthood of Kansas City v. Ashcroft* (1983); *Thornburgh v. American College of Obstetricians and Gynecologists* (1986). For analysis of the assumptions underlying this line of cases and their practical import, see Melton (1983b, 1987a); Melton and Pliner (1986); Melton and Russo (1987).

2. This may be true even if the parallel intrusion on the child's autonomy is not debated as actively.

3. Obviously, solicitude for parental autonomy and a protectionist philosophy need not overlap. Whenever the state intervenes, both parental and child autonomy necessarily give way. Paradoxically, even state action to protect the sanctity of the family inherently violates that special deference by entangling the state in family life. On the other hand, the legal tradition in this country generally is to use state power to enhance parental authority to fulfill the states' interest in protecting incompetent, vulnerable children. Thus, although parents are not "free . . . to make martyrs of their children," the tenet is "cardinal . . . that the custody, care and nurture of the child reside first in the parents, whose primary function and freedom include preparation for obligations the state can neither supply nor hinder" (*Prince v. Massachusetts,* 1944, pp. 170, 166).

4. The doctrine of the constitutional right to privacy has evolved almost exclusively in the context of reproduction decision making, an area of life consensually recognized as private in our society and in which consequences usually are profound and irreversible. No Supreme Court cases have explicated minors' right to privacy in any other context.

5. The age 16 is not derived doctrinally. Rather, it reflects an analysis of the characteristics of the cases in which a mature minor rule was recognized (see Wadlington, 1973).

References

Bakan, D. 1971. Adolescence in America: From Ideal to Social Fact. In J. Kagan and R. Coles (eds.), *Twelve to Sixteen: Early Adolescence,* pp. 73–89. New York: Norton.

Bellotti v. Baird I, 428 U.S. 132 (1976).
Bellotti v. Baird II, 443 U.S. 622 (1979).
Blum, R.W. 1982. Critical Care Decision-Making among Minnesota Physicians. *Minnesota Medicine* August:449–502.
Blum, R.W., M.D. Resnick, and T. Stark. 1987. The Impact of a Minnesota Parental Notification Law on Adolescent Abortion Decision-Making. *American Journal of Public Health* 77:619–620.
Board of Education v. Rowley, 458 U.S. 176 (1982).
Bonnie, R.J. 1985. The Efficacy of Law as a Paternalistic Instrument. In G.B. Melton (ed.), *Nebraska Symposium on Motivation*. Vol. 33, *The Law as a Behavioral Instrument*, pp. 131–211. Lincoln: University of Nebraska Press.
Carey v. Population Services International, 431 U.S. 678 (1977).
Citizens League. 1980. *Next Steps in the Evolution of Chemical Dependency Care in Minnesota*. Minneapolis.
City of Akron v. Akron Center for Reproductive Health, 462. U.S. 416 (1983).
Crane, D. 1975. *The Sanctity of Life*. New York: Russell Sage Foundation.
Department of Education. 1984. Student Rights in Research, Experimental Activities, and Testing. *Federal Register* 49:35, 318–335.
Division of Child, Youth, and Family Services, American Psychological Association. 1982. *Standards Regarding Consent for Treatment and Research Involving Children*. Washington, D.C.
Family Educational and Privacy Rights Act of 1974, U.S.C. 1232g (1982).
Felix v. Milliken, 463 F. Supp. 1360 (E.D. Mich. 1978).
Gephart, J., M. Egan, and V. Hutchins. 1984. Perspectives on Health of School-Age Children: Expectations for the Future. *Journal of School Health* 54:11–17.
Guttridge, P., and C.A.B. Warren. 1983. *Adolescent Psychiatric Hospitalization and Social Control*. Unpublished manuscript, University of Southern California, Department of Sociology.
H.L. v. Matheson, 450 U.S. 398 (1981).
Harris, J.E. 1982. Increasing the Federal Excise Tax on Cigarettes. *Journal of Health Economics* 1:117–120.
Harris v. McRae, 448 U.S. 297 (1980).
Hayes v. Shelby Memorial Hospital, 726 F.2d 1543, *reh'g denied,* 732 F.2d 944 (11th Cir.) (1984).
Hatch Amendment of 1978, General Educate Provision Act [ss] 439(b),20 U.S.C. [ss]1232h (1982).
In re Baby X, 97 Mich. App. 111, 293 N.W.2d 736 (1980).
In re Gault, 387 U.S. 1. (1967).
Jackson-Beeck, M. 1983a. *Effective Care '81 Program Status Report*. Minneapolis: Blue Cross and Blue Shield.
———. 1983b. *Juvenile Effective Care '81 Evaluation*. Unpublished manuscript.
Kett, J.F. 1977. *Rites of Passage*. New York: Basic Books.
Krisberg, B., and I.M. Schwartz. 1983. Rethinking Juvenile Justice. *Crime and Delinquency* 29:333–364.
Lerman, P. 1982. *Deinstitutionalization and the Welfare State*. New Brunswick, N.J.: Rutgers University Press.
Lewis, C.E. 1983. Decision Making Related to Health: When Could/Should Children Act Responsibly? In G.B. Melton, G.P. Koocher, and M.J. Saks (eds.), *Children's Competence to Consent*, pp. 75–91. New York: Plenum.
Lewis, D.E., and M.A. Lewis. 1983. Improving the Health of Children: Must the Children Be Involved? *Annual Review of Public Health* 4:259–569.

Lewitt, E.M., D. Coate, and M. Grossman. 1981. The Effects of Government Regulation on Teenage Smoking. *Journal of Law and Economics* 24:545–569.
Maher v. Roe, 432. U.S. 464 (1977).
Males, M.A. 1986. The Minimum Purchase Age for Alcohol and Young-Driver Fatal Crashes: A Long-Term View. *Journal of Legal Studies* 15:181–211.
Massachusetts Board of Retirement v. Murgia, 427 U.S. 307 (1978).
Melton, G.B. 1981. Effects of a State Law Permitting Minors to Consent to Psychotherapy. *Professional Psychology* 12:647–654.
———. 1983a. *Child Advocacy: Psychological Issues and Interventions.* New York: Plenum.
———. 1983b. Minors and Privacy: Are Legal and Psychological Concepts Compatible? *Nebraska Law Review* 62:455–493.
———. 1984. Family and Mental Hospital as Myths: Civil Commitment of Minors. In N.D. Reppucci, L.A. Weithorn, E.P. Mulvey, and J. Monahan (eds.), *Children, Mental Health and the Law,* pp. 151–167. Beverly Hills, Calif.:Sage Publications.
———. 1987a. Legal Regulation of Adolescent Abortion: Unintended Effects. *American Psychologist* 42:79–83.
———. 1987b. Special Legal Problems in Protection of Handicapped Children from Parental Maltreatment. In J. Garbarino, P. Brookhauser, and K. Authier (eds.), *Special Children, Special Risks: The Maltreatment of Children with Disabilities,* pp. 179–193. New York: Aldine.
Melton, G.B., and D.S. Hargrove. In press. Planning Mental Health Services for Children and Youth. New York: Guilford.
Melton, G.B., G.P. Koocher, and M.J. Saks (eds.). 1983. *Children's Competence to Consent.* New York: Plenum.
Melton, G.B., and A.J. Pliner. 1986. Adolescent Abortion: A Psychological Analysis. In G.B. Melton (ed.), *Adolescent Abortion: Psychological and Legal Issues,* pp. 1–39. Lincoln: University of Nebraska Press.
Melton, G.B., and N.F. Russo. 1987. Adolescent Abortion: Psychological Perspectives on Public Policy. *American Psychologist* 42:69–72.
Melton, G.B., and M.J. Saks. 1985. The Law as an Instrument of Socialization and Social Structure. In G.B. Melton (ed.), *Nebraska Symposium on Motivation.* Vol. 33, *The Law as a Behavioral Instrument,* pp. 235–277. Lincoln: University of Nebraska Press.
Melton, G.B., and W.J. Spaulding. In press. *No Place to Go: Civil Commitment of Minors.* Lincoln: University of Nebraska Press (Sponsored by Division 37, American Psychological Association).
Metropolitan Health Board of the Metropolitan Council. 1982. Phase IV Report on General Acute Hospital and Specialty Services. St. Paul.
Mosher, L.R. 1983. Alternatives to Psychiatric Hospitalization: Why Has Research Failed to Be Translated into Practice? *New England Journal of Medicine* 309:1579–1580.
New York State Association for Retarded Children v. Carey, 393 F. Supp. 715 (E.D.N.Y. 1975).
Parham v. J.R., 442 U.S. 584 (1979).
Pennsylvania Association for Retarded Children (PARC) v. Pennsylvania, 334 F. Supp. 1257 (E.D.Pa. 1971).
Pennsylvania Association for Retarded Children (PARC) v. Pennsylvania, 343 F. Supp. 279 (E.D.Pa. 1971).
Perry, G.S., and G.B. Melton. 1984. Precedential Value of Judicial Notice of Social Facts: *Parham* as an Example. *Journal of Family Law* 22:633–676.

Rawls, J. 1971. *A Theory of Justice.* Cambridge, Mass.: Harvard University Press.

Resnick, M.D. 1981. *Physician Attitudes and Practices Towards Confidentiality of Treatment for Youth.* Paper presented to the meeting of the Society for Adolescent Medicine, New Orleans, September.

Resnick, M.D. 1986a. *The Policy Dilemma of Confidentiality of Treatment for Youth.* Keynote address delivered to the annual meeting of Planned Parenthood, Eau Claire, Wis., May.

———. 1986b. *The Financing of Health Services for Youth: Trends and Implications.* Paper presented at the Health Futures of Adolescents National Invitational Conference, DHHS, Division of Maternal and Child Health, Daytona Beach, Fla., March.

Resnick, M.D., L. Bearinger, and R.W. Blum. Physician Attitudes and Approaches to the Problems of Youth: A Report from the Upper Midwest Regional Physicians Survey. *Pediatric Annals* 15(11):142–149.

Resnick, M.D., R.W. Blum, and D. Hedin. 1981. The Appropriateness of Health Services for Adolescents: Youths' Opinions and Attitudes. *Journal of Adolescent Health Care* 1(2):137–141.

Robertson, J.A. 1983. Procreative Liberty and the Control of Conception, Pregnancy, and Childbirth. *Virginia Law Review* 69:405–464.

Rodman, H., S.H. Lewis, and S.B. Griffith. 1984. *The Sexual Rights of Adolescents: Competence, Vulnerability, and Parental Control.* New York: Columbia University Press.

Rogers, C.M., and L.S. Wrightsman. 1978. Attitudes Toward Children's Rights: Nurturance or Self-Determination. *Journal of Social Issues* 34(2):59–68.

San Antonio Independent School District v. Rodriguez, 411 U.S. 1 (1973).

Starr, P. 1982. *The Social Transformation of American Medicine.* New York: Basic Books.

Tarlov, A.R. 1983. Shattuck Lecture: The Increasing Supply of Physicians, the Changing Structure of the Health Services System, and the Future Practice of Medicine. *New England Journal of Medicine* 308:1235–1244.

United Nations. 1959. *Declaration of the Rights of the Child.* Resolution adopted by the General Assembly.

Wadlington, W.J. 1983. Consent to Medical Care for Minors: The Legal Framework. In G.B. Melton, G.P. Koocher, and M.J. Saks (eds.), *Children's Competence to Consent,* pp. 47–74. New York: Plenum.

Wasby, S.L. 1976. *Small Town Police and the Supreme Court: Hearing the Word* Lexington, Mass.: Lexington Books.

Wechsler, H. 1980. *Minimum-Drinking-Age Laws: An Evaluation.* Lexington, Mass.: Lexington Books.

Weithorn, L.A. 1983. Involving Children in Decisions Affecting Their Own Welfare. In G.B. Melton, G.P. Koocher, and M.J. Saks (eds.), *Children's Competence to Consent,* pp. 235–260. New York: Plenum.

Williams, A.F. 1986. Comment on Males. *Journal of Legal Studies* 15:213–217.

Williams, A.F., M.J. Ginsburg, and P.F. Burchman. 1977. Motorcycle Helmet Use in Relation to Legal Requirements. *Accident Analysis and Prevention* 9:69.

Worsfold, V.L. 1974. A Philosophical Justification for Children's Rights. *Harvard Education Review* 44:142–157.

Youngberg v. Romeo, 457 U.S. 307 (1982).

II

Changes in the Financing of Health Services and Their Effects on Children's Health Care

4

A Children's Health Care Budget

Mary Jo Larson, M.P.A.

This chapter gives an overview of the flows of funds that finance health services for children in the United States. It is intended to provide a sense of the relative importance of different sources of funding and settings for treatment. It is also designed to convey some of the interrelationships between the roles of public and private sectors in the financing and delivery of health care for children. Health services are defined broadly here to include nutrition programs and certain social services as well as medical care.[1,2]

Financing Sources for Children's Health Care

The estimated personal and public health care expenditures for those under age 19 were $38.9 billion in 1984. Although persons under age 19 are 28 percent of the nation's population, they account for only 11 percent of all health expenditures (Levit et al., 1985). Average annual medical care spending for a young person is one-third of that for an adult under 65, and only one-seventh of that for an elder person (Fisher, 1980).[3]

Compared to that of other age groups, children's care is financed more by direct payments from families and health programs sponsored by state and local governments and somewhat less through private insurance (Table 4.1). Direct spending by families amounts to more than 35 percent of all payments, including the costs of uncovered services, copayments and deductions for those with insurance, as well as payments from those with no insurance.

Federal and state governmental sources each contribute 17 percent of the total payments for children's health care. The major portion of federal spending is through Medicaid.[4] The single largest source of state governmental financing for children's health care is also through the Medicaid program, though this represents only about 40 percent of state spending. States also provide substantial funding for children through their mental health, school health, and maternal and child health programs.

Spending on major children's health programs has not kept pace with major programs for other age groups (Table 4.2). Growing more slowly than the rate of inflation in the medical care sector, maternal and

Table 4.1 Estimated Health Expenditures for Children and Adults, 1984

Source of Funding	Expenditures (in $ millions) All Ages (Actual)	Expenditures (in $ millions) Under Age 19 (Estimated)	Percentage of Funds Spent on Persons under Age 19
Private funds	$206,500	$25,612	12.4
Direct payments	95,400	13,731	14.4
Private insurance	107,200	11,713	10.9
Philanthropy	2,000	168	8.4
Public funds[1]	146,100	13,284	9.1
Federal programs	102,500	6,622	6.4
State and local programs	43,600	6,662	15.3
All funds[2]	349,700	38,896	11.1

Source: Actual expenditures for all ages are reported in Levit et al. (1985). Estimated expenditures for persons under age 19 are based upon the 1984 National Health Accounts (Levit et al., 1985) and last published analysis of national age-group health care spending (Fisher, 1980). Estimates assume that the ratio of per capita spending between adults and children was the same in 1984 as in 1977.

[1] Includes federal and state public health programs; excludes expenditures for program administration.

[2] Does not include $19.6 billion paid for health premiums and program administration, $15.8 billion paid for research and construction of medical facilities, and $2.9 billion for industrial in-plant health programs.

child health and Medicaid programs, as well as child nutrition and welfare programs, have experienced real dollar declines. Only school health programs and spending from private sources have kept pace with increases in spending on other health programs such as Medicare.

Components of Private Spending on Children's Health Care

Families pay directly for nearly $4 out of every $10 of care for their children. Aggregate out-of-pocket expenditures for children's health services reached $13.7 billion in 1984 (see Table 4.1). Of the total $13.7 billion paid out-of-pocket, 85 percent is spent for dentist and physician visits and medicines.

Not surprisingly, families of children with no health insurance pay for the highest portion of care out-of-pocket, reportedly 75 to 83 percent of the total charges for care (presumably, providers receive subsidies or go uncompensated for the remaining portion). At the other extreme, the families of children eligible for Medicaid pay out-of-pocket only 4–15 percent of the total charges. Children covered by private insurance generally fall between these two extremes, with their families paying 30–37 percent of their medical expenses (Howell, Corder and Dobson, 1985) (Table 4.3).[5]

These direct payments for health care are most burdensome for low-income families (those at or below 150 percent of the poverty line). In 1980 about one-fourth of all children lived in such families. At least

Table 4.2 Trends in Expenditures for United States Major Health Programs, 1977–1984

Health Program	1977	1984	Annual Change
Child Health Programs	*Expenditure per Child*		
Medicaid (AFDC) (per recipient)	$279	$418	7.1%
Maternal and child health	10	16[1]	10.0
Personal health expenditures, all private sources	185	408	17.2
School health, education agencies	6	12[1]	16.7
Child nutrition	52	82[1]	9.3
Child welfare	13	3[1]	−12.8
Other Major Health Programs	*Expenditure per Recipient*		
Medicare (per recipient)	$1,889	$3,431[2]	16.3%
Medicaid, other programs[3] (per recipient)	1,034	2,603	21.7
Medical care price index	202.4	379.5	12.5

Sources: SSA (1985), tables 2, 8, 126, 127, 151, 153; SSA (1980), table 2. The 1977 private insurance estimates were taken from Fisher (1980). The 1984 private insurance estimate for all ages was taken from Levit et al. (1985).

Note: The 1984 private insurance estimates for children under age 19 were calculated using the method described in Table 4.1. The per child and per capita estimates for all other programs were calculated from the aggregate expenditures in the Social Security bulletin for 1977–79 and 1984–85 and estimates of the total population and the under-age-19 population.

[1] Data for 1983.
[2] Data for 1982.
[3] All Medicaid recipients and expenditures not part of dependent children's program.

Table 4.3 Percentage of Health Care Charges Paid Out-of-Pocket, by Type of Coverage

Insurance Coverage	Under Age 6	Age 6–21	All Persons under 65
Private insurance[1]	30	37	31
Medicaid	4	15	9
Other coverage[2]	8	12	15
No coverage	75	83	82
Average (all coverages)	24	36	27

Source: Howell, Corder and Dobson (1985), Tables 3 and 5. Both tables exclude costs of institutional care.

[1] The private insurance group includes only those with no Medicare and no Medicaid.
[2] Includes those persons covered by two sources, such as Medicaid and private insurance.

25 percent of these children were uninsured for part of 1980, and 16 percent were uninsured for the full year. Less than one-half (46 percent) of these children were covered by Medicaid for all or part of 1980; only 31 percent were enrolled in this program all year (Rosenbach, 1985).

Private insurance covered 38 million children in 1984, paying for $11.7 billion, or 30 percent of all child personal and public health costs

(Tables 4.1 and 4.4). Private insurance is the principal payer for children's hospital care and physician visits. Most private insurance policies, however, have limited coverage of the basic preventive health care commonly used by children, such as regular doctor and dentist office visits, immunizations, and prescriptions (Table 4.5).

The costs of care not covered by insurance or paid by insurance are largely borne by providers. While difficult to estimate precisely, free care and bad debt are undoubtedly important indirect sources of funding for children's health care. Based on evidence of health service use by uninsured patients, it appears that physicians provided about $1.5 billion of uncompensated care to children, and that hospitals provided between $3.2 and $4.6 billion of uncompensated children's care. These estimates include bad debt, free care, and reduced billings.

The scope of uncompensated care is not reflected in the previous tables, which are based on providers' payment sources rather than providers' total costs. Adding uncompensated care to this child health budget could increase expenditures on physicians' services by as much as 15 percent.[6]

Table 4.4 Children with Employer- or Union-Provided Health Coverage and CHAMPUS, March 1984 (in thousands)

	Number with Employer or Union	Number with CHAMPUS[1]
Children under age 6	12,599	760
Children 6 to 17	25,456	1,564
Percentage covered	61%	4%

Source: U.S. Census Bureau, Current Population Reports, Series 60, No. 150.

[1]CHAMPUS is the Civilian Health and Medical Program of the Uniformed Services, a Department of Defense program to cover medical care costs of wives and children of active military personnel, and retired military personnel and their dependents when government medical facilities are unavailable.

Table 4.5 Percentage of Children with Some Private Insurance, by Type of Service Covered, 1977

Service	Under Age 6	Age 6–18
Any service covered	75%	78%
Inpatient services	73	77
Physician office	62	66
Prescribed medicines	62	65
Mental health care	67	71
Dental care	21	21
Out-of-hospital nursing	39	43
Vision or hearing	10	9

Source: Farley (1985), based upon NMCES Health Insurance/Employer Survey data for 1977.

Pediatricians are more likely than other physicians to serve patients with no third-party coverage. Analysis of unpublished AMA survey data shows that almost one-half of pediatricians, compared to only 16 percent of all physicians, had more than one-third of their patients without any third-party coverage. These self-paying patients contributed substantially to uncompensated care.

There exist no comprehensive statistics on the proportion of uncompensated hospital care attributable to children. But children certainly accounted for a significant share of the $8–$9.5 billion spent on uncompensated hospital care in 1984 (Fackleman, 1986; Sulvetta and Swartz, 1986). Of the 3.6 million discharges for those under age 15 from short-term, nonfederal hospitals, 9 percent had no public or private insurance (NCHS, 1984). A case study of Vanderbilt Hospital found that patients in nursery, pediatrics, and obstetrics-gynecology accounted for 47 percent of the total unpaid charges. Nearly one-fourth the uncompensated care at Vanderbilt involved neonatal intensive care for sick newborns (Sloan, Valvona, and Mulner, 1986). Other studies indicated that maternity care represented a substantial source of uncompensated care. Nationwide, among annual hospital discharges, fully 22 percent of deliveries had no insurance source (National Center for Health Statistics, 1984). Forty percent of uninsured clients were discharged for deliveries (Sloan et al., 1986).

Although governmental grants subsidize public hospitals to provide some of this care, most uncompensated hospital care is cross-subsidized by other third-party payers (such as commercial insurance, Blue Cross/Blue Shield, and Medicare), and thus represents a source of private financing of services. Private hospitals provide care that accounts for 60 percent of the total charges for uncompensated care (Sulvetta and Swartz, 1986).[7] A study by the National Association of Children's Hospitals and Related Institutions discovered that in general hospitals nearly one-third of children's nursing costs are subsidized by adult patients (NACHRI, 1986).

Foundation gifts, private fundraising, and other charitable giving are a small portion of total health spending. Although a complete accounting is difficult, estimates suggest that in 1984 less than 1 percent of the total child health budget was from charitable sources. Even among nonprofit child-serving agencies, the level of private giving is relatively low. One study of a sample of agencies found that 21 percent of funding to children's nonprofit health and mental health agencies came from private charitable giving sources (Kimmich, Gutowski, and Salamon, 1985). Although a number of philanthropic foundations focusing on children's health are among the largest national health charities, much of this support is for research, health promotion activities, and facilities, not direct health services,[8] though private foundations do finance some medical treatment, mental health, and public health programs (Foundation Center, 1985).

Public Sources of Health Spending

When public health activities are included, such as disease control, prevention programs, and school health clinics, public funds provide for 34 percent of all children's care. More than $2.2 billion, or 17 percent of all governmental expenditures, are for such public health activities. In addition, public funds finance 30 percent of all personal health care for those under age 19. Of all age groups, only the elderly rely more heavily on government-subsidized health care (Waldo and Lazenby, 1984).

Although equal portions of children's health care are financed by federal and local sources, the major governmental programs are administered by state or local health agencies and governed by state health priorities rather than federal initiatives. Federal support for services to persons under 19 was estimated to be $6.6 billion in 1984, or 17 percent of all children's personal and public health care. Five major programs comprised most of these funds.

The federal share of the Medicaid program accounts for nearly 50 percent of federal child health expenditures. While children under age 21 comprise more than 40 percent of the recipients, they received only 19.4 percent of Medicaid expenditures, for an average $418 per recipient (Gornick et al., 1985). The second largest federal program for children's health care is CHAMPUS, the health insurance program financed by the Defense Department for civilian family members and retirees of the military. Together, CHAMPUS and Medicaid provide more than $8 of every $10 of federal support to children's care, or about 14 percent of all health spending for this age group (Table 4.6).

The federal block grant for maternal and child health is the third largest source of federal expenditures. Nearly $400 million in 1984 was appropriated to states through this block grant, the product of a 1981 consolidation of eight categorical programs. Although infrequently recognized as such, the Indian Health Service has the fourth largest federal expenditures for child health care. This program provides personal health care and public health services to nearly 1 million Indian and Alaskan natives, through 47 hospitals, 80 health centers, and more than 500 federal health stations and clinics (Levit et al., 1985).[9] We estimate that it serves roughly 400,000–500,000 children.

A fifth important federal program is the grant support to more than 800 community and migrant health clinics (financed through sections 330 and 329). Children are disproportionate users of these centers, which

Table 4.6 Federal Expenditures for Personal and Public Health, 1984 (in $ millions)

Federal Program	All Ages	Under 19
Medicaid, federal only[1]	19,820	3,140
Medicare	63,100	64
Veterans Administration	8,200	0
Workers' Compensation	300	0
CHAMPUS–Defense Department	6,800	1,871
Indian Health Service	607	218
Health Resources and Services Administration[3]		
Maternal and child block grant	399	399
Community Health Centers[3]	351	154
Family Planning	140	62
Migrant Health	42	18
National Health Service Corps	65	29
Centers for Disease Control	365	146
Alcohol, Drug Abuse, Mental Health block grant	462	185
Public Health Service Management		
Adolescent	15	15
Other health initiatives	7	6
Other federal sources not identified[4]	427	315
All funds	$101,100	$6,622

Sources: 1984 actuals for all ages are from Levit et al. (1985), table 8 and page 25; Office of Management and Budget (1985); estimates for under age 19 are the author's.

[1] Medicaid payments are reported for under age 21.

[2] Assumes that 44% of recipients are under age 18.

[3] Includes $1 million allocated to primary care block grant.

[4] A residual category that includes amounts not separately reported, such as Public Health Service and other federal hospitals.

receive Medicaid and other third-party reimbursements in addition to the grant support. Based upon 1984 utilization statistics, it appears that 44 percent of the $351 million in federal funds for all community and migrant health centers were spent for child health services (Bureau of Health Care Delivery and Assistance, 1986).

Other governmental public health programs include two block grants and other small federal health initiatives. The Alcohol, Drug Abuse, and Mental Health Block Grant provides about 14 percent of the total funding for community mental health centers, an estimated $185 million in 1984 for children's care. Health initiatives of the Centers for Disease Control (CDC), including the preventive health block grant, are used by local and state health departments to run health promotion programs (frequently in local schools) and programs for sexually transmitted disease, infectious disease, and childhood immunizations (Office of Disease Prevention and Health Promotion, 1985). In 1984, CDC spent an estimated $146 million on children's health care.

State-operated health programs are extensive, ranging from the Medicaid entitlement program to nurses in local schools. In 1984, state and local expenditures for personal and public health programs were estimated at $6.66 billion, equal in size to federal expenditures for this age group (Table 4.7).

While Medicaid is the primary state program for financing children's health care, spending nearly $2.7 billion for children under 21, it actually serves a relatively small proportion of young Americans. This is true even among children in low-income families—only 31 percent of poor and near-poor children are enrolled in Medicaid on a full-year basis (Rosenbaum and Johnson, 1986).

Health expenditures of local school districts are the second largest governmental source for child health care. Approximately $2.4 billion is spent for nurses in schools, an amount that disregards any additional and unidentifiable contractual spending with public health departments.[10] These estimates also do not include spending on health curricula or extra services for special education students.

Public mental health programs are estimated to be the third largest category of state health care spending for children, involving nearly $1.8 billion in 1984. These mental health programs include operation of state hospitals and financing of community-based services, research, and training. A survey of state mental health program directors found that 16 percent of the expenditures identifiable by the age group of the recipients were for child or adolescent programs (Glover et al., 1984). There are several components to these programs, including inpatient and outpatient care. Taube and Barrett's (1985) analysis of 1980 utili-

Table 4.7 State and Local Expenditures for Personal and Public Health, 1984 (in $ millions)

State and Local Programs	All Ages	Under 19
Medicaid, state match[1]	16,880	2,674
State-only medical assistance	2,000	169
State and local hospitals	8,400	143
Maternal and child health	273	273
Crippled children's programs	154	154
School health programs	900	900
Other state health agency	562	202
Other state mental health	4,797	1,777
Other state programs[2]	4,372	370
All programs	$43,638	$6,663

Sources: 1984 actuals for all age groups from Levit et al. (1985), Table 8 and page 26. Estimates for under age 19 are the author's.

[1] Medicaid expenditures are for under age 21.

[2] Total for all age groups includes sources not separately reported here when the source does not finance children's health services.

zation data indicated that children accounted for 10 percent of the days of care in state and county mental hospitals.[11]

The remaining major source of state spending takes the form of state funding of maternal and child health (MCH) programs and crippled children's (CC) programs.[12] These are discussed in more detail in Chapter 12.

Health-Related Services and Research

More than $10.8 billion are annually spent on food stamps, food commodities, and subsidized meals for children (Table 4.8). These programs are targeted to the poor and near-poor.[13] As with other programs for low-income groups, these programs lost funding under the Reagan Administration. Between fiscal years 1982 and 1985, coverage was reduced 29 percent in four school-based programs: school breakfast, school lunch, special milk, and summer feeding (Children's Defense Fund, 1987).

The special supplementary food program for women, infants, and children (WIC) promotes health outcomes through food, health care access, and nutrition counseling for pregnant women, new mothers, and children up to age 5. About 1,500 local WIC projects are operated by the U.S. Department of Agriculture. Allocations have increased in recent years, in 1984 totaling over $1.36 billion (Children's Defense Fund, 1987). There is, however, considerable variation in the extent to which states have implemented WIC. The proportion of the eligible population actually served by the state ranges from 23 percent in Hawaii to 77 percent in Vermont (Children's Defense Fund, 1987).

Table 4.8 Federal and State Programs for Child Feeding or Nutrition, 1984 (in $ millions)

Nutrition Program	All Ages	Under 19
Food stamps	11,726	5,324
School lunch	2,507	2,507
School breakfast	365	365
Special milk	12	12
Women, infant, child	1,360	1,360
Child care food program	378	378
Summer feeding program	105	105
Needy family	44	44
Commodities	862	391
Commodities to charities	194	88
Emergency feeding	1,091	495
All Funds	$28,389	$10,815

Sources: Children's Defense Fund (1987), SSA (1985), and author's estimates.

Several governmental social service and education programs may improve health outcomes and increase access to health services for children. Spending on these programs is summarized in Table 4.9. Head Start, the nation's early childhood development program for low-income children, arranged for health services such as screening and referrals for preschool-aged children. The total federal appropriation to finance these compensatory services was more than $995 million in 1984. The program now benefits about 451,000 children (CDF, 1987). The program also arranges for free medical care and enrollment in Medicaid of eligible children, though only a small portion of Head Start expenditures actually pays for medical care. The Social Services Block Grant (formerly Title XX) is a federal appropriation to assist states in the provision of a wide range of services to public assistance recipients and low- or middle-income children and families. Certain program goals are directed to preventing or remedying child abuse or neglect, and to preventing inappropriate institutional care. Other health and family-planning services can be provided at state option. For example, states may provide health-related home-based services, information and referral, or daycare programs. A national report on the Title XX program found that 50 percent of the funds in 1978 were to a broad range of child welfare services (Office of Human Development Services, 1980). Although residential care and treatment and health-related programs are known to be important program goals, the total scope of spending for children's services could not be calculated because of the limited reporting on these state-managed programs.

Research funding makes a significant indirect contribution to children's health care. Clearly children may benefit from virtually any form of medical research, though some is explicitly targeted to children. At the National Institutes of Health, the largest program on behalf of child health received $274 million in 1984 (Table 4.9). Located at the National

Table 4.9 Expenditures for Health-Related and Research Services, 1986 (in $ millions)

	All Ages	Under 19
Social Services Block Grant (Title XX)	$2,700	unknown
Head Start	995	$ 995
Federal Health Research Programs		
Mothers and Children	276	276
Other National Institutes of Health	2,515	unknown
Federal Child Abuse	25	25
Federal Family Violence	8	unknown
Federal Foster Care and Adoption (1986)	885	885
Federal Child Welfare Services	198	198
Handicapped Education (P.L. 94-142)	1,349	1,349

Source: Based upon appropriations reported by Children's Defense Fund.

Institute on Child Health and Human Development, the program is for research on mothers, children, and other population issues. Children certainly also benefit from other research conducted or funded by NIH.

The Organization of Child Health Services

In Table 4.10 we estimate that $37.2 billion financed hospital, physician, and other personal health services for children in 1984. Not shown in this table is $2.5 billion spent on other activities of public health agencies, which is not disaggregated in reports of national health expenditures but includes some mental health and prevention services, immunization, and disease-detection programs.

Hospital care captures the largest portion of expenditures, although hospital costs among children are small compared to those of other age groups. Although nonprofit or church-operated hospitals are the principal providers, an increasing number of hospitals are proprietary.[14] Public funding is important to child hospital services, with public financing programs paying for nearly 45 percent of all hospital services for children and a significant portion of hospital services provided in government-operated facilities (Table 4.11). Of the $1.8 billion spent on children by state mental health authorities, more than 63 percent funds institutional care.

In contrast to hospital care, spending on dentists and medicines is disproportionately high for children. These costs can be particularly burdensome to families, since nearly all such care is financed by out-of-pocket spending.

Children's care is predominantly delivered by private providers. More than 60 percent of the treatment by hospitals, physicians, and dentists occurs under private auspices (Table 4.10). Public providers take a variety of forms, including school health programs, public hospital outpatient clinics, and other local health clinics.

Physicians, dentists, and other ambulatory professionals provide the core of children's services, about two-thirds of all care (Table 4.12). However, the extent of physician care delivered in hospital settings is large. More than $2.7 billion is estimated for visits to emergency rooms and hospital outpatient departments; another $2.4 billion could not be identified by site, and most likely represents inpatient physician billings.[15] Of the $10 billion spent on physician services, only $4.5 billion can be attributed to visits in private physician offices.

Public sites for ambulatory care can take a variety of forms. A substantial portion of health services are delivered by school nurses and school psychological personnel. Nurses' salaries at local school districts

Table 4.10 Public and Private Expenditures, by Type of Personal Health Care, for Persons under Age 19, 1984 (in $ millions)

	Type of Expenditure						
	Hospital	Physician	Dentist	Other Health Professionals	Drugs and Medicines	Eyeglasses	Nursing Home	Other
Private expenditures	7,671	8,568	4,524	326	4,162	752	5	171
Direct payment	520	3,929	4,041	291	3,718	672	5	153
Private insurance	7,123	4,639	397	29	365	66	0	15
Other private[2]	28	0	86	6	79	14	0	3
Public expenditures	6,125	1,731	192	542	274	77	115	2,007
Medicaid	3,373	1,343	82	232	117	33	49	859
Other public expenditures	2,752	388	110	310	157	44	66	1,148
All funds[1]	$13,797	$10,300	$4,716	$868	$4,436	$830	$121	$2,178

Note: The expenditure categories follow the definitions used by the Health Care Financing Administration to construct national health accounts.

[1] The total for all funds differs slightly from the sum of the columns because of rounding error.

[2] Spending by philanthropic organizations and privately financed construction.

Table 4.11 Estimated Expenditures for Child Hospital Care, 1984

	Short-term General Private	Short-term General Public	Short-term General Mental Health	Private Psychiatric	State and County Mental Hospital
Expenditures (in thousands)	9,193,245	2,298,311	228,001	305,402	543,158
Patient days	17,055,200	4,263,800	610,330	602,460	897,048
Number of visits	31,840,000	7,960,000	N/A	N/A	N/A
Funding Sources					
Private insurance	60%	60%	N/A	85%	41%
Self-pay	10	10	N/A	9	8
Medicaid	22	22	N/A	—	35
Other government	—	—	N/A	3	16
Other and unknown	8	8	N/A	3	0
Estimated % of charges uncompensated	4%	11%	N/A	N/A	11%

Source: Author's estimates based on Taube and Barrett (1985), and Levit et al. (1985).

Table 4.12 Estimated Expenditures[1] by Physicians and Other Ambulatory Care Providers of Child Health Care, 1984 (in $ millions)

Providers in private settings	
Physicians' payments	
M.D. offices	$ 4,555
Emergency rooms or OPDs	2,706
Inpatient or unknown	2,225
Health centers, other	775
Dentist offices	4,716
Psychologist or social worker	176
Subtotal private	$15,153
Providers in public settings	
Physicians' payments	
Emergency rooms or OPDs	675
Inpatient or unknown	556
School nurses	2,400
School psychologist	1,116
Community mental health center	951
Community and migrant health center	791
Residential treatment centers	676
State and local health department clinics	1,348
Federal public health	1,400
Head Start	995
Subtotal public	$10,908

Sources: Author's estimates based upon Rosenbach (1985), Taube and Barrett (1985), Kimmich (1985), and Levit et al. (1985).

[1] Includes CHAMPUS payments to private providers that could not be separately calculated.

were estimated to be more than $2.4 billion in 1984. While more difficult to calculate, the costs of personnel delivering mental health services, such as psychologists, social workers, psychometrists, and others, were about $1.2 billion.[16] This estimate, based on a national salary survey of professional positions employed at public schools, excluded the educational components of Special Education programs operated in local districts for students with chronic physical or psychological disabilities (ERS, 1986, 1987). Taube and Barrett (1985) included these special services in their estimates and reported that more than $2.7 billion of direct costs for mental health care were delivered to students in schools in 1980. Still higher estimates would include the costs of health education. Statistics on these expenditures are not currently available.

Local school district policy governs the scope and extent of these health services. In some districts, nursing services may include: dental, vision, hearing, and scoliosis screenings; health screenings for children entering kindergarten; services to students who become sick or injured at school; and health education. Other services include the diagnoses, casework, and groupwork services of school social workers, and a variety of psychological services such as administration and interpretation of tests; and counseling and other services for behavioral or psychological problems.

Local health department clinics, public health programs, and community and migrant health centers provide an estimated $6.1 billion in services. More than 900 primary care centers are funded by a federal categorical grant, with an equal amount of financial support from state sources and fees. These centers include rural and urban community health centers, migrant health programs, National Health Service Corps sites, maternal and child health projects, and urban Indian health programs. Forty-four percent of the 4.3 million medical care patients at these federally sponsored programs are under age 19. Additionally, local health departments sponsor well-child clinics and maternal and child programs that offer immunizations, screenings, WIC certification, and other preventive measures.

Conclusions

Although somewhat crudely constructed, this budget for child health care helps identify the distribution of health services. Many of the consequences of this distribution are discussed in subsequent chapters. Several points are worth noting here.

First, children are often in the families least capable of paying for large medical bills. They comprise a significant portion of the nation's uninsured, and are overrepresented among the families in poverty. Children's care will thus be disproportionately affected by policies or programs that reduce cross-subsidies between sources or across patients.

Second, $4 out of every $10 spent on children's care are direct family expenditures. Therefore, health care purchases for this age group are more income dependent than purchases made for other populations. A corollary is that children are significant users of subsidized settings such as neighborhood health clinics.

Third, children's care relies heavily on governmental providers and governmental financing. Past history suggests that this public financing is vulnerable to competing priorities, and budget pressures on the national and state levels could lead to a further decline in the proportion of funding going to children's care. Because current reporting requirements are insufficient to monitor adequately the impact of budget cuts or shifts, it may prove difficult to devise timely policy responses.

Fourth, unlike the Medicare program for the elderly, the states and local agencies operate much of the public programs with large number of child beneficiaries, such as Medicaid and maternal and child health clinics. This fragments children's health financing along state boundaries. Even more fragmented is the provision of health care through local school districts. For low-income children in particular, who may depend upon these governmentally organized services, their access to adequate care is thus dependent upon where they live: in generous or penurious Medicaid states, in school districts with or without health programs, nearby or distant from a government-subsidized clinic.

Finally, a broad array of mental health providers and other nonmedical professionals apparently deliver a significant amount of services to children. Since they are not traditionally recognized as providers of care to children, further study could identify more precisely the nature and extent of such services and their coordination with primary care providers. If public policies are to be effectively designed, they must be guided by an understanding of this distribution of resources.

Notes

1. Studies suggest that these services significantly affect children's access to health care and health status (Physician's Task Force, 1985; U.S.D.A., 1986; Children's Defense Fund, 1987).

2. The appendix to this chapter describes the data sources and calculations used to make the estimates presented here. The basic method was to take per capita spending ratios for the under 19 age group and all age groups presented in Fisher (1980) and to create 1984 estimates using the National Health expenditures reported by Levit et al. (1985).

3. Fisher's (1980, p. 65) estimates of age group spending in 1978.

4. Not included in these estimates, however, are federal income tax subsidies to individuals for medical care expenditures, estimated at $50 billion annually for all age groups. Roughly $5 billion of these subsidies pay for the care of children.

5. Table 5.3 presents 1980 estimates based upon a household survey that shows a lower portion of out-of-pocket expenses than our estimates for 1984 based upon analysis of national health expenditures.

6. An American Medical Association survey in 1982 of fee-for-service physicians found that uncompensated care reduced physicians' total billings by 15 percent: 6 percent reduction from bad debt and 9 percent reduction from charity care (Ohsfeldt, 1985).

7. Public hospitals, however, are disproportionately burdened by free care and bad debt, when taken in the context of the total amount of their charges (Sulvetta and Swartz, 1986). The growing prevalence of for-profit medical care, prepaid health plans, and price competition among providers is likely to threaten this source.

8. National child health agencies that received more than $10 million in total contributions in 1984 include: March of Dimes Birth Defects, National Easter Seal Society, ALSAC St. Jude's Hospital, United Cerebral Palsy Association, National Association for Retarded Citizens, Cystic Fibrosis Foundation, and Juvenile Diabetes Foundation (AAFRC, 1986).

9. If the experiences of these Indian Health Service programs are similar to that of other community and migrant health centers, children make up 44 percent of the recipients of care.

10. These estimates are based on the number of nurse and psychological personnel on salary at local schools, and calculating a budget based upon their reported median salaries. They do not include an estimated $1.16 billion for school psychological personnel who provide counseling and therapy for certain students (Educational Research Service, 1986, 1987).

11. Although children account for only 4.5 percent of all admissions, the median length of stay for these youth is 54 days, more than twice as long as the median for all age groups (23 days) in state and county mental hospitals (Taube and Barrett, 1985).

12. The allocation of state funds to MCH versus CC programs is an estimate based on the reported expenditures of state health agencies.

13. According to governmental household surveys, about 45 percent of food stamp recipients are children (CPR, 1985). This statistic was used to estimate child nutrition expenditures for the programs that serve all age groups.

14. Hospital care expenditures shown here include all inpatient and outpatient care in public and private hospitals and all services and supplies provided by hospitals. Except for services of hospital staff physicians, expenditures for physician care provided in hospitals are included in the physician category (Levit et al., 1985).

15. These calculations were made by using Rosenbach's data (1985) on the distribution in 1980 of physician visits of low-income children and the author's estimates of total physician spending based upon national health expenditure data from Levit (1985).

16. The national reporting on school system positions and salaries combines these providers with other nonhealth providers.

References

American Association of Fund-Raising Council Trust for Philanthropy. 1986. *Giving USA: Estimates of Philanthropic Giving in 1985 and the Trends They Show.* New York.

Association of State and Territorial Health Organizations Foundation. 1984. *An Inventory of Programs and Block Grant Expenditures: Public Health Agencies 1982,* Vol. 4. McLean, Va.

Bureau of Health Care Delivery and Assistance, DHHS. 1986. Summarized BCRR Table Submissions from Pat Mather. Unpublished.

Children's Defense Fund. 1987. *A Children's Defense Budget: FY 1988.* Washington, D.C.

Committee on Finance, United States Senate. 1979. *Materials Relating to Existing Federal Programs Providing or Financing Health Care for Mothers and Children.* Washington, D.C.: G.P.O.

Dennison, C.F. 1985. 1984 Summary: National Hospital Discharge Survey. *NCHS Advance Data,* Number 112. Washington, D.C.: Division of Health Care Statistics, Vital and Health Statistics of the National Center for Health Statistics, Public Health Service. Washington, D.C.: G.P.O.

Educational Research Service. 1986. *Educational Research Service Report: Salaries Paid Professional Personnel in Public Schools, 1984–85: Part 2 of National Survey of Salaries and Wages in Public Schools.* Arlington, Va.

―――. 1987. *Educational Research Service Report: School Staffing Rations, 1986–1987.* Arlington, Va.

Executive Office of the President, Office of Management and Budget. 1985. *Budget of the U.S. Government, Fiscal Year 1986, Appendix.* Washington, D.C.: G.P.O.

Farley, P.J. 1985. *Private Insurance and Public Programs: Coverage of Health Services, Data Preview 20.* National Health Care Expenditures Study. DHHS Publication No. (PHS) 85-3374. DHHS, National Center for Health Services Research and Health Care Technology Assessment. Washington, D.C.: G.P.O.

Fisher, C.R. 1980. Differences by Age Groups in Health Care Spending. *Health Care Financing Review* 1(4):65–90. Office of Research, Demonstrations, and Statistics, HCFA. Washington, D.C.: G.P.O.

Foundation Center. 1985. *The Foundation Directory,* 10th Edition. New York.

Glover, R., N.A. Mazade, T. Lutterman, and H.C. Schnibbe. 1984. *Final Report: Funding Sources and Expenditures for State Mental Health Agencies: Revenue/Expenditure Study Results.* Washington, D.C.: National Association of State Mental Health Program Directors.

Gornick, M., et al. 1985. Twenty Years of Medicare and Medicaid: Covered Populations, Use of Benefits, and Program Expenditures. *Health Care Financing Review* 1985 Annual Supplement:13–59. Office of Research, Demonstrations, and Statistics, HCFA. Washington, D.C.: G.P.O.

Graves, E.J. 1983. Utilization of Short-Stay Hospitals by Adolescents: United States, 1980. *NCHS Advance Data,* Number 93. Division of Health Care Statistics, Vital and Health Statistics of the National Center for Health Statistics, Public Health Service. Washington, D.C.: G.P.O.

Health Care Financing Administration. 1986. *Medicare and Medicaid Data Book, 1984.* Health Care Financing, Program Statistics, HCFA Pub. No. 03210. Washington, D.C.: G.P.O.

Howell, E., L. Corder, and A. Dobson. 1985. *Out-of-Pocket Health Expenses for Medicaid Recipients and Low-Income Persons, 1980.* National Medical Care Utilization and Expenditure Survey. Series B, Descriptive Report No. 4. DHHS Publication No. 85-20204. Office of Research and Demonstrations, HCFA. Washington, D.C.: G.P.O.

Kimmich, M.H., M. Gutowski, and L.M. Salamon. 1985. *Child-Serving Nonprofit Organizations in an Era of Government Retrenchment.* The Nonprofit Sector Project. Washington, D.C.: Urban Institute.

Levit, K.R., H. Lazenby, D.R. Waldo, and L.M. Davidoff. 1985. National Health Expenditures, 1984. *Health Care Financing Review* 7(1):1–35. Office of Research and Demonstrations, HCFA. Washington, D.C.: G.P.O.

McCarthy, E., and L.J. Kozak. 1985. Hospital Use by Children: United States, 1983. *NCHS Advance Data,* No. 109. Division of Health Care Statistics, Vital and Health Statistics of the National Center for Health Statistics, Public Health Service. Washington, D.C.: G.P.O.

National Association of Children's Hospitals and Related Institutions, Inc. 1986. *NACHRI Urges Congress to Adopt New Patient Classification System for Use in Determining Payment to Hospitals Treating Children.* News Release, September 17.

National Center for Health Statistics, L. Lawrence. 1986. Detailed Diagnoses and Procedures for Patients Discharged from Short-Stay Hospitals, United States, 1984. *Vital and Health Statistics,* Series 13, No. 86. DHHS Publication No. (PHS) 86-1747. Washington, D.C.: G.P.O.

National Institute of Mental Health, DHHS, Public Health Service. 1986. *Use of Inpatient Psychiatric Services by Children and Youth under Age 18, U.S., 1980.* Mental Health Statistical Note No. 175. Division of Biometry and Epidemiology. Washington, D.C.: G.P.O.

National Institutes of Health. 1984. *1984 NIH Almanac.* Public Health Services, NIH Publication No. 84-5. Washington, D.C.: G.P.O.

Office of Disease Prevention and Health Promotion, DHHS, Public Health Service. *Prevention '84/'85.* Washington, D.C.: G.P.O.

Office of Human Development Services, DHHS. 1980. *Annual Report to the Congress on Title XX of the Social Security Act: Fiscal Year 1979.* Washington, D.C.: G.P.O.

Ohsfeldt, R.L. 1985. Uncompensated Medical Services Provided by Physicians and Hospitals. *Medical Care* 23(12):1338–1344.

Perrin, J.M. 1986. High Technology and Uncompensated Hospital Care. In F.A. Sloan, J.F. Blumstein, and J.M. Perrin (eds.), *Uncompensated Hospital Care: Rights, and Responsibilities.* Baltimore: Johns Hopkins University Press.

Rosenbach, M.L. 1985. Insurance Coverage and Ambulatory Medical Care of Low-Income Children: United States, 1980. *National Medical Care Utilization and Expenditure Survey.* Series C, Analytical Report No. 1. DHHS Publication No. 85-20401. National Center for Health Care Statistics, Public Health Service. Washington, D.C.: G.P.O.

Rosenbaum, S., and K. Johnson. 1986. Providing Health Care for Low-Income Children: Reconciling Child Health Goals with Child Health Financing Realities. *Milbank Memorial Fund Quarterly* 64(3):442–478.

Sloan, F.A., J. Valvona, and R. Mullner. 1986. Identifying the Issues: A Statistical Profile. In F.A. Sloan, J.F. Blumstein, and J.M. Perrin (eds.), *Uncompensated Hospital Care: Rights, and Responsibilities.* Baltimore: Johns Hopkins University Press.

Social Security Administration. 1980. *Social Security Bulletin: Annual Statistical Supplement, 1977–79.* Washington, D.C.: G.P.O.

———. 1985. *Social Security Bulletin: Annual Statistical Supplement, 1984-85.* SSA Publication No. 13-11700. Washington, D.C.: G.P.O.

Sulvetta, M.B., and K. Swartz. 1986. *The Uninsured and Uncompensated Care: A Chartbook.* Washington, D.C.: National Health Policy Forum, George Washington University.

Taube, C.A., and S.A. Barrett. 1985. *Mental Health, United States 1985.* National Institute of Mental Health. DHHS Publication No. 85-1378. Washington, D.C.: G.P.O.

U.S. Bureau of the Census. 1986. Consumer Income, *Current Population Reports,* Series P-60, No. 150. Washington, D.C.: G.P.O.

———. 1986. Economic Characteristics of Households in the U.S.: Fourth Quarter 1984, *Current Population Reports,* Series P-70, No. 6. Washington, D.C.: G.P.O.

———. 1984. *Federal Expenditures by State for Fiscal Year 1983.* Washington, D.C.: G.P.O.

———. 1985. *Statistical Abstract of the United States: 1986,* 106th edition. Washington, D.C.: G.P.O.

U.S. Department of Health and Human Services. 1980, February. *Annual Report to the Congress on Title XX of the Social Security Act, Fiscal Year 1979.* Washington, D.C.: G.P.O.

U.S. General Accounting Office. 1984. *Maternal and Child Health Block Grant: Program Changes Emerging Under State Administration.* Publication No. GAO/HRD-84-35. Washington, D.C.: G.P.O.

Waldo, D.R., and H.C. Lazenby. 1984. Demographic Characteristics and Health Care Use and Expenditures by the Aged in the United States: 1977–1984. *Health Care Financing Review* 6(1):1–29. Office of Research, Demonstrations, and Statistics, HCFA. Washington, D.C.: G.P.O.

Waldo, D.R., K.R. Levit, and H.C. Lazenby. 1986. National Health Expenditures, 1985. *Health Care Financing Review* 8(1):1–21. Office of Research, Demonstrations, and Statistics, HCFA. Washington, D.C.: G.P.O.

Appendix

Note on Data Sources and Estimation Methods

Tables 4.1 and 4.10. These estimates are based upon the 1984 National Health Accounts (Levit et al., 1985) and last published analysis of national age-group health care spending (Fisher, 1980). The estimates for private and public expenditures in Table 4.10, for care to those under age 19 for each expenditure category, were generated first using this method: First, per capita total expenditures in each category were calculated by dividing aggregate spending by the 1984 total population (232 million). Second, an under age 19 spending ratio was calculated for categories of care, equal to the 1978 per capita spending for persons under 19 divided by the 1978 per capita spending for all persons (Fisher, 1980). This ratio was then multiplied by the 1984 per capita expenditure to yield a 1984 per capita amount for children. This per capita amount was then multiplied by the population under age 19—the result was an estimated aggregate expenditure for children.

After total private and total public expenditures for each category were estimated, the amounts funded by direct payments, private insurance, Medicaid and other sources were estimated. The total expenditures were distributed to funding sources using the percentage break out reported by Fisher for the under-19 age group.

Table 4.2. The private insurance estimates for 1977 were taken from Fisher (1980). The author calculated 1984 private insurance estimates for under 19 using the method described in Table 4.1. The 1984 private insurance estimate for all ages was taken from Levit et al. (1985). The per-child and per-capita estimates for all other programs were calculated from the aggregate expenditures reported in the Social Security Bulletin for 1977–79 and 1984–85 and estimates of the total population and under age 19 population.

Tables 4.6 and 4.7. Whenever possible, estimates of spending by various funding sources were based upon reports from those sources. For the many programs that do not segregate spending on children from spending on all recipients, estimates were based upon the proportion of child recipients in the program. Expenditures for the following sources were based on reports of the sources: Medicaid (distribution between federal and state was estimated), maternal and child block grant, Crippled Children's programs, and school health programs.

When data on expenditures were not available for a particular funding source, estimates were calculated by using the per capita spending ratio method described in the note to Table 1.2. The exceptions are programs within Health Resources and Services Administration, where children were assumed to be 44 percent of all recipients and hence were allocated 44 percent of expenditures. The following expenditures were estimated in this fashion: Medicare, CHAMPUS, all HRSA programs, Center for Disease Control, Alcohol, Drug Abuse, Mental Health Block Grant, Public Health Service Management, adolescent and other health initiatives, state and local hospitals, and other state health agency programs.

Table 4.8. The Children's Defense Fund (1987) presents total spending for these programs. Spending for under age 19 was crudely estimated to be equal to the proportion of total recipients that was children. The age group of recipients was based upon a U.S. household survey, reported in *Consumer Population Reports.*

Table 4.9. Based upon appropriations reported by the Children's Defense Fund.

Table 4.10. See description under Table 4.1.

Tables 4.11 and 4.12. Estimates are the author's based upon utilization data reported in Rosenbach (1985), Taube and Barrett (1985), Kimmich et al. (1985), and expenditures reported in Levit et al. (1985). Physician's billings were allocated to various settings based upon Rosenbach's analysis of the number of visits made by near-poor children to physicians in 1980. School personnel estimates were made by multiplying the number of nurse and psychologist positions by the average salary for these positions, as reported to the Educational Research Service. The number of psychologist positions was estimated because they are one portion of a broader category. The estimated CHAMPUS expenditures are all shown under public hospitals, although this program also provides reimbursements to private providers and ambulatory settings, because no data were available to disaggregate these expenditures.

Definitions of Health Care Categories. The definitions and concepts used in Table 4.10 are those used to construct the National Health Accounts as reported in Levit et al., 1985:

Hospital care spending includes both inpatient and outpatient care, all drugs, supplies and salaries at hospitals, including physicians salaried at hospitals and home health agencies that are hospital based.

Expenditures for *physicians, dentists* and *other health professionals* are based primarily on Internal Revenue Service statistics, and expenditures on independent laboratory services, and nonprofit group practice dental clinics. Salaried physicians, dentists, and other personnel are included with expenditures for the employing provider (such as hospitals).

Other health personnel includes private-duty nurses, chiropractors, optometrists, home health agencies that are not hospital based and others.

Drugs and Medicines and *Eyeglasses* include only those expenditures for outpatient drugs and appliances purchased from retail trade outlets by consumers, and excludes those goods provided in hospitals and nursing homes and physicians' offices.

Nursing homes includes all nonhospital facilities.

Other personal health care expenditures are those for unspecified purposes or those that do not fit any category. Public expenditures include school health services, ambulance services, and others.

5

Children and Private Health Insurance

Sara Rosenbaum, J.D.

The purpose of this chapter is to assess the role private health insurance plays in financing children's health care. The chapter will analyze major trends in eligibility, benefits, cost sharing, and methods of administration and will assess the feasibility of various approaches to improving children's health coverage.

There are many reasons why policy makers must be concerned about children's relationship to the private health insurance system. A number stand out as most important for public policy considerations. First, millions of families need assistance in underwriting the cost of their children's health care. Virtually all families, whether poor or nonpoor, need financial assistance in ensuring access to health care. Given children's need for a wide range of health services and the proven effectiveness of many types of pediatric health procedures, strong efficacy, fiscal, and ethical considerations exist for adequately financing children's health care (Select Panel, 1980; President's Commission, 1983; U.S. Congress, Office of Technology Assessment, 1988).

Even routine pediatric health care is expensive. The medical, vision, and dental care necessary to meet a child's basic health needs can easily amount to between $500 and $600 over the course of a year. For lower-income working families, even basic health expenditures create large financial burdens.

Additionally, approximately 10 percent of all children suffer from at least one chronic disability requiring additional medical attention, while 3 percent can be classified as severely disabled (Gortmaker and Sappenfield, 1984). Even relatively well-to-do families cannot realistically accommodate these children's long-term costs without substantial financial assistance.

Childhood poverty in America appears to be both entrenched and long term. As a result of several factors, including higher unemployment rates, the minimum wage's failure to keep pace with inflation, and taxation of low wage earners, the percentage of children living in poor families grew significantly during the early 1980s: from 10 million to 13 million children (Congressional Research Service, 1985). It maintained its high levels throughout the mid-1980s even as the economy generally improved (Children's Defense Fund, 1987). Thus, there exist a large number of families that need substantial assistance in financing health care.

A second concern for policy makers relates to the fact that the employer-based health insurance system excludes millions of families. In 1977, employer-provided health insurance covered 93 percent of all privately insured children (Kasper, 1986), but the employer-based insurance system denies coverage to millions of children. It excludes families in which no one works. It excludes or shortchanges millions of working families whose employers do not offer benefits at all or who fail to provide affordable and appropriate family coverage. Since the cost of employees' insurance is underwritten primarily by excluding employer premium payments as taxable income, the system most heavily benefits those families in upper income tax brackets who are less in need of subsidy.

It is in great part because the employer-provided health insurance system is so generous to some that its failings for so many others pose such a stark contrast. Many employees are substantially insured, even against health costs that carry little or no risk. This tendency to substantially underwrite even relatively routine medical care costs reflects both the high cost of medical care and the financial attractiveness of employer-provided insurance and other health-related tax shelters to salary and wage earners, especially those in higher tax brackets.

The enormous cost of private health insurance alone justifies a close examination of its adequacy as a financing mechanism for children's health care. In 1983, Americans spent more than $300 billion on personal health services (Gibson, Levit, Lazenby and Waldo, 1984). Of this amount, $100 billion was paid by private health insurance. Families, businesses, and others spent $110 billion to purchase this coverage. The cost of health insurance to American industry is substantial. In 1984, American businesses spent about $90 billion on employee health insurance premiums, an amount equal to 38 percent of their pretax profits (Califano, 1986).

The cost of private insurance to government is also enormous. Excluding employer-paid health insurance benefits as taxable income costs the United Stated Treasury about $27 billion in tax revenues foregone (Congressional Budget Office, 1983). When all federal tax subsidies for employment-related or individual personal health expenditures are considered, the total annual federal price tag was estimated at approximately $50 billion in 1985—double the amount the the federal government spent to provide Medicaid coverage to the poor that year (Enthoven, 1985). These federal "tax expenditure" estimates do not take into account states' tax expenditures for personal health care that result from the parallel nature of the two tax systems in many jurisdictions. Thus, private health insurance requires a huge investment of individual, governmental, and business resources.

Private health insurance thus constitutes the nation's primary health care financing mechanism and thus determines children's access to health care.[1] The absence of health insurance coverage has a sizable impact on children's access to health care. Low-income children, whose health status is poorer to begin with (Egbuono and Starfield, 1982), are disproportionately likely to be completely uninsured. The absence of insurance coverage among lower-income children has been shown to result in as much as 40 percent differential in poor children's use of health services (Blendon, et al., 1986).

Equally as disturbing, perhaps, is the fact that private insurance, even when available, is not an effective subsidy for many children. These gaps are clearly illustrated by comparing coverage in private insurance to that under Medicaid. Only 4 percent of privately insured children are covered for preventive medical care and only 21 percent have preventive dental coverage (Kasper, 1986). Yet all persons under age 21 covered by the Medicaid program have complete preventive coverage under the Early and Periodic Screening Diagnosis and Treatment program for comprehensive medical, dental, vision, and hearing care. Privately insured low-income children use fewer health care services than do their publicly insured counterparts. Publicly insured low-income children under age 6 are 1.5 times more likely to have at least one preventive health exam during a year than either their privately insured or uninsured counterparts (Rosenbach, 1985). In spite of these gaps, privately insured low-income children, whose families can ill afford to pay the cost of their care, nonetheless have out-of-pocket health costs four times higher than those of their publicly insured counterparts (Rosenbach, 1985).

The nation is experiencing a period of major retrenchment in private health coverage that exacerbates these limitations. Between 1977 and 1984, the number of uninsured Americans grew from 26.2 million to more than 35 million (Sulvetta and Swartz, 1986). Between 1982 and 1985 alone the number of uninsured children grew by 16 percent even as unemployment declined (Employee Security Research Institute, 1987). Retrenchment in private coverage is occurring for several reasons, including the growth of single-parent-headed households, changes in employment patterns that have led to more employment in firms that offer no coverage, and efforts by employers who do offer health insurance to shift costs to employees, who in turn cannot afford to absorb them (Sulvetta and Swartz, 1986).

The past several years have witnessed a major shift away from employment in higher-paid manufacturing jobs with good fringe benefits toward poorer-paying jobs with few or no benefits (Swartz, 1984). Simultaneously, those employers who continue to offer health insurance have reduced their subsidies for employee premiums and have incorporated additional cost-sharing requirements, such as larger deductibles and co-insurance.

This retrenchment in private health insurance has coincided with a burgeoning child poverty. Indeed, many of the trends that are causing childhood impoverishment are simultaneously leading to children's loss of health insurance, because of the close link between poverty, employment and health insurance coverage.

At a time when private insurance coverage is shrinking, residual public health financing programs are inadequate to take up the slack. The erosion of public coverage has occurred as a result of both covert Medicaid reductions arising from stagnating state welfare assistance levels in the face of inflation (Budetti, Butler and McManus, 1982) and overt restrictions on Medicaid eligibility for poor working families imposed by Congress in 1981 (Rosenbaum and Johnson, 1986).

Low-income children in working families face a particularly acute situation. The fastest growing sector of the employment market is currently in the area of low-paid service jobs that carry few or no fringe benefits (U.S. Department of Labor, 1984). But because of Medicaid's historic exclusion of the working poor from coverage (Rosenbaum and Johnson, 1986), children in low-income employed families are significantly less likely to be eligible for benefits than those in nonworking families. As a result, children of the working poor are substantially more likely than those of the nonworking poor to be completely uninsured (Table 5.1).

To make matters worse, in 1981 Congress enacted a series of changes in the Aid to Families with Dependent Children (AFDC) and Medicaid programs. Their impact was to further restrict working families' eligibility for Medicaid (Rosenbaum and Johnson, 1986). A 1985 governmental study of the effects of these 1981 changes on working families' eligibility for AFDC and Medicaid found that on average, the percentage of the AFDC caseload with earned income, already less than 15 percent of the entire AFDC caseload, dropped by an additional 50 percent in the cities surveyed (U.S. General Accounting Office, 1985). Thus, with limited exceptions for pregnant women and extremely young children (Children's Defense Fund, 1987; Rosenbaum, 1987), the Medicaid program provides virtually no relief for the increasing numbers of poor children living in working families who fall through the private health insurance net. Those Medicaid expansions which did occur during the 1980s were insufficient to offset the significant erosion in children's private coverage (Hughes, et al., 1988).

For all these reasons, the adequacy of private insurance coverage is becoming an ever more important determinant of access to care for

Table 5.1 Children's Insurance Status by Characteristics of Child's Family, 1977

Characteristics of Child's Family	Population (in thousands)	Uninsured All Year	Private Insurance All Year	Private Insurance Part Year[1]	Medicaid All Year	Medicaid Part Year[1]	Other[2]
All children under 18 years	64,216	8.8	70.3	3.9	8.9	4.4	3.8
Sex of head by age of child							
Male head							
<6 years	15,433	8.9	72.5	6.3	5.2	2.8	4.3
6–17 years	38,063	9.0	78.6	3.0	3.6	2.3	3.5
Female head							
<6 years	2,746	7.0	21.2	2.8	45.9	18.7	4.4
6–17 years	7,966	8.0	43.0	3.9	28.6	12.9	3.7
Poverty level by sex of head							
Poor[3]	25,605	13.0	49.9	3.5	19.5	9.3	4.7
Male head	17,693	15.5	60.4	3.8	9.5	5.5	5.2
Female head	7,912	7.4	26.4	2.9	41.9	17.9	3.5
Not poor[4]	38,611	5.9	83.8	4.1	1.9	1.2	3.1
Male head	35,811	5.7	85.0	4.0	1.4	0.9	3.0
Female head	2,800	8.6	68.6	5.6	7.7	4.6	5.0
Employment status of head by poverty level of family[5]							
Works full time							
Poor	14,404	10.6	61.4	4.9	11.6	6.0	5.5
Not poor	31,333	4.4	86.2	4.1	1.3	0.8	3.2
Works part time							
Poor	1,629	19.7	24.4	3.4*	32.3	13.2	6.9*
Not poor	994	6.2	67.7	5.9*	8.7	5.3	6.3*
Self-employed							
Poor	1,643	29.1	57.0	3.6*	6.6*	2.6*	1.1*
Not poor	4,015	13.8	78.0	4.7	1.1*	0.9*	1.4*
Not working							
Poor	6,706	12.4	28.3	0.6*	37.6	17.8	3.3
Not poor	1,037	14.3	56.0	1.9*	14.3	9.4*	4.1*

Source: National Medical Care Expenditure Survey, household survey, 1977. In Kasper (1984).

[1] Otherwise uninsured.

[2] Includes children covered by CHAMPUS and children who when covered by private insurance or Medicaid only part of the year were otherwise insured.

[3] Poor < 201% of the poverty level (poor, near poor and other low income)

[4] Not poor ≥ 201% of the poverty level (middle and high income)

[5] Income adjusted for family size.

*RSE > 30%.

children. Even as it is, gaps in private insurance coverage are creating greater threats to children's well-being.

Assessing the Adequacy of Private Health Insurance for Children

In evaluating how the private health insurance system treats children, four separate issues must be considered. These are: children's eligibility for benefits; the nature and content of benefit plans; cost-sharing requirements; as well as administrative and structural issues. Each issue can significantly affect the adequacy and appropriateness of children's coverage.

Many of the statistics discussed in this chapter are taken from two major surveys conducted by the federal government. These are the 1977 National Medical Care Expenditure Survey (NMCES) and the 1980 National Medical Care Utilization and Expenditure Survey (NMCUES). Both surveys are national probability studies of a representative sample of the United States population that were designed to measure the scope and extent of health insurance coverage and utilization of health services.[2] In addition, NMCES included a Health Insurance/Employer Survey (HIES), which provides researchers with information about the characteristics of employers' health insurance plans.

While both surveys are dated, their contribution to knowledge about health insurance is unparalleled. NMCES and NMCUES probably present an overly optimistic picture of the health insurance situation for children, since insurance benefits in private plans have generally declined in the past decade (Jensen et al., 1987).

The data reviewed in this chapter lead to four central conclusions. First, the private insurance system does not cover enough children. Second, private insurance plans by and large cover neither the range of preventive care that children need nor the amount or scope of services essential to children with particularly heavy health care needs. Third, private insurance does an inadequate job of underwriting the cost of even covered care and services. And finally, the very structure of many private insurance plans is incompatible with the financial needs of lower income families with children.

Eligibility

Table 5.1 indicates that in 1977, 70.3 percent of all children under 18 had full-year private health insurance, while 8.8 percent lacked any coverage, public or private. Among low income families, only 49.9 percent of the children had private coverage, and 13 percent were completely uninsured that year. NMCUES data reveal a similar pattern in 1980 (Butler, Winter, Singer and Wenger, 1985).

Children's limited eligibility for private insurance arises from the nature of the system itself. Children's private insurance coverage hinges upon whether they reside with an adult family member who works for an employer who offers family health insurance at an affordable rate.[3] Since the vast majority of all privately insured children are insured through employer-provided health insurance, a discussion of private health insurance and children is in reality a discussion of the adequacy for children of an employer-based health insurance system.

Children's eligibility for private health insurance coverage is thus dependent upon: (1) the employment status of the family head; (2) whether group health insurance is available as an employee benefit; (3) whether the employer's plan offers family coverage at all; (4) whether the employer subsidizes the cost of the premium; and (5) whether the child bears the type of relationship to the family worker that permits the worker to declare the child as a dependent under the plan. The relationship between children and private health insurance is thus particularly fragile and complex. Indeed, it has been estimated that the number of uninsured children could be reduced by 25 percent if every child who lived with an insured household head was also insured (Congressional Budget Office, 1979). And this relationship appears to be growing more fragile over time—the proportion of children covered by a family member's employment-based plan fell from 67 percent in 1979 to 65 percent in 1986 (Congressional Research Service, 1988).

1. Employment status of household head as a key factor. In 1984, 86 percent of all children under 18 had at least one parent who was currently employed (U.S. Bureau of the Census, *Current Population Survey,* 1985). However, about 8.7 million children that year lived in households in which neither parent worked (1985). NMCES data indicate that the unemployed are only slightly less likely to have private coverage than the employed (89 percent versus 91 percent) (Monheit, Hagan, Berk and Wilensky, 1984). However, the unemployed are much less likely than the employed to have full-year private coverage (74 percent versus 84 percent). Moreover, NMCES shows that the unemployed poor and near-poor are more than 3 times less likely than unemployed, non-low-income persons to have access to alternative sources of private coverage (such as spouse's coverage during periods of unemployment [Monheit, Hagan, Berk and Wilensky, 1984]).

The NMCES data presented in Table 5.1 show that in 1977, *regardless of family income levels,* children living in families in which the household head was unemployed were significantly less likely to have full or part-year private insurance than children living in households in which the family head was employed. However, these data also show that children living in poor unemployed families that year were somewhat *more* likely to have full-year private insurance than children living in poor households in which the family head worked part time. In 1977, the unemployed included many individuals temporarily laid off by smokestack and manufacturing industries during the recession of the mid-1970s. Unlike those employed part-time, these were not long-term poor families. Moreover, many of the health insurance plans offered by such industries included coverage extensions for the unemployed (Chollet, 1984).

Unemployed families in the 1980s may be less likely to be insured than their counterparts in the 1970s because today's unemployed workers are younger, have less real income, are less likely to live with a spouse who is working, and are experiencing longer periods of unemployment (Monheit, 1984). This increasing lack of health insurance among the unemployed means that children in unemployed families are also more likely to be uninsured.

2. *The availability of group health insurance as an employee benefit.* The availability of an employer-provided health insurance plan is the key determinant of an employee's insurance status. NMCES data indicate that in 1977, more than 87 percent of employees insured for a full year worked for an employer who offered health insurance (Monheit, Hogan, Berk and Farley, 1985).[4] Among employees who were uninsured all year or who relied on public insurance for all or part of a year, 66.9 percent and 44.0 percent, respectively, worked for employers who offered no health insurance plan (Monheit, Hogan, Berk and Farley, 1985).

NMCES data also show that workers with no employer-provided coverage are disproportionately likely to work at low-paying jobs. Table 5.2 indicates that in 1977, two-thirds of poor/near-poor workers were privately insured on a full-year basis, while a slightly over 93 percent of workers who received a high hourly wage rate were privately insured on a full-year basis.

A key question is whether uninsured family members in the work force are without health insurance because no plan is available or because the family chooses not to purchase coverage. Among America's 9.2 million poor/near-poor workers in 1977, about one-quarter (2.3 million workers) were completely uninsured (Monheit et al., 1985). Of these, two-thirds (1.5 million workers) were uninsured because their employers offered no coverage. Thus, the majority of uninsured working families are uninsured not because they have elected not to purchase coverage, but because a plan is simply not available through an employer. Moreover, as will be discussed below, a sizable proportion of

Table 5.2 Employment and Insurance Coverage by Family Income Level and Hourly Wage Rate, 1977

Characteristics	Total Employed (thousands)	Private Insurance All Year	Private Insurance Part Year	Public Insurance All or Part Year	Uninsured All Year
Family income					
Poor/near-poor[1]	9,244	50.8	4.4	21.6	23.3
Low income	12,317	67.8	6.0	8.7	17.5
Middle income	41,282	85.8	3.8	2.4	8.0
High income	43,400	93.3	1.9	3.7	3.7
Hourly wage rate					
$2.50 or less	10,816	67.9	3.7	11.0	17.4
$2.51 to $5.00	42,890	79.3	4.0	5.2	11.4
$5.01 to $7.50	19,346	91.8	2.9	1.1	4.2
$7.51 to $10.00	9,058	93.8	1.4	1.7	3.1
$10.01 and above	5,640	92.6	2.2	1.9	3.3

Source: National Medical Care Expenditure Survey. In Monheit et al. (1985).

[1] Defined as 125% of the federal poverty level.

those families who do elect not to purchase group insurance may be foregoing coverage because of its cost.

3. The availability of family coverage under an employer plan. Even firms that offer their employees insurance coverage may not offer coverage for dependents. This is particularly true among firms of 100 or fewer employees and firms engaged in nonmanufacturing industries. More than 9 percent of firms employing fewer than 20 persons and offering any health insurance at all offer no family coverage (Chollet, 1984).

The probability that a child will reside with a family head employed by a firm that does not offer family health insurance coverage has increased in recent years. For example, in 1982, 55.7 percent of America's 89.5 million persons employed on nonagricultural payrolls worked in nonmanufacturing, service industries other than government (U.S. Bureau of Labor Statistics, 1986). By 1985, that percentage had risen slightly to 57.7 percent, a growth in jobs that are less likely to offer coverage of dependents as an employee health benefit.

Table 5.1 illustrates that 34 percent of poor children living with a full-time employed household head were without any private health insurance in 1977. The situation was far more serious for poor children living with self-employed or part-time workers or with an unemployed household head. It should also be noted that in 1977, children of poor self-employed or part-time workers were more likely to be completely uninsured than poor children living with an unemployed family head. This phenomenon results in great part from the fact that public insurance programs such as Medicaid are generally unavailable to poor families that work.

4. The availability of an employer subsidy for employees' health insurance premiums. In assessing the adequacy of the employer-based health insurance system, one must determine not only whether an employer offers family coverage but also what proportion, if any, of its employees' annual family premiums the employer pays. Certainly the mere existence of an employer plan is beneficial, since a group plan will ensure more affordable premium rates. However, unsubsidized group premium rates for comprehensive medical and hospital coverage, especially if an employee chooses to purchase family coverage, can amount to as much as $3000 per year. Moreover, unless an employee works for a firm offering a flexible spending account,[5] he must bear his share of the premium cost with posttax dollars. Thus, unless an employer pays most, or all, of the employee's premium, employer-based family insurance coverage may be beyond the reach of many working families.

Data from a major employer-provided health insurance survey show that in 1980, 84 percent of employers offering health insurance paid the full cost of their employees' health insurance, but that only 60 percent paid the full cost of insurance coverage for employees' dependents (Chollet, 1984). Table 5.3 shows that manufacturing firms and larger firms were significantly more likely to contribute to dependent coverage. As Table 5.4 shows poorer families are far more likely than high-income families to bear the full cost of coverage and are substantially less likely to have all premium costs (both for individual and family coverage) borne by the employer.

5. *Eligibility among children living with family members other than parents.* In March 1984, 1.2 million children under 18 lived with rel-

Table 5.3 Employer Contribution to Dependents' Coverage as a Percentage of Plan Cost by Industry Group and Establishment Size, 1980

	No Coverage of Dependents	Employer Contribution as a Percentage of Plan Cost			
		0	1–49	50–99	100
All establishments	4.2	18.0	3.0	14.7	60.1
Industry group					
Manufacturing	2.5	8.3	1.5	12.2	75.5
Nonmanufacturing	5.3	23.7	4.0	16.2	50.9
Establishment size (number of employees)					
1–19	9.5	27.4	2.8	11.5	48.7
20–49	6.9	27.8	3.2	16.1	46.0
50–99	7.3	27.7	3.0	16.6	45.5
100–249	—	12.3	8.8	24.0	54.9
250–499	—	11.4	2.0	14.8	71.8
500–999	—	6.7	2.0	14.8	76.5
1,000–2,499	—	4.9	1.5	12.1	81.4
2,500 or more	[a]	2.8	0.4	9.0	87.8

Source: Employee Benefit Research Institute. In Chollet (1984).

[a] Less than 0.05 percent.

Table 5.4 Number and Percentage Distribution of Multiple-Person Families with Heads under 65 Years of Age and with Private Health Insurance, by Family Income and Premium Payment Status

			Premium Payment Status		
Characteristic	Number (in thousands)	Total	Family Pays None of Premiums	Family Pays Part of Premiums	Family Pays All of Premiums
All families	30,379	100.0%	42.1%	41.0%	16.8%
1979 family income					
Less than $10,000	2,974	100.0	32.2	34.1	33.7
$10,000–$19,999	9,875	100.0	39.9	41.5	18.5
$20,000–$34,999	11,262	100.0	45.7	43.9	10.4
$35,000 or more	4,043	100.0	43.1	39.3	17.6

Source: Dicker (1983).

atives other than their parents (U.S. Department of Commerce, 1985, pp. 29–31). This living arrangement is disproportionately common among black children. Such living arrangements can pose great difficulty with respect to health insurance if the relative's employer-provided plan does not permit the employee to claim a child as a dependent unless the employee is the child's parent. It is unclear how widespread this limitation is, but anecdotal evidence suggests that it is not an uncommon one (Health Insurance Association of America, 1986).

The Nature and Content of Benefit Plans

In assessing the adequacy of insurance coverage for children, the nature and content of benefit plans is as crucial a consideration as whether a family is able to obtain coverage at all. Indeed, the high cost of insurance necessitates the provision of comprehensive benefits, particularly in the case of lower-income families, since the premium cost itself may consume virtually all of a family's available resources for health expenditures.

The content of benefit plans. Over the past decade insurers have substantially expanded the range of benefits in their plans. For example, in recent years there has been growth in the coverage of preventive and maintenance services, such as vision, hearing and dental care, outpatient mental health services, and "well child" examinations (Hansen, 1986).

However, each benefit adds something to the cost of a plan, even though the additional cost may be relatively modest. As a result, one would expect that, as in the case of employer subsidization of insurance premiums, the generosity of the benefit plan will vary in accordance with the willingness of a firm to invest in its work force.

Employers' insurance premium subsidy practices are also indicative of the breadth and depth of coverage offered under their plans, and lower-paid workers in turn have less generous plans. For example, Tables 5.5 and 5.6 show that small firms are less likely to include routine dental care or outpatient physician mental health care for children.

Data from the NMCES Health Insurance Employer Survey underscore the relative deficiency of private coverage for many low-income children. Table 5.7 indicates that poor and nonpoor children's health insurance plans do not differ greatly for hospitalization or diagnostic benefits but do vary considerably on the basis of family income with respect to coverage of preventive and health maintenance benefits. Poor children are less likely to be covered for prescribed medicines, vision and hearing care, home physician visits, outpatient mental health services, and preventive and restorative dental care.

Table 5.5 Benefits for Routine Dental Examinations

	All Children with Private Insurance (in thousands)	With Coverage for Routine Exam (Number in thousands)	Percentage	Full Coverage, No Deductible	Limited Coverage	All Other
All children under 18 years	49,463	12,386	25.0	32.9%	32.8%	34.3%
Size of group coverage[1]						
25	3,821	455	11.9	22.4	40.3	37.3
26–250	9,585	1,508	15.7	23.4	32.2	44.4
251–2,500	11,981	3,779	31.5	18.7	38.8	42.5
2,500+	14,371	5,550	38.6	41.5	29.9	28.6

Source: Kasper (1986).

[1] Excludes about 6 million children for whom group size was unknown and 3.4 million with nongroup coverage.

Table 5.6 Benefits for Outpatient Physician Mental Health Care

	All Children With Private Insurance (in thousands)	With Mental Health Benefits (Number in thousands)	%
All children under 18 years	46,463	35,975	72.7
Type of coverage			
Nongroup	3,443	659	19.1
Group*			
<25	3,821	2,633	68.9
26–250	9,585	7,630	79.6
251–2,500	11,981	9,201	76.8
2,500+	14,371	11,576	80.6

Source: Kasper (1986).
*Excludes about 6 million children for whom group size was unknown.

In short, poorer families are not only less likely to have employer-subsidized insurance plans but also more likely to have less generous plans that are limited in their scope of coverage. It should be emphasized, however, that insurance has significant gaps even for nonpoor children, particularly for dental care and physical exams (see Table 5.7).

The availability of benefit plans that include HMO coverage. The Health Maintenance Organization Act of 1973 requires that firms with 25 or more employees offer enrollment in a "qualified" health maintenance organization as a health benefit option if one is available (42 USC Sec. 300e et seq.). Since this statute was enacted, enrollment in HMOs and other forms of prepayment plans has increased markedly, in part because of federal legislation encouraging their growth and in part because the private sector, believing that such plans deliver comprehensive health care in a more cost-effective and efficient fashion, has embraced them.[6]

The proliferation of health maintenance organizations and other prepayment systems has further popularized the notion of comprehensive insurance coverage for routine health care needs, not merely catastrophic services. By 1985, 21 million Americans were enrolled in HMOs, a 26 percent increase over 1984 enrollment levels (Sorian, 1986). The number of HMOs grew by 43 percent in the second half of 1985 alone. As HMOs claim a greater share of the insurance market, traditional insurance plans may be increasingly forced to broaden their scope of coverage in order to become more competitive.

However, NMCES data indicate that in 1977, lower-income employees were only half as likely as upper-income employees to have employer insurance plans that offered HMO enrollment (Farley and Wilensky, 1983a). Wide differences in HMO enrollment options were

Table 5.7 Type of Services Covered for Privately Insured Children by Group and Nongroup Coverage and by Income

Type of Service	All Children with Private Insurance	Type of Coverage Group[1]	Type of Coverage Nongroup	Income Poor[2]	Income Not Poor
All children under 18 years					
(in thousands)	49,376	45,933	3,443	11,886	37,490
(percent)	100.0%	93.0%	7.0%	24.1%	75.9%
Hospital inpatient services					
Room and board	97.7%	98.2%	91.9%	98.7%	97.4%
Surgery	97.0	97.3	93.2	97.3	96.9
Inpatient medical	98.5	98.6	96.8	99.2	98.3
Outpatient physician services[3]					
Office visits	84.1	97.3	41.5	79.8	85.3
Home visits	78.2	83.5	19.3	70.0	80.6
Routine physical exam	6.2	6.5	2.8	4.0	6.9
Outpatient diagnostic services[3]	94.0	95.6	71.9	93.9	93.9
Outpatient surgery[3]	95.0	96.0	83.1	99.5	93.7
Outpatient emergency services[3]	81.5	84.0	53.5	82.0	81.4
Prescribed medicines[3]	82.1	85.9	30.1	78.8	83.0
Vision or hearing care[3]	11.5	12.3	1.4*	9.6	12.2
Mental health care					
Inpatient hospital	83.6	84.6	70.1	83.7	83.5
Outpatient physician	72.7	76.8	19.1	68.7	74.0
Dental care					
Any dental	28.0	30.1	—	21.7	29.9
Routine maintenance	25.9	27.8	—	21.0	27.4
Orthodontics	15.2	16.3	—	11.8	16.2

Source: Kasper (1986).

[1]Includes about 6 million children for whom group size was unknown.
[2]Poor = Income < 200% of federal poverty level.
[3]The percentage of privately insured children with nongroup coverage was slightly larger for these services, 8.2% or about 4 million children.
*RSE > 30%.
— No cases.

also evident by geographic location and by number of subscribers in the employer's group plan (Farley and Wilensky, 1983a). Because HMOs and prepaid plans tend to market their services to certain types of populations and in certain geographic areas (Johnson and Aquilana, 1986; Luft, Maerki and Trauner, 1986), it is likely that these uneven development patterns will continue.

Prepaid health plans may be an attractive option for many young families with children, because in some instances they provide better coverage for routine and predictable health care needs and because, unlike many traditional fee-for-service plans, HMOs pay providers directly rather than by indemnifying enrollees (reimbursing enrollees at a later date for out-of-pocket payments made for covered services). This eliminates the need for families to lay out cash on an "up-front" basis for otherwise covered services. Prepaid care also has, however, some important liabilities, as described in Chapters 7 and 8 of this volume.

Limits on the amount and scope of benefits. A health insurance plan may be apparently broad, yet be seriously limited if restrictions are placed on the amount or scope of covered benefits. These limitations can work a particularly serious hardship on severely ill or disabled children, regardless of family income. Common limits include annual visit maximums on outpatient mental health services, dental services, home health and rehabilitation therapy services.

Insurance plans routinely impose either annual or lifetime maximums on payment levels or the amount of benefits they will cover under their plans. Table 5.8 shows that, in 1977, only 8.7 percent of all privately insured persons who were members of even large group plans had coverage for unlimited lifetime medical benefits, and children were disproportionately in plans that had benefit maximums in 1977 of $25,000 or less. While upper-income persons were more likely to have maximum benefit levels of $250,000 or higher, only 52 percent of all insured high-income individuals and only 48 percent of children under age 19 residing in families with major medical plans had such coverage.

Additionally, many health insurance plans impose maximum benefit limits for specific services—for example, no more than $2,000 in any given year for dental care, no more than $1,000 per year for outpatient mental health services, or no more than $100,000 for inpatient hospital services. Such benefit limits, whether imposed service-by-service or on an overall basis, limit protection against unexpectedly high, or catastrophic, medical costs.

To put the concept of benefit maximums into some perspective, consider the fact that 9,600 infants born in the United States annually have first-year costs exceeding $50,000, while another 9,600 children

Table 5.8 Maximum Major Medical Benefits of the Privately Insured under Age 65: Percentage Distribution According to Population Characteristics

Characteristic of Person	Number (in thousands)	$1–25,000	$25,000–50,000	$50,001–249,999	$250,000	Over $250,000	Unlimited
All persons	153,315	12.8	10.3	10.8	23.9	15.9	8.7
Age in years							
Less than 19	53,332	13.5	11.3	10.9	25.2	14.6	8.3
19–24	17,003	10.8	10.0	11.3	22.8	19.3	9.4
25–34	26,772	12.3	9.7	10.8	24.2	16.8	10.0
35–54	39,080	12.7	10.5	10.8	23.6	15.9	8.7
55–64	17,128	13.4	7.9	9.7	21.0	15.2	7.0
Family income							
Poor and near poor[1]	9,979	17.1	7.5	9.0	21.4	12.3	9.0
Low[2]	19,462	14.5	10.9	9.1	24.8	13.5	5.2
Middle[3]	65,789	13.7	11.4	11.4	24.5	15.1	7.9
High[4]	58,084	10.4	9.3	11.0	23.2	18.2	10.7
Type of insurance							
Nongroup	14,815	19.3	*0.9	2.5	9.7	2.4	4.3
Any group	138,500	12.2	11.3	11.6	25.4	17.3	9.1
25 or fewer members	12,130	8.4	5.3	5.3	30.0	24.3	9.2
26–250 members	28,154	13.5	9.7	6.7	28.5	22.1	10.5
251–2500 members	36,331	16.4	14.0	12.4	24.8	17.0	5.9
More than 2500 members	43,020	9.3	13.3	15.4	26.2	13.1	8.9

Source: Farley and Walden (1983 Public Health Association).

[1] Poor/nearpoor = < 1.25 of the federal poverty level.
[2] Low = 1.25–2.0 of the federal poverty level.
[3] Middle = 2–4 of the federal poverty level.
[4] High = More than 4 of the federal poverty level.

over age one have similar costs (NACHRI, 1987). Ten percent of all high-cost hospitalized infants and children will continue to have annual costs exceeding $10,000, thereby exposing approximately 20,000 families annually to the risk of extraordinary medical care expenditures.

One of the most troubling of all insurance limitations is the preexisting condition exclusion. Much has been written about the alleged practice by some HMOs of screening out applicants who have medical problems (Luft, Maerki and Trauner, 1986). In fact, however, exclusion of high-risk individuals is a common practice among all types of insurers, whether traditional fee-for-service or prepaid. Moreover, this practice is common among both groups of individually purchased plans. A recent comprehensive survey of 861 corporations and other organizations that was designed to determine what cost-containment practices they were utilizing to control health insurance expenditures found that 73 percent use preexisting condition clauses to contain costs (Hansen, 1986).

Preexisting condition exclusions can work a tremendous hardship on children. For example, nearly all insurance plans used to impose a waiting period before a newborn child's coverage began, resulting in the denial of health benefits when they were needed most. Preexisting condition clauses also make it difficult for families to adopt disabled children, because the children's conditions are not covered under their adoptive parents' plan.[7]

In summary, the majority of private insurance plans fail to cover the services that children need and use most, such as routine health exams, and vision and dental care. Moreover, many plans include limitations that seriously affect their adequacy and appropriateness in the case of severely disabled children. Finally, while HMOs and other forms of prepaid plans appear to emphasize coverage of primary and preventive pediatric care, there exists conflicting evidence regarding the ease with which families can gain access to these benefits.

Patient Cost-sharing

Extensive patient cost-sharing can greatly diminish the value of comprehensive coverage and deter utilization (Liebowitz et al., 1985). Among children, this deterrent effect may be felt even in the case of medically necessary services, thereby posing a threat to their health and well-being. Indeed, recently published results from a landmark patient cost-sharing experiment showed that the most dramatic impact of patient cost-sharing on poor families is demonstrated when children's use of medical care is considered (Ball and Roskamp, 1986). The study determined that even income-adjusted cost-sharing requirements reduced by more than 40 percent the probability that low-income children would seek effective medical care.

Cost-sharing is a traditional feature of private health insurance. In addition to premium charges, the insured must commonly pay a deductible before coverage begins and must also pay co-insurance each time they use a covered service. Traditional fee-for-service plans make use of both deductibles and co-insurance, while HMOs are particularly likely to use co-insurance (Washington Report on Medicine and Health, 1986).

In a recent nationwide study of employer's health care cost containment practices, 54 percent of companies surveyed indicated that their plans now require employees to pay deductibles for both medical and hospital expenses (Hewitt Associates, 1985). Moreover, as Table 5.9 indicates, the deductible and co-insurance burdens faced by children insured under a group plan may be small in comparison to those borne by children insured under nongroup coverage.

As a result of benefit limitations and high cost-sharing requirements, many families bear high out-of-pocket burdens despite their health insurance coverage. As in the case of premiums and benefits, the least well-off families who are most in need of comprehensive coverage face the highest out-of-pocket burdens. In 1980, the percentage of family income consumed for out-of-pocket health costs for children was second only to that for the elderly and near-elderly (Howell et al., 1985). Moreover, poor families were 10 to 30 times more likely than families with incomes over 200 percent of the federal poverty level to have out-of-pocket expenditures equal to more than 15 percent of their annual incomes.

NMCES statistics indicate that low-income and upper-income, privately insured families face identical cost-sharing burdens with no adjustment made for their relative economic positions (Farley and Wilensky, 1983b). The poor and nonpoor are also equally likely to be covered by the plans that place no limit (either income-related or service-related) on their out-of-pocket costs (Farley and Walden, 1983).

High out-of-pocket burdens, combined with limited coverage of key benefits mean that families can be faced with an economic crisis if serious illness strikes a child. Moreover, heavy patient cost-sharing plus limited benefits also leaves privately insured low-income children in a worse position than their Medicaid-insured counterparts. NMCUES data indicate that in 1980, while low-income, privately insured children were less likely than uninsured children to incur out-of-pocket expenditures for physician services, they were nearly equally as likely as completely uninsured children to experience annual out-of-pocket costs of $100 or more (Rosenbach, 1985). In 1980, low-income, privately insured children were twice as likely to experience out-of-pocket cost-sharing burdens as low-income children with full-year Medicaid coverage (Howell et al., 1985).

Table 5.9 Major Medical Coverage, Deductibles, and Coinsurance

	All Children with Private Insurance (in thousands)	With Major Medical Coverage (Number in thousands)	Percentage	Standard Deductible/ Low Coinsurance	Standard Deductible/ High Coinsurance	High Deductible
All children under 18 years	49,463	41,401	83.7	21.5%	71.5%	7.1%
Type of coverage						
Nongroup	3,443	1,454	42.2	10.1	46.0	43.8
Group size:*						
25	3,821	3,217	84.2	27.2	65.8	7.0
26–250	9,585	8,718	91.0	18.2	77.1	4.7
251–2,500	11,981	10,860	90.6	18.6	77.1	4.3
2,500+	14,371	12,319	85.7	28.3	64.5	7.2

Source: Kasper (1986).

*Excludes about 6 million children for whom group size was unknown.

The deterrent effect of this out-of-pocket burden can be seen in utilization of preventive services by privately insured, low-income children under age 6. NMCUES data indicate that in 1980 young, privately insured, low-income children were one-third less likely than their Medicaid-insured counterparts to utilize preventive services (Rosenbach, 1985). Disabled low-income children with high out-of-pocket burdens are more likely to receive less remedial care than their publicly-insured counterparts (Butler, 1986).

Structural and Administrative Constraints

In the case of HMOs, prepaid plans, and preferred provider organizations (PPOs),[8] payments are made directly to a provider, thereby eliminating the need for an individual to first pay the provider and then seek indemnification from his or her insurer. However, most traditional, employer-provided fee-for-service plans are indemnity plans. An indemnity plan requires that an insured person first pay for medical care and then seek recovery from the insurer. Thus, unless a provider accepts "assignment" of the enrollee's indemnification and bills the enrollee only for the difference between the charges imposed and the payments actually made under the plan, the enrollee must bear the full charge out of pocket. Indemnity was originally a feature only of commercial insurance, but the indemnity model came to dominate the marketplace after World War II (Law, 1976).

Although many indemnity plans contain an "assignment" feature, providers may be increasingly unwilling to accept assignment of benefits for fear that high deductibles and co-insurance, lack of coverage for certain procedures, and long payment delays mean that they will recover very little from the plan itself.

For several reasons, providers' fears may be particularly borne out in the case of children. First, families' insurance plans normally do not cover preventive and health supervision services. Second, the cost of each pediatric encounter is low enough[9] that, in the case of plans without first-dollar coverage for pediatric services, a child's office visit might not cost nearly enough to exhaust a family's annual deductible. Thus, pediatric providers may commonly reject assignment of benefits in all but costly pediatric cases.

Indemnification is an irritant to any insured family, since it can regularly find itself in the position of having to pay for health services "up front" and seek coverage later. But for low-income families, indemnification can prove disastrous, because these families do not have the resources to pay for their care on an "up front" basis. Medicaid, the major public insurance program for poor children, expressly recognizes and requires all participating providers to accept direct payment of benefits (42 CFR Section 447.205). There exists no similar requirement for private health insurance.

Trends in Health Insurance Coverage

Evidence indicates that the nation is in the midst of a weakening of employer-provided and underwritten private insurance. The rise in the number of uninsured Americans during the early 1980s reflected employers' desire to reduce burgeoning health insurance expenditures, which grew from $18.3 billion in 1973 to $97.1 billion in 1984 (Employee Benefit Research Institute, 1986). Moreover, the increased number of uninsured reflected the loss of highly paid, unionized jobs and the growth of low-paying service jobs that command far less compensation in the form of salary and fringe benefits. Additionally, the rise in the number of uninsured most likely will be accompanied by increasing *under*insurance, as employers, in the face of rising insurance costs, limit coverage by raising deductibles and coinsurance.

Several surveys of employers' insurance cost containment practices show that the effect of many of the most popular practices is not merely to contain costs but to actually reduce both utilization of covered services and coverage itself. A 1985 survey of 861 corporations and organizations stated that "a revolution is well underway that will substantially reorganize the business of health care before the end of this decade" (Hansen, 1986). Nearly 90 percent of those surveyed classified cost containment as "considerably important," and a "typical" goal was to experience either *no* cost increase, or one that was less than the increase in the consumer price index.

Those surveyed noted that four cost-containment approaches, including increased employee cost-sharing, outpatient incentives, employee education, and utilization review and precertification programs, appeared promising, but they classified cost-sharing as the most effective measure. Forty-three percent indicated that they had increased deductibles in the preceding two years, 33 percent had altered co-insurance features, and 33 percent had increased employee contributions. Cost sharing, whether in the form of premium increases or heightened deductibles and copayments, saves money by shifting the cost of coverage and care from the employer to the employee.

Other surveys have found a similar trend away from extensive employer underwriting of employee health insurance costs (Chollet, 1984; Swartz, 1984; Health Research Institute, 1986). Especially important, are surveys showing that employers are increasing employee contribution requirements for dependent coverage (Chollet, 1984). This increase could encourage lower-paid employees to drop dependent coverage altogether.

Some believe that simply switching from the current financing system to one that significantly increases individuals' cost-sharing responsibilities will reduce real health expenditures by deterring unnecessary utilization. However, a key finding of the Rand Corporation's 10-year cost-sharing study, which studied the effects of imposing various levels of cost-sharing on persons enrolled in traditional fee-for-service insurance plans, was that regardless of the level of cost-sharing imposed, the content of care furnished individuals who actually made contact with the health care system remained virtually constant (Ball, 1986). This finding suggests that among actual recipients of care, there is little evidence that cost-sharing will reduce unnecessary or inappropriate utilization.

The Rand experiment also demonstrated that the effect of cost-sharing is to deter persons without adequate resources from entering the health care system at all as a result of high copayment requirements (Ball, 1986). Untargeted cost-sharing appears to be a poor way to reduce unnecessary care, since those who can afford to pay for unnecessary care will still receive it. Cost-sharing's only real effect may be to discourage those who really do need care from seeking it. To the extent that increased patient cost-sharing reduces access to necessary health care by shifting payment obligations to those who cannot afford it, access to medical care may be compromised. Since lower-income families already face sizeable cost-sharing burdens, any further cost shift appears to be particularly unwarranted.

With respect to coverage of benefits, some employers are beginning to improve coverage of certain types of outpatient and preventive benefits (Chollet, 1984; Hansen, 1986; Health Research Institute, 1986). These benefits include outpatient mental health care, home health care, hospice benefits, preventive health exams, fitness programs, and patient counseling and case management programs. But while some employers may have expanded their plans to include coverage of "wellness" benefits, many are simultaneously reducing their share of payment for covered benefits by raising deductible and coinsurance obligations and increasingly are excluding persons with health problems. Expanded benefit packages will be of little use to children if their families cannot overcome greater cost-sharing requirements or enroll them in the plan at all.

Almost no American family is immune from the effects of a shrinking health insurance system. The federal tax system does offer families several ways of coping with declining coverage, but as a practical matter, only upper-income families who have disposable resources are in a position to take advantage of these additional tax subsidies.

The skewing of medical benefits under the tax system toward the well-to-do begins with the employer-subsidized premium itself, which in 1977 was worth an average of $92 to a family with income of less than $10,000 but $395 to a family with an annual income of $50,000 or more (Wilensky, Farley and Taylor, 1984). The disparity in the value of this benefit was lessened but by no means eliminated by the 1986 Tax Reform Act. This skewing of tax benefits also applies to the medical expense deduction. This deduction amounted to $2.451 billion in lost federal revenues in 1982, but only $516 million went to families earning less than $20,000 per year (Joint Committee on Taxation, 1984).

Employees with disposable resources can also offset higher health costs resulting from rising premiums and deductibles by setting up flexible spending accounts (FSAs) through their employers. A flexible spending arrangement permits an employee to set aside a portion of pretax income to meet health care costs, including his or her portion of the annual insurance premium, as well as deductibles and copayments (Enthoven, 1985). FSAs can thus reduce the economic burden of rising health expenditures. For example, $100 worth of uninsured medical care costs only $60 when a wage earner in the 40 percent tax bracket pays for the care out of an FSA.

However, most of these tax-sheltered expenditures are made by upper-income households with higher marginal tax rates (Enthoven, 1985). Lower-income families do not have the same ability either to shelter income or to make sizeable medical outlays that can later be taken as a deduction. For these families, the tax system provides little protection from the effects of eroding employer-provided coverage.

Governmental Responses to the Limitations of Private Insurance

Government might respond to the private insurance system's deficiencies in four ways. First, government might do nothing to remedy the problem and instead permit health care coverage and utilization to be market-responsive, as is utilization of other goods and services. Policy makers have rejected this path, particularly in recent years, as evidenced by expanded Medicaid coverage and aggressive efforts to broaden and regulate the private coverage system, as discussed below.

Second, government might attempt to *regulate* employers' and insurers' practices to make insurance more accessible and appropriate.

Third, government might create *financial incentives* designed to make private insurance more accessible and appropriate. Government might use the tax code, for example, to create financial incentives that would encourage employers to offer affordable plans, or to subsidize employees' purchase of private coverage through their place of employment or through some other pooling arrangement.

Fourth, policy makers might conclude that the political, structural, and systemic problems raised in trying to repair and improve the private insurance system are so great, and the benefits that realistically could be achieved so marginal, that a preferable approach would be establishment of a supplementary, public insurance program for families with children. The parallel for this approach is the 1965 enactment of Medicare.

The selection of remedial options depends significantly on the legal and political contexts in which the private health insurance system operates. The next section of this chapter will review the various activities recently undertaken by federal and state policymakers and the constraints they have faced.

Regulating the Availability and Content of Private Insurance

At least three central issues must be taken into account in discussing governmental approaches to regulating private health insurance: (1) the longstanding delegation to state government of the authority to regulate private insurance; (2) the enactment in 1974 of the Employer Retirement and Income Security Act (ERISA) and its attendant impact on states' ability to regulate insurance; and (3) the United States Tax Code's regulation of employers' and employees' ability to exclude payments for health insurance as taxable income.

State regulation of private insurance. State law traditionally has been the primary source of insurance regulation. The 1945 McCarren Ferguson Act has been construed by the Supreme Court as delegating to the exclusive domain of the states the power to regulate the "business of insurance," which involves the relationship between insurer and insured, the type of policy which could be issued, its reliability, interpretation and enforcement" (*Securities and Exchange Commission v. National Securities, 1969*).[10] Thus, issues pertaining to the financial solvency of insurers, the spreading and underwriting of policy holders' risks, and the required scope and content of plans have traditionally fallen within the purview of state regulation. The states' role as regulators was restated by the court as recently as 1985, when it reaffirmed states' right to establish minimum content standards for employer-purchased health insurance (*Metropolitan Life Insurance Company v. Commonwealth of Massachusetts,* 1985).

States are increasingly regulating the content and availability of private group health insurance plans. By 1987, over 600 mandated benefit laws were in existence for a variety of benefits.[11] For example, the previous practices by insurance companies of imposing a "newborn waiting period," that denied coverage to thousands of sick infants, is now virtually a thing of the past as a result of state regulation.

Additionally, the Child Support Enforcement Amendments of 1984 (P.L. 98-378, 1984) require state child support agencies to pursue absent parents for not only financial support but also health insurance for the custodial spouse and dependent children "when health care coverage is available to the absent parent at reasonable cost" (42 U.S.C. Section 652(a), 1984). Enforcement of this requirement potentially can mean ordering an employed parent to acquire employer-provided medical insurance for his or her family and may thus in time diminish the chilling effect that separation and divorce have on a child's insurance status.

To ensure that coverage is actually made available to the custodial parent and children, a state's child support order might require an employer to deduct the cost of an absent parent's family coverage premium from his or her pay and administer the benefit plan on behalf of the absent family. Administrative responsibilities might conceivably entail ensuring that custodial parents receive full disclosure of their plans' benefits and are assured a speedy and efficient procedure for submitting provider claims for services rendered. Evidence suggests that anywhere from 25 percent to 34 percent of absent parents under the jurisdiction of a state's child support enforcement system have access to health insurance (Haskins, 1985). Thus, full enforcement of the Child Support Enforcement Act could significantly reduce the number of uninsured children with absent parents.

The impact of ERISA on states' ability to regulate the business of insurance. The longstanding authority of states to regulate the "business of insurance" was severely curtailed by passage of the Employee Retirement Income Security Act (ERISA). Enacted in 1974, ERISA had two purposes: to protect employer-provided pension and health and welfare benefits; and to encourage employers who had not already done so to set up such plans. Employers have responded extensively to ERISA, not only by setting up pension plans but also by converting from a system of *purchased* health insurance to one in which the employer "self-funds" by maintaining a reserve pool to pay employee health costs (Intergovernmental Health Policy Project, 1986). While these self-funded pools may be administered by private insurers, the employer, not the insurer, retains the actual revenues. As of 1986, more than 40 percent of employees covered by employer-provided insurance plans were insured under self-funded plans (Intergovernmental Health Policy Project, 1986). By self-funding for health insurance and using outside firms only for plan administration, employers can avoid both payment of costly insurance premiums and virtually all state regulation.

The impact of ERISA's health and welfare provisions on states' power to regulate insurance has been enormous. First, ERISA has cost states potentially billions of dollars in insurance revenues, since taxation of employer *self-funded,* as opposed to *purchased,* plans has been held to violate ERISA's provisions (*Franchise Tax Board of State of California v. Construction Laborers Vacation Trust for Southern California,* 1982). Since employers that self-fund pay no premiums to an insurance company, no taxable transaction is involved.

Second, while ERISA purports not to preempt state laws governing the "business of insurance,"[12] the statute also supersedes all state regulation with respect to any "employee benefit plan" established pursuant to the Act.[13] An "employee benefit plan" includes self-funded health insurance plans. As a result, states' insurance regulations, including laws governing the content and scope of group health insurance, laws pertaining to the underwriting and spreading of risk, and laws governing administration of insurance plans, have been held to apply to employer-*purchased* health insurance plans but not to employers' *self-funded* plans.[14]

The limits of ERISA's preemption of state authority to regulate the "business of insurance" in the case of employer self-funded plans are still being tested. Many courts have been unwilling to invalidate state health and welfare laws on a wholesale basis merely because they also amount to regulation of a self-funded employer health benefit plan. For example, courts have affirmed that state domestic relation laws that ensure a divorcee's entitlement to a portion of a divorced spouse's ERISA pension plan, are not preempted by ERISA (*Stone v. Stone,* 1980; *Pacific Maritime Association Pension Plan v. Stone,* 1985).

Key to the issue of whether ERISA preempts a particular state law that has the effect of regulating a self-funded plan is a determination of whether the "conduct sought to be regulated by the state law is part of the administration of the employee benefit plan" and therefore constitutes an activity within the sole regulatory purview of ERISA (*Martori Brothers* at 1358). If a state law is in fact intended to regulate the administration of a plan it is preempted. If, however, a state law affects an ERISA plan in a "tenuous, remote and peripheral a manner" and does not *purport* to regulate an ERISA plan, it should not be preempted.[15]

For example, were a state to impose a general tax on employer payrolls (rather than on employers' benefit plans) as a revenue generating device in order to underwrite the cost of a public insurance plan for the working poor, such a tax should not be in violation of ERISA, even if funds were ultimately used to fund services for the uninsured. Similarly if, pursuant to the Child Support Enforcement Amendments, a state were to establish insurance coverage and recovery procedures affecting all firms employing absent parents subject to a child medical support order, these procedures should be considered part of a state's authority to ensure the well-being of families under its domestic relations laws and therefore binding on both employer-purchased and self-funded plans. It seems unlikely that Congress would have mandated that states implement broad child medical support recovery procedures under the Child Support Enforcement Act if it had considered such recovery programs to be preempted by ERISA legislation in the case of self-funded employer benefit plans. Indeed, state courts have traditionally addressed issues such as health insurance coverage in fashioning divorce decrees. The 1984 child support amendments appear to simply codify and make uniform this traditional state and common law practice of providing for the health and welfare of children in domestic relations disputes, and ERISA in this context should not be read as overturning the longstanding fabric of state domestic relations laws.

Using the power of the Fair Labor Standards Act and tax code to indirectly regulate insurance plans. The federal tax code grants employers the right to exclude the cost of health insurance payments from employees' taxable income, Similarly, the Fair Labor Standards Act regulates labor conditions for over most working Americans. Thus, Congress could add a minimum health benefit requirement to the FLSA, similar to the minimum wage, which establishes minimum content and structural requirements that all employer insurance plans must meet. Congress could also establish minimum content and structural requirements which employer plans would have to meet in order to qualify for tax deductibility. These major congressional changes would supersede ERISA and apply to both purchased and self-funded plans.

In recent years the Congress has become somewhat more willing to consider legislation to establish minimum federal standards for private insurance. In 1986, for example, federal protections were added to the tax code to require employers to continue to make group coverage available to widows, divorced spouses, and children of deceased or divorced employer-insured workers. Federal legislation that would provide insurance protections for laid-off workers and their families in the case of bankruptcies was considered and rejected in 1986 (H.R. 5300, 1986). In addition, legislation has been introduced that would mandate inclusion of well-child benefits and home health benefits for severely disabled children in private plans (S. 376, 1985; S. 1783, 1985) and to foster the growth of state-based insurance pools for individuals unable to purchase coverage because of preexisting conditions (H.R. 5300, 1986).

Finally, in 1987, in the most sweeping proposal of the decade, Senator Edward Kennedy and Congressman Henry Waxman introduced legislation to require all firms employing full or part-time workers and subject to the requirements of the FLSA to include a minimum health benefit plan as part of their employees' compensation (S. 1265, 1987). The bill establishes certain basic standards governing eligibility, premium contributions, covered benefits, and beneficiary costsharing. It also would preempt all state mandated benefit laws. If enacted, the Kennedy/Waxman plan would reduce by two-thirds the number of completely uninsured Americans.

Creating Incentives to Furnish Private Insurance

If employers and insurers cannot be regulated into furnishing more affordable and appropriate coverage, they might be provided with financial incentives to provide such coverage. Several experts have discussed the potential for offering tax credits and other incentives in exchange for better employer coverage of health insurance for their employees (Monheit et al., 1985). However, little federal legislation introduced to date has included financial incentives.

A number of states are considering the establishment of programs to help the working poor pay for their insurance, while others in 1987 either enacted or began developing public insurance plans for uninsured poor and near-poor residents ineligible for Medicaid.

Expanding Public Insurance to Fill the Gaps in the Private System

Both federal and state governments have responded to the insurance crisis in recent years primarily by enacting modest improvements in public health financing programs, particularly Medicaid. Examples of federal and state actions within the past several years include:

1. Expansion of Medicaid in 1980 to cover disabled adopted children with preexisting conditions and without regard to the income levels of their adoptive families.

2. Expansion of Medicaid in 1984, twice in 1986, and again in 1987, to broaden coverage for certain low-income children and pregnant women, many of whom were previously ineligible for coverage because of their families' employment status or their income levels, which, even if low, were too high to qualify for cash assistance.[16]
3. Expansion of Medicaid coverage for children, pregnant women, and (in a few cases) unemployed families by approximately 20 states (Children's Defense Fund survey, 1982–1987). These expansions occurred independently of Congressional actions in 1984 and 1986.
4. Creation in 9 states of health insurance pooling systems, financed through general and dedicated revenues and individual premiums, for individuals who are medically uninsurable (Intergovernmental Health Policy Project, 1986).
5. Development in 7 states of ratesetting or pooling systems designed to reimburse hospitals for the uncompensated care they provide (Intergovernmental Health Policy Project, 1986).
6. Creation by some states of public, primary health service programs for the medically indigent (Rosenbaum, Hughes and Johnson, 1986).

Additionally, officials in at least 5 states (Massachusetts, Minnesota, Michigan, Washington, and Wisconsin) are considering the development of or have enacted public health insurance plans, funded through general revenues, dedicated taxes, and individual premiums, for working families whose employers do not offer health insurance and who cannot afford to purchase private coverage. In all cases, officials are considering subsidizing policy holders' premium payments to place coverage within families' financial reach. Such a subsidy would be analogous to that provided insured employees by the federal tax system.

Some of these expansions are relatively ambitious. For example, if states were to take advantage of all of the new Medicaid options for covering low-income pregnant women and children that were enacted in 1986 and 1987, the number of uncovered children under age 5 would be reduced by about 40 percent, and the number of uncovered pregnant women would be reduced by two-thirds.[17] While states historically have been slow to take advantage of options for covering additional families under Medicaid,[18] by December 1987, 24 states and the District of Columbia had in fact implemented the 1986 option (Hughes, 1988).

But the erosion of private health insurance coverage is occurring so rapidly that states' public health insurance improvements simply cannot keep pace. For example, expansions in the Texas Medicaid program in 1984 and 1985 led to a near tripling of the number of infant deliveries paid for by the program by 1986 (Texas Department of Human Services,

1986). Yet over the same time period, the totally uninsured poor grew from 28 percent to 40 percent of that state's poor population.

Remedying the Private Health Insurance Problem

The current approach to financing health care for children suffers from major gaps and failures. It is relatively easy to identify the outlines of a health financing system that would reasonably accommodate children's needs. But the major questions are whether to structure such improvements as private insurance, public insurance, or according to some other model, and how to finance them. Some possible answers are presented below.

What Should a Children's Health Financing Program Look Like?

Any health financing system for children should contain several features. First, it should be open to all children, regardless of where they live, regardless of whether they live in employed or unemployed families, regardless of where the family head is employed, and regardless of the degree of relationship to their caretaker relative. Second, coverage should be available at affordable rates, with family contributions limited to an income-adjusted premium payment. Nominal copayments (if necessary) should be limited to services, such as inpatient care, whose utilization in the case of pediatrics has been demonstrated to be unaffected by cost-sharing (Liebowitz et al., 1985).

Third, the financing arrangement should pay for the range of medical, dental and related health services that children need. Particularly important are a basic schedule of routine medical and dental examinations, immunizations, restorative dental care, emergency medical care, vision care, and treatment for physical, developmental, or mental health problems that are either detected during the routine exam process or that develop episodically.

Fourth, a financing arrangement should not set lifetime limits in the case of children, and preexisting condition exclusion clauses should be prohibited. Additional "wraparound" catastrophic coverage should be included to ensure access to medically appropriate care for chronically ill and disabled children who require care and services beyond the maximum benefit level. Moreover, community-based health and remedial benefits should be covered to avoid unnecessary skewing of pediatric long-term care toward inpatient services.

Fifth, provider reimbursement should take into account price, medical and technological advances, and the characteristics of the child population. Very young children and adolescents are more expensive than other children. Poor children may be more expensive to care for than nonpoor children. Providers' fees should reflect these variations.

Finally, the plan should provide for direct reimbursement of providers and mandatory assignment of benefits, so that families are not required to pay cash in advance of care.

What Form Should Reforms Take?

Various approaches might be taken in remedying private insurance's inadequacies. In the author's opinion, any approach must be national in scope, in part because of the myriad barriers that restrict states' ability to respond to the insurance crisis, in part because the problem is national in scope, and in part because the cost of financing reforms should be borne nationally.

Regulating the employer-based system. One approach to improving private insurance would be a wide-ranging regulatory effort designed to address the system's failings for families with children, similar to the legislation introduced by Senator Kennedy. This approach would be consistent with Congressional efforts in recent years to use the federal legislative framework to make employer-based plans more responsive to the needs of employees and dependents who have fallen through the gaps of the "private ordering" system that underlies employer/employee relations.

Through federal legislation, Congress might mandate employer coverage and condition the deductibility of employee health benefit costs to employers who make available a health plan that contains the features described above. Some of the benefit and structural features that have been recommended (such as coverage of preventive services and direct payment of providers) are in fact hallmarks of prepaid plans and other managed care systems that have grown in popularity. Thus, to this extent, such regulation would not be inconsistent with the current direction in which employee health benefits are evolving.

However, insofar as the minimum standards affect the level and extent of employers' *contributions to the cost of their employees' health coverage,* Congressional regulation would directly oppose current trends by increasing employers' share of cost. This contradiction might be lessened if regulatory reforms were tied to additional tax credits or other economic advantages for employers offering such benefits.

The primary advantages of this regulatory approach are first, that it builds upon the existing system for privately insuring most Americans, and second, that it is compatible with current attitudes regarding the primacy of the employer/employee relationship and the appropriateness of an interstitial government role within a basic "private ordering system."

However, this approach also has a number of disadvantages. First, while it is ostensibly consistent with recent Congressional efforts to legislate private insurance benefits that have not been achieved through the private employer/employee bargaining process, these past improvements are extremely modest in comparison to those that would be needed to adequately insure millions of working families with children. Congress has not taken the important step of requiring employers to make group-rate health insurance available to all employees, nor has it required employers to subsidize the cost of their enrollment. Even modest mandated benefit legislation that would require employer plans to include "well-child" and other care has met with intense opposition. Thus, the changes that would be needed to ensure access to affordable, appropriate employer-provided health insurance for families with children are conceptually vast in comparison to Congressional precedent.

While the Kennedy bill has met with considerable support it has also encountered virulent opposition, not only from employees but also from the very insurance industry that theoretically stands to make billions from increased consumption of private insurance that the Kennedy bill would buy. At hearings on the Kennedy bill held in June 1987, major insurers testified that the cost of insuring millions of poor, previously uncovered persons would significantly exceed the cost of an affordable premium (Blue Cross, 1987; HIAA, 1987).

Second, this approach philosophically reaffirms the desirability of an employer-based insurance system. But unless employers were actually mandated to provide coverage this proposal would do nothing for the millions of Americans employed by firms that offer no benefits. Nor would this approach aid the millions of uninsured families who have no connection to the work force.

If Congress were to require all employers to offer health insurance to their employees, such a requirement could realistically be achieved only if employers' costs were underwritten. That would pose an enormous expense. The cost of such legislation might be underwritten in part if Congress were to place financial limits on the value of insurance benefits that could be excluded as taxable income and to dedicate the resulting revenues to subsidizing health benefit plans for employees whose firms currently offer no health benefits. However, opposition to limiting the value of employee health plans is enormous, since employee groups obviously fear the loss of key benefits.

Were Congress to establish a general subsidy program to aid the purchase of insurance by firms that currently offer none, those firms that do underwrite the cost of their employees' coverage might reduce or eliminate their subsidy. Once employers stopped funding their own plans and instead turned to the government for a subsidy, the whole rationale for the subsidy—namely, preservation of the employer-based system—would evaporate.

In sum, it is unclear whether the political struggle that would ensue over a regulatory/taxation-subsidy approach to remedying the employer-provided health insurance gaps would yield sufficient results to compensate for the shortcomings of the employer-based system. The task could not be achieved without considerable governmental underwriting of a system that, even if more broadly available, suffers from inherent structural problems. Health insurance as an employment-related fringe benefit may have once been a reasonable way to finance health care, but as employers limit their benefits, as the work force shifts to firms that traditionally have not offered such benefits, and as the need for more uniform controls over health costs and expenditures grows in the force of inflation, an aging society, and major epidemics such as AIDS, policy makers must decide whether a pluralistic, employer-based system is the type of insurance structure that should be preserved in the long run.

Supplementing the current employer-based system with a private insurance system supported by individual vouchers. Another approach would be to reject the notion of regulating the employer-based system and instead provide persons with insurance vouchers in the form of either refundable tax credits or direct payments. These vouchers could in turn be used to purchase "qualifying" private insurance that is offered at a group rate through some alternative pooling system (Enthoven and Kronick, 1989).

This approach has several benefits. First, it avoids direct regulation of employer-provided insurance. Second, it builds upon the private insurance system and is thus compatible with the existing insurance industry. Third, it avoids the exclusions and restrictions present in an employment-based system.

This approach has a number of problems as well. First, it, too, would need to be heavily regulatory to ensure the purchase of high-quality plans. In light of private industry's traditional opposition to federal and state efforts to regulate the content and design of plans, intense resistance could be expected.

Second is the question of where the funds to pay for the vouchers would come from. Limits on the tax exclusion of employer-provided benefits would be fiercely resisted. Employers who do not offer insurance would also resist any sort of surtax. The insurance and medical care industries, another potential source of special revenues, would also resist a tax. An additional source of taxation might be on employees themselves, but this would be inconsistent with recent Congressional efforts to lower individual tax burdens.

Third is the issue of cost. Assuming that revenues can be found, should they be used to subsidize the purchase of private insurance, which, even at group rates, is far more costly than a public benefit program?

Finally is the issue of oversight. There are thousands of private benefit plans. The enforcement machinery needed to monitor their adherence to coverage and quality standards would be considerable, and an entire new administrative and accountability structure would be required.

Expanding existing public benefit programs into insurance programs for families with children. In 1965 Congress created Medicare for the aged to compensate for the limitations of both the private insurance system and existing public benefit programs. Taking a similar approach for families with children—that is, modifying or replacing existing public programs—is an equally viable option.

Congress might create a companion to the existing Medicaid program, which through a variety of revenue sources would offer public insurance to families for a fixed annual premium adjusted for family income; legislation that would do precisely this was introduced in 1987 by Senator John Chafee (S. 1139, 1987). Indeed, the existing "medically needy" component of the Medicaid program was originally envisioned as ultimately operating, at least in part, as a similar type of premium-based program, but inherent structural defects and subsequent legislative erosion of the 1965 statute prevented this outcome.[19]

This approach has several benefits. First, a modified or "companion" Medicaid program is consistent with recent and repeated Congressional efforts to make the program more responsive to previously uncovered individuals and families. In recent years both Congress and state governments have been particularly interested in Medicaid improvements that aid women, children and the working poor, all of whom are disproportionately likely to lack private insurance coverage. Thus, limited philosophical acceptance of the need for, and appropriateness of, such an undertaking is in place at both federal and state levels of government.

Second, Medicaid is a basically sound and cost-efficient structure. Overall administrative costs represent less than 5 percent of total program outlays. Health insurance premiums *alone* exceed insurance outlays for all costs (benefits plus administration) by 10 percent. Medicaid benefits for families with children are far better in amount and scope than the great majority of private plans. Moreover, the notion of direct provider reimbursement in lieu of indemnity is firmly in place. Additionally, there is no preexisting condition exclusion clause. Furthermore, with a few exceptions, state Medicaid plans have avoided the use of "dollar maximums" on coverage in favor of other cost control efforts. Finally, eligibility determination, plan administration, and quality control procedures are either already in place or within reach.

This approach also has its shortcomings. As with the other two approaches, government would have to raise revenues to provide subsidized coverage, and the same political resistance to additional taxation would persist.

Another shortcoming may be resistance to viewing Medicaid as a public health rather than welfare benefit. Medicaid began as an adjunct to AFDC and related cash assistance programs for the very poorest Americans. Despite its evolution in recent years, it is still administered by state welfare agencies, and eligibility requirements are extraordinarily complex and cumbersome. If, however, eligibility is simplified and if Medicaid is modified to include coverage for working families, this traditional program characterization will begin to disappear.

An additional problem is that of heavy provider resistance to participation in Medicaid, which again might be overcome if fees were adjusted upward, administrative procedures modified, and the characteristics of enrollees changed.

Most significant, however, is the impact that the new program would have on the existing private insurance system. Some employers might continue to offer insurance as a benefit if employees continued to seek health coverage as part of their wage and benefit package. However, many other employers would no longer provide health benefits. Consequently, the insurance industry might oppose such an expanded public role, fearing a major loss of business. However, ERISA, by promoting employer self-funding, has and will continue to cost the industry billions of dollars in health plan business. The insurance industry has also thrived under Medicare by offering supplementary plans (popularly known as "Medigap" policies) and by playing a major role in administration of the program. Finally, if employers were to respond to an expanded public program by ceasing to provide insurance altogether, it would then be possible to simply impose a modest tax on employers to help underwrite the cost of an expanded public program.

None of the solutions outlined above is politically easy. All are legally and structurally extremely complex. Time is pressing, however. Each year brings more disinsured Americans, and the trend toward disinsurance appears to be a long-term one. Policy makers need to decide which approach makes the most economic and structural sense and proceed to develop a health care subsidy system that is equitable and that makes sense for families with children.

In the author's opinion, a long-term approach that focuses on the development of a supplementary public program may be the most economical and the most appropriate, given employers' diminishing desire to be the primary funders and maintainers of the private system, and given the profound difficulties involved in regulating the content, structure, and cost of private insurance.

Notes

1. It has been observed that the federal government's subsidization of private health insurance represents an investment of public funds for health care coverage second only to that made for the Medicare program (Enthoven, 1985).
2. For a more complete description of the NMCES and NMCUES surveys, see Berk, Wilensky and Cohen, 1984.
3. Eighty-five percent of all private health insurance is purchased through employer group plans (Sorian, 1984).
4. However, 22 percent of employees who were employed by firms offering insurance but were uninsured all year were ineligible for their employers' plans. Reasons for an employee's ineligibility might include a preexisting condition or his or her failure to fulfill the employer's service requirement. A service requirement is a provision in an employer plan that requires that an employee work a minimum period of time before coverage begins. In 1980, only one-third of employer plans had no service requirement. One-third had service requirements of 2–3 months, while nearly 9 percent had service requirements of 4–6 months (Chollet, 1984, p. 34).
5. See text, p. 33.
6. Recent reports suggest that employers are discovering that the savings to be achieved through conversion to prepaid plans may be somewhat illusory. In some instances plans have set their premium rates in accordance with prevailing fee-for-service plans, rather than at a lower level. In others, adverse selection by some plans resulted in the exclusion of sicker employees and higher attendant insurance costs to the employer on these employees' behalf through the fee-for-service system (Farley and Wilensky, 1983).
7. The Adoption Assistance and Child Welfare Act of 1980, P.L. 96-272, provided Medicaid coverage for adopted disabled children covered by the Act, regardless of the income levels of the adoptive families, for precisely this reason. The legislative history to the Act indicates that this Medicaid provision was adopted to encourage the adoption of children who, without Medicaid, would be unadoptable because of preexisting condition exclusions in private insurance plans. See H. Rep. 95-1481 to accompany H.R. 2831.
8. Preferred provider organizations are group practice arrangements which provide their services for a discounted fee.
9. NMCES data indicate that in 1977, the mean charge per physician office visit was $18.00 for children under 6 and 23.00 for children ages 6–18. (Wilensky and Bernstein, 1983).

10. The law was enacted in response to the United States Supreme Court's decision in *United States v. South Eastern Underwriters Association* (322 U.S. 533, 1944) holding that the "business of insurance" amounted to interstate commerce and was therefore not exempt from federal antitrust laws.

11. Intergovernmental Health Policy Project, 1986. The first mandated benefit laws regulating the terms of group health insurance appeared in 1971–72 before the enactment of ERISA, and were passed by the state of Arizona (*Metropolitan Life Insurance Company v. Commonwealth of Massachusetts*, 105 S. Ct. 2380, n. 3).

12. 29 U.S.C. Section 514(b)(2)(A). This provision is known as the "insurance saving" clause.

13. 29 U.S.C. Section 514(b)(2)(B). This provision is known as the "deemer" clause.

14. *Standard Oil Company of California v. Agsalud*, 1980, holding that Hawaii's *Prepaid Health Care Act*, mandating universal insurance coverage by employers, was preempted by ERISA. Congress subsequently amended ERISA to exempt Hawaii's statute from the preemption provision.

15. As a result, at least 3 states have imposed taxes on health providers themselves to reach insurance payments by employer self-funded plans that would otherwise be unreachable. These states include Florida, South Carolina, and West Virginia. State rate-setting laws such as those in effect in Maryland and Maine, which regulate hospitalization rates paid by insurers and incorporate the cost of uncompensated care into the rate, also appear not to be preempted.

16. *The Deficit Reduction Act of 1984*, P.L. 980369, 98 Stat. 494, See 2361 (Coverage of financially needy children under 5 and pregnant women whose children, if born, would qualify for AFDC of AFDC-Unemployed Parent Benefits); *The Consolidated Omnibus Budget Reconciliation Act of 1986* (requiring coverage of all financially needy pregnant women); *The Omnibus Budget Reconciliation Act of 1986* (providing for optional state coverage of pregnant women and children under age 5 with family incomes in excess of state AFDC payment levels but less than the federal poverty level; and *The Omnibus Reconciliation Act of 1987* (permitting coverage of pregnant women and infants with family incomes under 185 percent of the federal poverty level; extending mandatory coverage of financially needy children up to age 7; and permitting optional coverage of poor children up to age 8).

17. Estimates by Children's Defense Fund, based on current population survey data presented in Sulvetta and Schwartz, 1986, and Gold and Kenny, 1985.

18. For example, as of 1986, 20 state Medicaid programs still fail to cover all financially needy children under age 21, even though the option to do so has existed since 1965.

19. For example, the original Medicaid statute contained no upper limits on protected income levels for the medically needy and contemplated the use of premiums. Therefore, state "spend down" programs might have set far more generous eligibility thresholds, which would have permitted the program to act as a supplementary public insurer for middle class Americans. Fearing large budget costs, however, Congress in 1967 amended the statute to include upper limits on protected income levels under the medically-needy program of 133 percent of states' AFDC payment level (Section 220 of the Social Security Amendments of 1967). Because AFDC payment levels are so low, states' medically-needy income eligibility thresholds are likewise so low that the program is inaccessible to middle class Americans unless they have suffered catastrophic illnesses and have lost virtually all of their income and resources. As medically needy eligibility levels slipped to 50 percent of the federal poverty level in 1986, the notion of applying an income-adjusted premium has become moot. It is interesting to note, however, that Utah has for years administered its medically needy program as a premium program and is the only state

to do so. Similarly, the so-called "Ribicoff Amendment" of 1965 (granting states the authority to extend coverage to all financially needy children under 21) was envisioned by its sponsor as the first step toward "decategorization" of Medicaid. With the exception of coverage for pregnant women and young children in recent years (see note 17), this has not happened.

References

Alan Guttmacher Institute. 1987. *Blessed Events and the Bottom Line.* New York.
Ball, J.K., and J.A. Roskamp (eds.). 1986. *Medical Care* Supplement 24:9.
Berk, M., and G. Wilensky. 1984. Health Care of the Working Poor. *National Health Care Expenditures Study.* Washington, D.C.: National Center for Health Services Research. Presented at the Annual Meeting of the American Public Health Association.
Berk, M., G. Wilensky, and S. Cohen. 1984. Methodological Issues in Health Surveys: An Evaluation of Procedures Used in the National Medical Care Expenditure Survey. *Evaluation Review* 8(3):307–326.
Blendon, R., L. Aiken, H. Freeman, L.B. Kirkman-Liff, and J. Murphy. 1986. Uncompensated Care by Hospitals or Public Insurance for the Poor: Does It Make a Difference? *New England Journal of Medicine* 314:1160–1163.
Budetti, P., J. Butler, and M. McManus. 1982. Federal Health Program Reforms: Implications for Child Health Care. *Milbank Memorial Fund Quarterly* 60:155–181.
Butler, J., W. Winter, J. Singer, and M. Wenger. 1985. Health Insurance Coverage and Physician Use among Children with Disabilities. *Pediatrics* 76:495–506.
Califano, J. 1986. *America's Health Care Revolution: Who Lives? Who Dies? Who Pays?* New York: Random House.
Chavkin, D. 1977. California's Prepaid Health Plan Program: Can the Patient Be Saved? *Hastings Law Journal* 28:685–710.
Children's Defense Fund. 1986. *A Children's Defense Budget,* pp. 352–353. Washington, D.C.
———. 1986. Semi-annual survey of state Medicaid changes (Unpublished).
Chollet, D. 1984. *Employer-Provided Health Benefits: Coverage, Provisions, and Policy Issues.* Washington, D.C.: Employee Benefit Research Institute.
Congressional Budget Office. 1979. *A Profile of Health Insurance Coverage: The Haves and Have-Nots.* Washington, D.C.: G.P.O.
———. 1983. *Tax Expenditures: Current Issues and Five Year Budget Projections for Fiscal Years 1984–1988.* Washington, D.C.: G.P.O.
Congressional Research Service. 1988. *Health Insurance and the Uninsured: Background Data and Analysis.* Washington, D.C.: G.P.O.
Consolidated Omnibus Budget Reconciliation Act of 1986. Pub L. 99-272, 100 Stat. 82, Title X.
Deficit Reduction Act of 1984, Pub. L. 98-369, 98 Stat. 494, Sec 2361.
Egbuono, L., and B. Starfield. 1982. Child Health and Social Status. *Pediatrics* 69:550–557.
Employee Benefit Research Institute. 1986. *Employee Benefit Notes.* February. Washington, D.C.
Enthoven, A. 1985. Health Tax Policy Mismatch. *Health Affairs* 4:5–14.
Enthoven, A., and R. Kronick. 1989. A Consumer-Choice Health Plan for the 1990s. *New England Journal of Medicine* 320:29–37, 94–101.
Farley, P., and D. Walden. 1983. The Privately Insured under Age 65: Cost-Sharing, Depth of Benefits and Other Aspects of Their Health Insurance. *National Health*

Care Expenditures Study. Washington, D.C.: National Center for Health Services Research.

Farley, P., and G. Wilensky. 1983a. Options, Incentives and Employment-Related Health Insurance. *Advances in Health Economics and Health Services Research* 4:57–82. Reprinted by National Technical Information Service, Springfield, Va.

———. 1983b. Private Health Insurance: What Benefits Do Employees and Their Families Have? *Health Affairs* 2(1):92–101.

Franchise Tax Board of State of California v. Construction Laborers Vacation Trust for Southern California, 679 F 2d 1307 (9th cir., 1982); *Vac. on other gds.,* 103 S. Ct. 2841.

Freeman v. Jacques Orthopaedic and Joint Implant Surgery Medical Group, 721 F 2d 654 (9th Cir., 1983)

Gibson, R.M., K.R. Levit, H. Lazenby, and D. Waldo. 1984. National Health Expenditures, 1983. *Health Care Financing Review* 6:1–29. Baltimore: Health Care Financing Administration.

Gold, R., and A. Kenney. 1985. Paying For Maternity Care. *Family Planning Perspectives* 17:103–111.

Gortmaker, S.L., and W. Sappenfield. 1984. Chronic Childhood Disorders: Prevalence and Impact. *Pediatric Clinics of North America* 31:3–17.

Hansen, A.S., Inc. 1986. Health Care Survey, January 20, 1986. *Medical Benefits* 3:4. Charlottesville, Va.: Kelly Communications.

Haskins, R. 1985. *Estimates of National Child Support Collections Potential and the Income Security of Female-Headed Families.* Final Report, Grant no. 18-P-00259-4-01, Office of Child Support Enforcement, Social Security Administration.

Health Insurance Association of America. Discussion by author with employee, 1986.

Health Research Institute. 1986. Health Care Cost Containment Survey. *Medical Benefits* 3:1–2. Charlottesville, Va.: Kelly Communications.

Hewitt Associates. 1986. Salaried Employee Benefits Provided by Major U.S. Employers in 1985. *Medical Benefits.* June 15, p. 8. Charlottesville, Va.: Kelly Communications.

Howell, E., A. Corder, and A. Dobson. 1985. *Out-of-Pocket Health Expenses for Medicaid Recipients and Low-Income Persons, 1980.* National Medical Care Utilization and Expenditure Survey, Series B, Descriptive Report No. 4. DHHS Publication No. 85-20204. Office of Research and Demonstrations, HCFA. Washington, D.C.: G.P.O.

H.R. 5300, *The Omnibus Budget Reconciliation Act of 1986,* as reported by the House of Representatives on July 31, 1986.

H.R. 5300, *The Omnibus Budget Reconciliation Act of 1986,* H.R. 99-509.

H.Rep. 96-136, to accompany H.R. 3434 (reference #68, re: Adoption Assistance and Child Welfare Act of 1980). Washington, D.C.: G.P.O.

Hughes, D., K. Johnson, S. Rosenbaum, J. Simons, and E. Butler. 1988. *The Health of America's Children.* Washington, D.C.: Children's Defense Fund.

Intergovernmental Health Policy Project. 1986. ERISA and the States. *Focus On.* March. Washington, D.C.: George Washington University.

———. 1986. *States Show Interest in Risk Pools.* Washington, D.C.: George Washington University.

Jensen, G., M. Morrissey, and J. Marcus. 1987. Cost Sharing and the Changing Pattern of Employer-Sponsored Health Benefits. *Milbank Memorial Fund Quarterly* 65:521–551.

Johnson, A.N., and D. Aquilana. 1986. The Competitive Impact of Health Maintenance Organizations and Competition on Hospitals in Minneapolis/St. Paul. *Milbank Memorial Fund Quarterly* 60:659–674.

Joint Committee on Taxation, United States Congress. 1984. *Estimates of Federal Tax Expenditures for Fiscal Years 1984–1989.* Publication 98-227. Washington, D.C.: G.P.O.

Kasper, J. 1986. *Children at Risk: The Uninsured and Inadequately Insured.* Presented at the 114th meeting of the American Public Health Association, Las Vegas.

Law, S. 1976. *Blue Cross: What Went Wrong?* 2d ed. New Haven: Yale University Press.

Liebowitz, A., W. Manning, E. Keeler, N. Duan, K. Lohr, and J. Newhouse. 1985. Effect of Cost-Sharing on the Use of Medical Services by Children: Interim Results From a Randomized Control Trial. *Pediatrics* 75:942–952.

Lohr, K., R. Brook, C. Kamberg, et al. 1986. Use of Medical Care in the Rand Health Insurance Experiment. *Medical Care* 24(Supplement).

Luft, H., S. Maerki, and J. Trauner. 1986. The Competitive Effects of Health Maintenance Organizations: Another Look at Evidence from Hawaii, Rochester, and Minneapolis/St. Paul. *Milbank Memorial Fund Quarterly* 10:625–658.

Martori Brothers Distributors v. James-Massengale, 781 F 2d 1349 (10th Cir., 1986).

Metropolitan Life Insurance Co. v. Massachusetts, 106 S. Ct. 2380, n.3.

Monheit, A., M. Hogan, M. Berk, and P. Farley. 1985. *The Employed Uninsured and the Role of Public Policy.* Washington, D.C.: National Center for Health Services Research.

Monheit, A., M. Hogan, M. Berk, and G. Wilensky. 1984. Health Insurance for the Unemployed: Is Federal Legislation Needed? *Health Affairs* 3(1):101–111.

National Center for Health Services Research. 1986. *National Hospital Discharge Survey, 1985.* Rockville, Md.

Pacific Maritime Ass'n Pension Plan v. Stone, 453 U.S. 922.

President's Commission for the Study of Ethical Problems in Medicine and Biomedical and Behavioral Research. 1983. *Securing Access to Health Care,* Vol. 1. Washington, D.C.: G.P.O.

Rosenbach, M. 1985. Insurance Coverage and Ambulatory Medical Care of Low-Income Children: United States, 1980. *National Medical Care Utilization and Expenditure Survey,* Series C, Analytical Report No. 1. DHHS Publication No. 85-20401. Washington, D.C.: National Center for Health Statistics.

Rosenbaum, S., D. Hughes, and K. Johnson. 1988. Maternal and Child Health Services for Medically Indigent Children and Pregnant Women. *Medical Care* 26(4):315–332.

Rosenbaum, S., and K. Johnson. 1986. Providing Health Care for Low-Income Children: Reconciling Child Health Goals with Health Care Financing Realities. *Milbank Memorial Fund Quarterly* 64(3):442–478.

Rossiter, L.F. 1982. Dental Services: Use, Expenditures and Sources of Payment. *National Health Care Expenditures Study.* Washington, D.C.: National Center for Health Services Research.

Schlesinger, M. 1986. On the Limits of Expanding Health Care Reform: Chronic Care in Prepaid Settings. *Milbank Memorial Fund Quarterly* 64(2):189–215.

Scott v. Gulf Oil Co., 754 F 2d 569 (9th Cir., 1985).

Securities and Exchange Commission v. National Securities, Inc., 393 U.S. 453, 460 (1969).

Select Panel for the Promotion of Child Health, DHHS. 1980. *Better Health Care for Children.* DHHS Publication No. 79-55071. Washington, D.C.: G.P.O.

Sorian, R., ed. 1984. Access to Health Care: Who Are the Uninsured? 1984. *Washington Report on Medicine and Health* January 9, p. 1. New York: McGraw Hill.

———. 1985. *Washington Reports on Medicine and Health.* March 6, p. 2. New York: McGraw Hill.

———. 1986. *Washington Reports on Medicine and Health* June 9, p. 4. New York: McGraw Hill.

Spitz, B. 1979. When a Solution Is Not a Solution: Medicaid and Health Maintenance Organizations. *Journal of Health Politics, Policy, and Law* 4(2):497–546.

Standard Oil Company of California v. Agsalud, 633 F 2d 760 (9th Cir., 1980); *aff'd*, 454 U.S. 801.

Stone v. Stone, 632 F 2d 740 (9th Cir., 1980); *cert. den.*, 453US922.

Sulvetta, M.B., and K. Swartz. 1986. *The Uninsured and Uncompensated Care*. Washington, D.C.: National Health Policy Forum.

Swartz, K. 1984. *Who Doesn't Have Health Insurance, and What Is to Be Done?* New Orleans: Urban Institute.

Texas Department of Human Services. 1986. Conversation between author and officials.

U.S. Bureau of the Census. 1985. Money Income and Poverty Status of Families and Persons in the United States: 1984 (Advance Data from the March, 1985 Current Population Survey). *Current Population Reports* Series P60, No. 146. Washington, D.C.: G.P.O.

———. 1985. *Current Population Survey*. March. Washington, D.C.: G.P.O.

U.S. Bureau of Labor Statistics. 1984. *Employment Projections for 1995*. Bulletin no. 2197. Washington, D.C.: Department of Labor.

———. 1986. *Employment and Earnings*. January. Washington, D.C.: Department of Labor.

U.S. Congress, Office of Technology Assessment. 1988. *Healthy Children: Investing in the Future*. Washington, D.C.: G.P.O.

U.S. Congressional Research Service. 1985. *American Children in Poverty*. Washington, D.C.: G.P.O.

U.S. Department of Commerce. 1985. *Marital Status and Living Arrangements: March, 1984* series P-20, no. 399:29–31. Washington, D.C.

U.S. General Accounting Office. 1985. *An Evaluation of the 1981 AFDC Changes: Final Report*. Publication No. 85-4. Washington, D.C.

Wilensky, G.R., and A. Bernstein. 1983. Contacts with Physicians in Ambulatory Settings: Rates of Use, Expenditures, and Sources of Payment. *National Health Care Expenditure Study*. PHS, Data Preview #16. Washington, D.C.: National Center for Health Services Research.

Wilensky, G.R., P. Farley, and A. Taylor. 1984. Variations in Health Insurance Coverage: Benefits vs. Premiums. *Milbank Memorial Fund Quarterly* 62(1):53–81.

Ware, J., W. Rogers, A. Davies, G. Goldberg, R. Brook, E. Keeler, C. Sherbourne, P. Camp, and J. Newhouse. 1986. Comparison of Health Outcomes at a Health Maintenance Organization with Those of Fee-for-Service Care. *Lancet* 16:1017–1022.

322 U.S. 533 (1944).

15 USC Section 1011 et seq. 59 Stat. 34 (1945).

42 U.S.C. Section 652(a) (1984).

Pub. L. 93-406, 88 Stat. 829 (1974), codified at 29 U.S.C. Section 1001, et. seq.

Pub. L. 98-378, 98 Stat. 1305 (1984), codified at 42 U.S.C. Section 651, et. seq.

29 U.S.C. Section 514 (b)(2)(A) (1985).

29 U.S.C. Section 514 (b)(2)(B) (1985).

S. 376 (1985), *The Child Health Incentives Reform Plan;* S. 1783 (1985).

42 USC section 300e, et. seq., 1985.

42 CFR Section 447.205 (1985).

6

Medicaid as Public Health Insurance for Children

*Margaret A. McManus, M.H.S., and
Stephen M. Davidson, Ph.D.*

The American health care system is and, from its beginnings, has been primarily a private system. Physicians and other healers have for most of our history earned their livelihoods as independent practitioners, charging fees for their ministrations to people who were ill. For most Americans these fees were paid out-of-pocket or, for the past 35 years, in combination with private insurance purchased through their employers. The role played by government has been residual: tax money has been used to provide or pay for services used by groups who, for one reason or another, are unable to purchase care.

The boundaries between the public and private sectors in American medicine have been determined in large part by a tension between ideology and pragmatism. Americans have rejected European models of national health insurance or a national health service out of a belief in the greater efficiency of the private sector and a distrust of the centralized government. Yet this largely ideological stance is often tempered by characteristically American pragmatism. For many Americans, governmental funding for necessary goods and services, including housing, food, and medical care, is justified by the knowledge that many good people cannot get more stable, higher paying jobs because they are poorly educated in public schools and that sometimes they lose their jobs as a result of economic conditions outside their control.

Any discussion of the role of public insurance in paying for health care for children must be viewed in this context. Although our ideological beliefs have limited the overall scope of public financing of health care, many of the important characteristics of public spending programs have been shaped by more pragmatic considerations for compassion or fair play. This duality is reflected in the history of the Medicaid program, the major source of public sector spending for children's health. (See Chapter 4.) Expanding or changing Medicaid's role will require justification in light of this accepted role for public insurance. The fundamental purpose of this publicly financed health care coverage has been (1) to enable individuals and families to gain access to needed health care services, and (2) to protect them from the financial consequences of using those services, even when the cost is large or "catastrophic."

These goals replicated the initial concerns motivating the growth of private health insurance (Anderson, 1985).

As costs have become a greater concern in the health care system, additional attention has been focused on encouraging the most appropriate use of services and sites for treatment. For example, patients might use a hospital emergency department (ER) instead of a physician's private office for nonemergency treatment because the former was covered while the latter was not. An ER visit may be three or four times more expensive than an office visit, result in more intensive care than necessary, and increase the chance of an inpatient admission. One way to avoid this inefficiency is to provide coverage for a more comprehensive package of services without restriction as to the site of care and to encourage providers to select among these services in a conscientious fashion.

To achieve both of its historic goals while keeping an eye on total expenditures, a publicly financed health care program should (1) cover a comprehensive array of services, (2) encourage the use of the most appropriate, least costly level of care, and (3) encourage providers to exercise their clinical judgment in the most efficient manner. Clinical need thus becomes the governing criterion. Although the funds available for medical care are limited, and it is important to consider the cost of a service, we believe that the choices regarding the use of services should be made by people who, because of training, experience, and/or intimate knowledge of the clinical situation, are in the best position to determine their desirability. Typically, that means physicians acting in concert with patients and/or other physicians and taking into account the cost of services as well as their clinical benefits.

We believe that these criteria, taken together, provide the best chance that the services used will be both effective and relatively inexpensive. Moreover, they will do so without the intrusion of external regulators—whether claims examiners employed by insurance companies or officers of a government—into the decision-making process regarding a particular patient. We discuss in this chapter how these goals fit into the evolution of the Medicaid program and which future reforms seem worthwhile.

Medicaid's History

With the passage of Title XIX of the Social Security Act in 1965, the Medicaid program was created as a federal grant-in-aid program to the states. It offered federal funds to any state that created a program to pay for the use of a broad range of services by low-income citizens who received cash grants under any of the federally assisted welfare categories (then, Aid to the Aged, Blind, Disabled or Families with Dependent Children). It also offered funds, at state option, for services used by people (referred to as the medically needy) who, though not eligible for welfare based on their incomes, would become eligible when the cost of needed medical care was deducted from their somewhat higher incomes.

Medicaid has reduced the financial barriers to utilization and has become a major source of health care financing for many of America's low-income children (Wilson and White, 1977; Davis and Shoen, 1978; Aday, Andersen and Fleming, 1980). According to Newacheck and Halfon, "That poor children now receive similar or higher levels of physician services than children from more affluent families is a reversal of the patterns existing in the early 1960s" (1986, p. 5).

In 1985, 10.97 million children under 21 were Medicaid recipients as a result of their eligibility as dependent children under 21 (9.76 million) or as "other Title XIX" children (1.21 million).[1] An estimated 12 percent of blind and disabled Medicaid recipients, about 360,000 individuals, also were under 21 (HCFA, 1986). Another 12.5 percent of all Medicaid recipients (or 690,000) were adolescents ages 19–21, eligible for Medicaid as adults in families with dependent children (McManus, 1986). All totaled, in 1985 approximately 55 percent or 12 million Medicaid recipients were infants, children, and adolescents under the age of 22, meaning that 16 percent of all children under 21 in the United States participated in Medicaid in 1985. Forty-six percent of low-income children (defined as below 150 percent of poverty level) were covered by Medicaid for all or part of 1980 (Rosenbach, 1985).

Medicaid is the only public or private insurance program that has articulated principles of child health care with relatively well defined measures of comprehensiveness, cost effectiveness, and quality of care. Despite the lack of aggressive implementation of the Early and Periodic Screening, Diagnosis and Treatment Program (EPSDT), there exists in legislation and regulation and, in many cases, actual programs, a thoughtful embodiment of child health supervision, including continuity of care, aggressive outreach, and follow-up.

But Medicaid's effectiveness varies greatly from one geographic area to another. Key programatic decisions are made by the states, which pay between 17 percent and 50 percent of the program's cost.[2] These include (a) specific eligibility criteria for each welfare category; (b) whether to cover the medically needy; (c) which optional services to cover, if any; (d) whether to impose limits on any of the services that were covered; and (e) the prices at which providers were to be paid. These decisions determine the shape and scope of each state's program and, thus, the extent to which each meets the criteria described in the previous section.

Eligibility

Medicaid eligibility categories for children. Eligible children may fall into either a mandatory or an optional coverage group, depending not only on the income and assets of their families but also on their family composition, parents' employment status and their own health status.[3]

To receive federal support for their Medicaid programs, states must provide benefits to persons receiving cash assistance under the federally assisted welfare category, Aid to Families with Dependent Children (AFDC), and usually to recipients of the Supplemental Security Income (SSI) program, the federal welfare program for low-income individuals who are aged, blind, or disabled. When the adult welfare categories were consolidated under SSI in 1974, some states were permitted to impose more restrictive eligibility criteria (i.e., higher income or asset levels) for Medicaid than were used for SSI. Passage of the Consolidated Budget Reconciliation Act of 1985 (COBRA) added two mandatory groups who were not cash assisted: all financially eligible pregnant women (regardless of family composition) and children under 5 years of age who were born after September 30, 1983.

For children, the most important mandatory eligibility groups are: AFDC recipients, "Ribicoff children," newborn children of Medicaid-eligible women, and children for whom adoption assistance or foster care maintenance payments were made under Title IV-E. "Ribicoff children" are those in low-income, two-parent families. For adolescents, the coverage of all financially eligible pregnant women is also very significant.

States have the option to extend eligibility for Medicaid (but not cash assistance) to many more children and pregnant women. The three most important optional groups for children are: families with unemployed parents, the medically needy, pregnant women, and infants (subsequently raised to children under age 5) in families with incomes above the Medicaid eligibility cut-off but below the federal poverty line. Families with unemployed parents (AFDC-U) refers to children who live in two-parent families in which the principal wage earners were unemployed or underemployed. The medically needy are those whose families have incomes and assets above the cash assistance levels,[4] but incur medical expenses that bring them down to that payment level. The latest optional category, added in the Omnibus Budget Reconciliation Act of 1986 (SOBRA), provided states the option of covering pregnant women and infants (in subsequent years to be raised to age 5) in families with incomes between the Medicaid eligibility level and the federal poverty level. Medicaid eligibility is thus based on a complex set of criteria. The size of the child Medicaid population and their health spending for 1985 are presented in Table 6.1.

Policy changes affecting eligibility since 1980. The 1980s have brought the most dramatic changes in eligibility policy as well as well as in benefits, reimbursement and administration since the program's inception. Federal regulation led to first contraction, then expansion, of eligibility.[5]

The Omnibus Budget Reconciliation Act of 1981 (OBRA) mandated major changes in AFDC eligibility which affected primarily working, poor families (Hill, 1984). The intent of OBRA was to limit eligibility and to increase states' flexibility in imposing their limits. The legislation addressed these goals in two ways. First, it narrowed AFDC eligibility to the very poor, leaving a large pool of other low-income families, including some with employed heads of household, with no form of public or private insurance. Second, it eliminated requirements that program provisions be identical in all parts of the state and for all groups of eligibles (so-called comparability provisions).[6] This allowed states to expand or contract benefits for particular subpopulations of Medicaid recipients.

Table 6.1 Medicaid Recipients and Expenditures for Children under 21, 1985

Basis of Eligibility	Recipients	Expenditures (in thousands)	Expenditures/ Recipients
Total Medicaid Recipients	21,818,897	$37,524,890	$1,720
Total children	10,969,293	4,218,452	476
AFDC children	9,755,492	4,419,219	453
Other Title XIX	1,213,801	799,233	658
Total Categorically Needy (Cash)	16,464,790	19,329,847	1,173
Total children	8,159,209	3,643,266	447
AFDC children	8,159,209	3,643,266	447
Other Title XIX	0	0	0
Total Categorically Needy (Noncash)	2,613,650	7,849,275	3,003
Total children	1,097,441	620,301	565
AFDC children	771,933	308,101	399
Other Title XIX	325,508	312,200	958
Total Medically Needy	3,414,333	10,345,768	3,030
Total children	1,716,243	954,885	556
AFDC children	824,350	467,852	568
Other Title XIX	888,293	487,033	548

Source: Unpublished preliminary 1985 HCFA data.

OBRA's greatest impact was in reduced eligibility for working poor families. Although 16 states raised their need standards to protect AFDC families from losing eligibility in 1983 (Hill, 1984), more than 2 million low-income people lost Medicaid eligibility between 1981 and 1982 (Cromwell, 1984). A GAO (1985) study of five cities (Boston, Milwaukee, Syracuse, Dallas, and Memphis) found that between 16 percent and 63 percent of those who lost AFDC benefits remained without health insurance for 1½ to 2 years after their cases were closed.[7] Adolescents and young adults were also very much affected by OBRA. Before its passage, some 36 states had extended Medicaid benefits to persons 18–21 who were attending school. OBRA forced states to drop them from the eligibility rolls, resulting in the loss of coverage for approximately 200,000 Medicaid recipients (Hill, 1984).

The Tax Equity and Fiscal Responsibility Act of 1982 (TEFRA) included further limits on AFDC and SSI eligibility, but none was as far reaching as OBRA. States were permitted, with some restrictions, to impose cost-sharing requirements on categorically needy recipients using mandatory services.[8] Under TEFRA, however, some eligibility criteria were made more generous. States were given the option of covering severely ill children at home if the cost of care was less than or equal to that provided in an institution.

By 1984, Congressional attitudes had begun to shift in response to concern regarding the negative impact of OBRA and growing evidence of access barriers for pregnant women and children (IOM, 1985; Rosenbaum and Johnson, 1985; Fox, 1986a, 1986b; McManus, 1986). Provisions adopted in 1984, 1985, and 1986 strengthened the states' ability to target coverage and adopt more generous eligibility criteria for pregnant women, young children, and severely ill children.

The Deficit Reduction Act of 1984 (DEFRA) allowed states greater latitude in establishing Medicaid eligibility under AFDC and expanded Medicaid coverage to special targeted groups: first-time pregnant women who would be eligible for AFDC if the child were already born; pregnant women in two-parent families where the principal wage earner was unemployed; and financially eligible children up to age 5 who lived in two-parent families, were institutionalized, or resided in foster homes. This latter provision of DEFRA, termed the Child Health Assurance Program, allowed for receipt of Medicaid benefits by certain families not eligible for AFDC, introducing an important separation of eligibility for Medicaid from that for cash assistance.

The Consolidated Budget Reconciliation Act of 1985 (COBRA) further expanded coverage for pregnant women and young children with the goal that "by fiscal year 1990, all pregnant women and all children under five years of age, regardless of family status, will be covered by

Medicaid provided that their family incomes are below the state's payment standards" (Rodgers, 1986).[9] Specifically, COBRA mandated that pregnant women meeting the state's income eligibility criteria be covered by Medicaid regardless of their family structure (and thus their eligibility for AFDC). In addition, COBRA extended the period of Medicaid eligibility for pregnant women to 60 days after delivery and gave states the option of immediately covering Ribicoff children up to age 5.

States also were given the option of waiving (without HCFA approval) the comparability requirement for pregnant women. This permitted a state to offer such additional services as social work assessments, nutritional counseling, and health education to only their eligible pregnant population and not all Medicaid eligibles. For severely ill children, COBRA gave states more flexibility in operating home and community-based waiver programs under Section 2176. States were also allowed to provide case management services to selected populations, again waiving (without HCFA approval) both the statewideness and comparability requirements.[10]

The Omnibus Budget Reconciliation Act of 1986 (SOBRA) provided states the option of covering low-income, pregnant women and infants under age one (subsequently up to age five in future years), with family incomes above current state eligibility levels up to the federal poverty level. As under COBRA, the eligibility extended for 60 days following the infant's birth, regardless of changes in family income. States were also permitted to offer short-term Medicaid coverage to pregnant women based only on preliminary family income information—called "presumptive eligibility"—to avoid delays in timely and appropriate prenatal care while the application is being processed. By May 1987, more than half of all states had implemented these options or had bills pending in their state legislature to do so.

Summary and implications of eligibility policy. Changes in Medicaid eligibility during the first half of the 1980s can be thought of either as adjustments designed to fine-tune the program so that only the "truly needy" were covered or as overreactions to perceived fiscal problems. In the first part of this period, these changes took the form of cuts in AFDC eligibility, coupled with policies designed to expand state flexibility ostensibly to experiment with new arrangements free of the heavy hand of rigid federal policies. The clear intent on the part of federal officials was to save money by freeing the states to ratchet down their own programs. Unfortunately, at the same time that AFDC families were being dropped, the size of the child poverty population grew 38 percent between 1979 and 1983 (CRS and CBO, 1985).[11]

Although subsequent budget reconciliation acts—as well as efforts by some of the states—restored some of this lost eligibility, today a smaller proportion of poor children, particularly those of working poor parents and adolescents, are eligible for Medicaid than at the start of the period (see CRS and CBO, 1985).

In response to state and federal concerns about OBRA's impact on the working poor, several of the budget reconciliation bills passed by Congress during the 1980s offered the states more flexibility and provided assurances that certain populations would be included in a "safety net." During that period, however, only a few states attempted to increase significantly their AFDC payment standards and, in the process, to extend Medicaid coverage. States were reluctant to do more because they feared that major new budget outlays would be required to pay for the services used by a larger group of covered poor children. Instead, many more states expanded their eligible populations only to comply with DEFRA in particular or to assure a "safety net" for targeted high-risk groups, such as pregnant women or infants.

A surprisingly large number of states have taken advantage of these opportunities under DEFRA and SOBRA to increase eligibility for pregnant women and infants. But while this represents an important expansion of Medicaid eligibility, state income eligibility policies for other women and children still reflect excessively low and variable standards—a situation that exacerbates existing inequities in the Medicaid program.

In 1984, although the federal poverty line was $884 per month for a family of 4, no state set its payment standard (the amount that determines Medicaid eligibility) as high as that amount. (The mean for all states was about $380.) Except for Alaska, which at $775 per month was an exception, the highest payment standards were in Connecticut ($617), New York ($602), and California ($601). At the other end of the spectrum, five states established payment standards below $200 a month for a family of 4. They were Alabama ($147), Tennessee ($154), South Carolina ($174), Texas ($178), and Arkansas ($191). Families in those states with incomes above those amounts had too much income to be eligible for Medicaid benefits in 1984 even if they met the other criteria. In 60 percent of the states, families become eligible for Medicaid only at incomes below those the state itself has designated as necessary for subsistence.

The size of these inequities highlights an important outstanding question: does the recent trend toward allowing states greater flexibility in establishing eligibility represent a net gain or loss for low-income families and children? The answer depends partially on how one values the groups that gain (pregnant women and children) versus those that lose (families with working parents). It also depends on the longer-term political consequences of dividing Medicaid's recipients into more fragmented groups. These issues will be explored further later in the chapter.

Benefits

Title XIX of the Social Security Act mandates that all state Medicaid programs provide a range of benefits to its categorically needy and medically needy recipients, including inpatient and outpatient hospital services, physician and laboratory services, family planning services, rural health clinic services, and, particularly important for children, screening, diagnosis and treatment services for individuals under 21 years of age. The states decide, however, what conditions, if any, to place on the use of these services, including limits on the amounts or frequency, provisions for copayment, or requirements for prior authorization.

States have the option of providing any number of additional benefits to supplement their mandatory services. These can be offered to only their categorical eligibles or to those who qualify under either categorical or medically needy provisions. The following 21 (out of a total of 32) optional Medicaid services have been recommended by the American Academy of Pediatrics (AAP, 1986) as important for comprehensive delivery of health care services to children. (Those services marked with an asterisk are relevant primarily for children with special health care needs.) These include (1) practitioner services, such as optometrist's services, other practitioners' services*, dental services*, physical therapy*, occupational therapy*, speech, hearing, and language disorders*, and rehabiliative services; (2) drugs and devices, such as prescribed drugs*, prosthetic devices*, and eyeglasses; (3) outpatient services, such as screening services, preventive services, diagnostic services, clinic services, and emergency hospital services; (4) intermediate care facilities (ICFs), including ICF services*, ICFs for the mentally retarded*, and inpatient psychiatric services for those under age 22*; (5) skilled nursing facilities (SNFs) for those under age 21*; and (6) personal care services* and private duty nursing*.

Of the 21 optional services listed above, clinic services and intermediate care facilities for the mentally retarded (ICF-MR) are two of the most important to children, but for very different reasons. Because of the limited availability of office-based physician services for Medicaid children in some areas of the country, clinic services are used by a large proportion of Medicaid children for some or all of their care. Since ambulatory care is relatively inexpensive, however, clinics consume only a limited amount of total Medicaid dollars. ICF-MRs, on the other hand, are used by very few children but consume a disproportionately high and increasing share of Medicaid payments for children. According to Rymer et al. (1984), "the increasing proportion of Medicaid expenditures spent on nursing homes is entirely attributable to the growth in expenditures for ICF-MRs" (p. 9).

State policies regarding coverage of optional services have important implications for children with special health care needs, because so many are health-related support services that supplement mandatory physician and hospital care. The optional services that almost all state Medicaid programs reimburse are intermediate-care facilities (offered in all 50 states), ICF-MR (all but Wyoming), optometrist services (all but South Dakota and Tennessee), prescribed drugs (all but Alaska and Wyoming), skilled nursing facilities for children under 21 (all but Florida and Missouri), and clinic services (all but Mississippi, Rhode Island, and Texas) (HCFA, 1985). Table 6.2, shows which are most and least likely to be covered by states. While there appears to be no fully consistent pattern, some of the most costly optional services (ICFs, SNFs, emergency hospital services, clinic services, and prescribed drugs) are more likely to be covered than the less expensive services. (The exception is inpatient psychiatric services.) Only 16 states cover screening services, for instance. It also appears that states are more likely to cover hospital or institutional-based optional services and are less likely to cover home-based services such as private duty nursing or personal care services.

Medicaid generosity can also be examined by comparing the number of optional services covered by different states, as shown in Table 6.3. Ten states cover fewer than 14 optional services. Half of these are in the South, two each in the West and Northeast, and one in the North Central region of the country. More than half of the states (27) cover 15 to 24 optional services. Twelve states with the most comprehensive

Table 6.2 Probability of Optional Services Coverage by State, 1985

Services Offered by 29 or Fewer States	Services Offered by 30–39 States	Services Offered by 40 or More States
Occupational therapy (29)	Other Practitioners' Services (36)	ICF (50)
		ICF-MR (49)
Personal Care Services (26)	Physical Therapy (36)	Optometrists' Services (48)
Diagnostic Services (24)	Rehab. Services (35)	Prescription Drugs (48)
Preventive Services (23)	Speech, Hearing, and Language Disabilities (34)	SNF (48)
Private Duty Nursing (18)		Clinic Services (47)
Screening Services (16)	Dentures (34)	Prosthetic Devices (45)
	Inpatient Psychiatric Services (33)	Emergency Hospital Services (42)
		Dental Services (40)

Source: HCFA, unpublished 1985 data.

Table 6.3 State Generosity Related to Optional Service Coverage, 1985

Least (<14 services)		Moderate (15–24 services)		Generous (26+ services)	
(10 STATES)		(27 STATES)		(12 STATES)	
AL	(13)	AR	(22)	CA	(31)
AK	(13)	CO	(16)	CT	(25)
DE	(14)	DC	(23)	IL	(26)
GA	(12)	FL	(16)	IN	(27)
MS	(9)	HI	(21)	MA	(32)
MO	(13)	ID	(17)	MI	(25)
OK	(14)	IA	(22)	MN	(31)
RI	(11)	KS	(24)	MT	(26)
TX	(14)	KY	(22)	NH	(26)
WY	(8)	LA	(19)	NJ	(27)
		ME	(21)	WA	(26)
		NB	(23)	WI	(25)
		NM	(15)		
		NV	(22)		
		NY	(24)		
		NC	(20)		
		ND	(24)		
		OH	(24)		
		OR	(24)		
		PA	(17)		
		SC	(16)		
		TN	(22)		
		UT	(23)		
		VT	(21)		
		VA	(18)		
		WV	(18)		

Source: HCFA unpublished data for 1985.

coverage offer 26 or more optional services. Five of these are from the North Central region, four from the Northeast, and three from the West.

Trends in benefit management. Despite budgetary pressures, many states have expanded benefits somewhat in recent years. Between 1984 and 1985, several states that previously offered optional services only to categorically needy recipients extended them to medically needy Medicaid recipients, as well. During this same period, some states also increased their coverage of additional optional services. Those showing the greatest expansion were rehabilitative services (5 states), other practitioners' services (4 states), occupational therapy (4 states), and diagnostic and personal care services (with 3 states each). The Intergovernmental Health Policy Project (1986) reported that states also expanded coverage of clinic services and other practitioners' services. For example, under clinic services, several states added coverage of developmental and mental health clinic services. Similarly, under other practitioners' services, nurse midwives and nurse practitioners were added by some states.

Rather than setting limits on benefits, state Medicaid programs have instead focused their attention on utilization controls and managed care systems for controlling the use of their benefits. Cost-sharing requirements and prior authorization are commonly used for a variety of benefits ranging from emergency room services to prescription drugs (IHPP, 1986). As of June 30, 1985, about 774,000 Medicaid recipients were enrolled in HMO-type plans in 25 states (Neuschler, 1986).

Federal legislation in the 1980s provided states with new flexibility to waive statewideness and comparability requirements for both mandatory and optional benefits offered to their eligible populations. This flexibility has been too recently introduced to be able to assess its consequences for the Medicaid program and its recipients. However, the history of the Early and Periodic Screening, Diagnosis and Treatment (EPSDT) component of Medicaid, offers some insights into the possible consequences of more flexible benefit management by the states.

Twenty years have passed since Congress added a mandatory preventive child health benefit to Medicaid, called the Early and Periodic Screening, Diagnosis and Treatment Program (EPSDT). For many years, EPSDT has been a source of frustration and unfulfilled potential. The major criticisms of Medicaid include: (1) its historic emphasis on screening with minimal attention to diagnosis and treatment, (2) inadequate screening methods to identify and refer children with special health care needs, (3) limited involvement of primary care providers to offer continuous care, (4) weak links between health departments and clinics and physicians in private practice, (5) limited outreach and case management for high-risk children, and (6) a very low portion of the Medicaid budget (Foltz, 1982; McManus, 1986; Rosenbaum and Johnson, 1986).

Originally EPSDT was primarily a screening program to detect health care problems among underserved school-age Medicaid children. Diagnosis and treatment were lower priorities, and frequently the provider who screened the child was not the one to diagnose and treat him or her. In many states, Medicaid program does not pay for the services that the screening examination determined to be needed because they are not covered services under the state's Medicaid plan. Thus, the links of EPSDT to Medicaid and between local health departments and private physicians were difficult to maintain. In fact, as recently as 1985, HCFA reported that the majority of EPSDT users were between the ages of 5 and 6 in need of immunization, vision and hearing examinations, and treatment for other health problems (McManus, 1986).

In 1984, a coalition of children's health organizations succeeded in persuading HCFA to change its EPSDT regulations from their historical orientation favoring screening toward one that encourages comprehensive and continuing care. The goal was to make EPSDT services part of a continuum of care so that the child's screening services are delivered by someone familiar with his or her episodes of acute illness and who has an ongoing relationship with the family as the regular source of the child's care (Federal Register, 1984).

The basic changes included in the 1984 regulations were as follows. (1) EPSDT services are required to meet standards of medical and dental practice, including a periodic schedule of services established by expert professionals for children of all ages. (2) The EPSDT screening package is expanded to cover comprehensive health, developmental history, and physical examinations; vision, hearing, and laboratory tests; and dental referrals. States are required to provide immunizations. (3) States have flexibility to use continuing care providers to deliver EPSDT services. (4) States can now provide additional services under EPSDT which are not included in the state Medicaid plan (termed "discretionary services").

With these reforms, EPSDT can be used in conjunction with existing state Medicaid benefits to create an enriched primary care package of services for low-income infants, children and adolescents. However, before EPSDT is able to reach its full potential, several additional areas require attention. First, EPSDT medical and dental standards need to be consistent with recognized professional standards. As noted by Rosenbaum and Johnson of the Children's Defense Fund (1986), many states fail to meet them. In a 1985 survey conducted by the Children's Defense Fund, only the state of New York met the AAP's recommended periodicity schedule of 20 health supervision visits from infancy through age 21. In Wyoming, for example, the number of recommended visits was only 5.

The articulation of these standards along with periodicity schedules is increasingly important because of the growth in managed care arrangements. As noted in Chapters 7 and 8, prepaying providers in managed care settings may create incentives that lead to provision of inadequate health care. If states perform medical audits of HMOs, continuing care providers, and local health departments, they could use the EPSDT periodicity schedule and standards as quality of care indicators and a strong negotiating tool.

Second, efforts to link EPSDT benefits with ongoing Medicaid benefits need to be more fully developed. This can most readily be accomplished by having the same provider deliver EPSDT and Medicaid services. To this end, local health departments and state Medicaid offices should also examine strategies for maintaining continuing care arrangements when children lose their Medicaid eligibility. For example, rather than being the new providers of care to the uninsured children, state or local health departments may be able to subcontract the continuing care of uninsured children to the physician who had been the primary provider.

Even if Medicaid and EPSDT services are provided in different settings, a management information system that links the two settings will allow states to obtain federal matching funds for outreach and follow-up, to examine their utilization patterns of preventive as well as acute health services; to evaluate the effectiveness of providers delivering continuing EPSDT and Medicaid services; to reimburse more appropriately for the provision of cognitive as well as procedural services; and to better use the discretionary service component of EPSDT.

Another new direction that only a limited number of states are experimenting with is the design of EPSDT benefit packages and outreach components that are targeted to different subgroups of children. Some special populations that might be considered are adolescents (many of whom are sexually active, pregnant, substance abusers, at risk for accidents or injuries, or with other special health problems), chronically ill children, SSI-eligible children, children ages 0–3, children in foster care, state hospitals, and residential or criminal justice facilities. States already have the authority to enact an EPSDT waiver of comparability by making a state plan change to enrich benefits and to expand limits on mandatory and optional services (McManus, 1986). Further refinement and dissemination of innovative EPSDT programs can now be attempted with the new flexibility in the regulations.[12]

The history of EPSDT and optional Medicaid benefits reflects the conflicting pressures for further reform of Medicaid. On one hand, greater state flexibility in benefits creates the opportunity to better target particular services to the children who most need them. On the other hand, flexibility may undermine the goal of guaranteeing at least a minimal range of services that children in all states and groups need. For twenty years now, Medicaid has been in the forefront of offering preventive benefits for all children. Despite the problems previously outlined, EPSDT continues to represent an exciting benefit that enhances the health of children.

Medicaid's Relationship with Physicians

Medicaid was intended to make medical services financially accessible to low-income people in the mainstream of American medicine. Usually this means having a relationship with a private physician such that, when a person is in need of medical services, he or she calls that doctor, receives primary care services, and is referred to other physicians or services as needed. This system is thought to have provided continuity of care, efficiency in the use of services (by avoiding self-referral to unnecessary services), and lower expenditures (by using office-based physicians instead of more expensive hospital services.) In practice, it does not always work that way. Medicaid patients have not always had easy access to office-based physicians. The fee-for-service method of payment tends to lead to the provision of more services than might otherwise be the case, including some that are unnecessary. Nonetheless, it is true that office-based physicians provide primary care services at prices that are substantially less than hospital emergency departments and offer at least the potential for continuity of care. For those reasons, office-based physicians are the preferred providers of primary care services.

Yet, state policies have tended to discourage physicians from treating Medicaid patients for two reasons. First, physicians' professional autonomy (that is, their ability to act independently on the basis of their knowledge and the ethics of their profession) is compromised by eligibility provisions that promote turnover and thereby reduce the opportunity for continuity of care, as well as by benefit provisions that require prior authorization or place limits on the amount of a service that is covered. While some states cover unlimited amounts of physician or hospital services, others restrict coverage to 7 physician visits annually, for example, or 21 days in the hospital. These are essentially arbitrary limits designed to save the state money. The extent to which they actually accomplish that purpose is unclear, since relatively few people actually come up against these limits. Those that do, most often newborns in neonatal intensive care and chronically ill children, tend to need more services than are covered by Medicaid, hampering clinicians' efforts to provide them with needed services.

Inadequate, unpredictable, or slow compensation under Medicaid also leads physicians to prefer privately insured patients who pay higher prices and have fewer externally imposed constraints on the use of services (Davidson, 1982; Davidson et al., 1983). Prices for physician services vary widely from state to state, but tend to be at the low end of the pricing structure. In 1984, the price paid to a general practitioner for a brief office visit, a common service, varied from $4.20 in Mississippi to $16.40 in Indiana, a four-fold difference, with 2 outliers ($28.41 in Alaska and $20 in Delaware). The mean was $10.73, and the median was $10.45 (Table 6.4).

When a physician has as many patients as he needs or wants, and those patients pay the prices the physician charges and tend to follow his recommendations regarding care, the doctor is likely to limit the extent to which he treats Medicaid patients. When that occurs, access

Table 6.4 Maximum Allowable Fees, General Practioners, by State, 1984

State	Brief Office Visit	Appendectomy	Obstetrical Care
AL	$11.70	$405	$450
AK	28.41	N/A	N/A
AR	12.00	275	500
CA	12.00	312	450
CO	11.75	280	392
CT	6.75	240	289
DE	12.66	390	N/A
DC	20.00	315	N/A
FL	10.00	198	310
GA	12.36	340	340
HI	9.06	413	287
ID	10.50	336	450
IL	10.50	250	375
IN	14.40	356	489
IA	16.40	280	437
KS	7.00	268	332
KY	10.50	402	N/A
LA	11.70	350	600
ME	8.00	218	268
MD	10.00	191	266
MA	6.00	225	168
MI	7.00	259	373
MN	12.10	370	350
MS	4.20	255	446
MO	10.00	220	220
MT	11.30	343	577
ME	10.00	462	650
NV	13.16	513	539
NH	6.00	225	214
NJ	10.40	368	306
NM	7.00	184	210
NY	7.00	160	200
NC	11.40	378	400
ND	9.90	390	336
OH	10.00	225	225
OK	11.75	487	750
OR	10.24	359	464
PA	11.00	100	100
RI	12.00	186	300
SC	6.30	307	323
SD	10.00	345	325
TN	10.30	446	441
TX	11.03	368	382
UT	10.04	313	401
VT	6.00	N/A	275
VA	6.30	236	263
WA	12.34	283	474
WI	10.00	230	255
WV	15.00	400	530
WY	12.50	464	545
High	28.41	513.00	750.00
Low	4.20	100.00	100.00
Mean	10.73	299.36	345.70

to mainstream medical care for Medicaid eligibles is reduced, and program expenditures increase.

Data from a recent two-and-a-half-year experiment confirmed that the generosity of Medicaid payment affects physicians' willingness to participate in the program (Davidson et al., 1987). As part of the experiment, fees paid to primary care physicians were doubled (Table 6.5), and the effects on the amount and distribution of services were dramatic. The study compared the behavior of four groups of children: two experimental groups and two comparison groups. Each mother of a child in one of the experimental groups chose a participating office-based primary care physician to assume responsibility for providing or ordering any care the child needed during the project. The comparison groups were selected to include similar children who continued to use Medicaid and the medical care system in Suffolk County without modification.

The findings show that children in the experimental groups had substantially more visits to office-based physicians than did either group of comparison children. Table 6.6 reports visit rates to office-based physicians of 4.7 and 5.1 visits per year of eligibility for the 2 experimental groups and only 3.3 and 3.2 visits per year for the comparison children. Similar differences were observed for visits to all sites. Of even greater significance is that children in the experimental groups received approximately 20 percent more of their ambulatory visits from office-based physicians than the comparison children. The conclusion is that, even in a time-limited demonstration, physicians treated Medicaid patients to a much larger extent than normally is the case, primarily because of higher fees. Several physicians who had not previously accepted patients in the regular Medicaid program did participate in the demonstration, in part because of the higher fees.

Implications of Recent Changes in Medicaid

Early in this chapter, we identified goals for a publicly financed health care program: that it should provide the poor with protection against

Table 6.5 Payments to Physicians in the Fee-for-Service Group for Primary Care Services

New Code	Service	Old Fee	New Fee
99880	Comprehensive exam, incl. treatment	$14.50	$28.00
99881	Routine office visit	9.00	17.00
99882	Initial hospital visit	7.00	28.00
99883	Follow-up hospital visit	7.00	17.00

Table 6.6 Visit Rates per Year of Eligibility, Suffolk County Demonstration, 1983–1985

Category of Service	Experimental Groups Capitation	Experimental Groups Fee-for-Service	Comparison Groups In-area	Comparison Groups Out of area
Physicians*				
Rate	4.709	5.088	3.276	3.168
Percent users	84.4%	83.4%	62.5%	65.8%
Clinic/OPD*				
Rate	0.504	0.528	0.852	1.176
Percent users	13.2%	15.0%	25.6%	30.2%
Emergency Department*				
Rate	0.336	0.372	0.348	0.684
Percent users	29.6%	30.0%	29.1%	47.5%
Total Physician Visits*				
Rates	5.549	5.988	4.476	5.028

*Statistically different at 2-tail .05 alpha level.

Note: Number of visits reported by capitated physicians for their children in the demonstration has been inflated by 9% to correct for underreporting.

financial catastrophe, offer a comprehensive array of services, encourage use of the most appropriate, least costly level of care, and encourage providers to exercise their best clinical judgment in the most efficient manner. Title XIX of the Social Security Act, which created the Medicaid grant-in-aid program, makes possible a program that can meet these criteria. It permits states to cover virtually any other recognized service and receive federal reimbursement for some of the cost.

The discretion allowed states under Medicaid, however, inhibits the realization of this potential. While all states must cover mandatory services, they may set limits and prior authorization requirements on them which arbitrarily deny coverage to the sickest enrollees. State discretion arbitrarily limits the proportion of the poor who are entitled to Medicaid benefits: while 12 states set their AFDC payment standards at 60 percent of poverty or above, 19 others set theirs below 40 precent of the poverty line (U.S. Congress, 1986). When states set artificially low ceilings on physician fees, they not only reduce continuity of care but also indirectly drive patients to more costly settings for treatment (e.g., the hospital emergency room) (Holahan, 1982; Long et al., 1986).[13]

This experience raises a number of important questions for policymakers:

1. Can a program tied to welfare cover sufficient numbers of the poor? To receive Medicaid benefits, one must be eligible for welfare (except for pregnant women and infants), which depends on criteria related to income and family characteristics, which in turn are set by each of the 50 states. Three possibilities for reform are to (a) sever the tie between welfare and Medicaid, (b) limit the scope of state decision-

making by establishing federal minimums for welfare eligibility at higher levels than presently, and (c) create a national welfare program with a uniform set of eligibility and coverage criteria set at a level that approaches the poverty line and a comprehensive package of services.

2. Can a program that leaves so many decisions to the states provide comprehensive coverage to those who are eligible? The answer depends on the reasons states make the choices they do. Since the program is, in reality, 50 different state programs, it is virtually certain that some states will move away from comprehensive coverage, because they are responding to other policy goals.

3. Can a program that combines payment of acute medical care for children and long-term care for the elderly achieve a fair and sensible balance of funding? The aged, blind, and disabled recipient population amounted to 27 percent of all Medicaid recipients in 1980, falling to 24 percent in 1982 and 1984. Vendor payments for this group, on the other hand, accounted for 70 percent of the total in 1980, 72 percent in 1982, and 73 percent in 1984.

While child Medicaid recipients represented more than 50 percent of all Medicaid recipients, only 16 percent of vendor payments went for their care in 1980 and 14 percent in both 1982 and 1984 (Table 6.7). The overall pattern appears to be that long-term care is obtaining a greater share of the Medicaid dollar despite the tremendous size of the child Medicaid population.

Children do not vote, but the elderly do (and are politically well organized). Moreover, the interests of hospitals and nursing homes regarding Medicaid are much more concentrated than those of physicians and other practitioners (Marmor et al., 1983). For all these reasons, the needs of children tend to receive less attention from Medicaid policy makers than those of the elderly. Not surprisingly, in a climate of budgetary restraint, it is easier to adopt policies that have the effect of curtailing ambulatory services.

4. Can a program with the present structure encourage the exercise of sound clinical judgment and efficiency? The answer is that it probably can but will not, again, largely because the priorities of the 50 states will not equally value this goal, as reflected in the growth of arbitrary limits on coverage. To ensure against this, reforms that either restrict or remove the state role in decision making have a better chance of achieving the goals discussed earlier. To reach this position, however, would require us as a nation to reassert that pragmatism requires a national articulation of purpose, acknowledging that the present structure has resulted in widespread inequities and fragmented care.

There is little evidence that policymakers are at the point of being ready to reconsider the basic structure of Medicaid. We can, however,

Table 6.7 Trends in Medicaid Recipients and Medical Vendor Payments by Basis of Eligibility, 1980, 1982, and 1984

Basis of Eligibility	1980 Recipients No. (mil)	1980 Recipients %	1980 Vendor Payments Amt. (mil)	1980 Vendor Payments %	1982 Recipients No. (mil)	1982 Recipients %	1982 Vendor Payments Amt. (mil)	1982 Vendor Payments %	1984 Recipients No. (mil)	1984 Recipients %	1984 Vendor Payments Amt. (mil)	1984 Vendor Payments %
Dependent Children < 21	9.3	43	$3,123	13	9.6	44	$3,473	12	9.7	45	$3,979	12
Adults in Families with Dependent Children	4.9	23	3,231	14	5.4	25	4,093	14	5.6	26	4,421	13
Other Title XIX	1.5	7	596	3	1.4	7	689	2	1.2	5	699	2
Aged, Blind, and Disabled	5.9	27	21,361	70	5.2	24	21,144	72	5.1	24	24,796	73
Total	21.6	100	$23,311	100	21.6	100	$29,399	100	21.6	100	$33,894	100

Source: HCFA unpublished data.

identify several areas of promise associated with the Medicaid reforms of the 1980s.

One possible direction for additional reform is to separate further eligibility for Medicaid from eligibility for welfare and to offer an extended period of guaranteed eligibility. SOBRA represents a step in this direction by giving states the option of extending Medicaid to pregnant women and children under 1 (up to 5 in subsequent years) who fall below the federal poverty level even if they are above the state's AFDC criteria. A guaranteed period of eligibility for pregnant women was also part of COBRA and SOBRA. Extending these reforms would have several potential benefits. First, if eligibility were based on income and guaranteed for a year, it would increase the stability of the Medicaid population and encourage office-based physicians to treat more Medicaid patients. Second, it would simplify administration of the Medicaid program by eliminating the need for a link with AFDC, which is the province of another large and complex organization. Third, it might save welfare money because Medicaid is such a substantial benefit that fear of its loss leads some welfare mothers to refrain from looking for work. If the opportunity to keep Medicaid benefits were guaranteed, at least for their children, some additional women would seek employment. To the extent they found it, they would no longer need AFDC payments.

Another critical, though neglected, issue involves the large number of children potentially eligible for Medicaid but not enrolled. According to Rodgers (1986), Medicaid participation rates for children are estimated to be between 50 and 65 percent. In other words, almost half the children who are eligible for Medicaid are not enrolled.

Medicaid is a very complex program to understand. Providers, eligibles, and even Medicaid administrators readily admit to the complexities, confusions, and misinterpretations associated with the program. Some of these difficulties would be eliminated or reduced if (1) Medicaid eligibility were separated from that for welfare; (2) it were based on income alone and not family composition, too; and (3) the benefits were more comprehensive, so that whether a particular patient had used his full allotment would not be an issue for a provider. Program simplification must be accompanied by an aggressive community marketing and education effort. This would be of particular value to the large numbers of non-English-speaking families who currently are unaware of their eligibility.

But the greatest challenge facing Medicaid reform is the program's interstate variability, which has increased in recent years as states have been given increased discretion by Congress. Wide state variation in Medicaid services is never more apparent than in its effects on families with severely chronically ill children. Fox and Yoshpe (1986) aptly described such variation in a series of case studies of technology-dependent children in five different states. For these children, the amount, duration, and scope of mandatory and optional services bear special significance. Take the case of Michael Jones, an 18-month-old toddler who had been hospitalized since birth because of numerous metabolic and developmental problems. These included insulin-dependent diabetes mellitus, congenital heart failure, seizures, liver dysfunction, and failure to thrive (p. 45).

Michael's mother, who was divorced and had no other children, earned an annual salary of $14,500. She wanted to bring her child home. Monthly costs of home care would have been $4,320 ($3,700 for nursing, $70 for equipment, $280 for supplies, $250 for medications, and $20 for a physician visit). Michael's mother's employee benefits had been exhausted. In California, Georgia, Kansas, and Maryland, Michael would have been eligible for SSI and, thus Medicaid. Missouri would not have covered Michael under SSI because he was not a resident of an intermediate care facility. Also because Missouri has no medically needy program or Section 2176 waivers for this population, he would not have qualified for Medicaid under those eligibility options.

While few children are as seriously ill as Michael, the situation in Missouri is not uncommon for states or for families with chronically ill children. The presence or absence of medically needy components in Medicaid programs, waivers, and selected optional benefits (particularly private duty nursing and personal care services) can force families into untenable situations, including moving to another state, uprooting them from established social support systems, and keeping children hospitalized or institutionalized when home care or group homes are a much more reasonable option.

The challenge of Medicaid to provide preventive and acute services for more than 50 percent of all Medicaid recipients, namely, children, will continually be balanced against states' budget constraints and the need to finance long-term care services, especially for the elderly and disabled. The context that pits several groups in need against each other might result in the formation of new coalitions that will find viable ways of achieving the maximal amount possible for each. As with all public issues, these are essentially political questions and will be resolved by political means.

The following recommendations are offered as means of improving the extent to which Medicaid serves low-income children and others. In the process, they will bring Medicaid policy closer to the model health insurance plan articulated early in this chapter.

1. Separate Medicaid eligibility from welfare eligibility. One way to reduce the extent to which low-income children are denied access to medical services is to establish eligibility criteria that are independent

of welfare. Then, assuming the programmatic structure remained the same (see Recommendation #2), a state would be able to grant eligibility to needy families and children without committing itself to cash welfare grants, too.

Another potential benefit to separating eligibility for the two programs derives from the fact that some mothers remain on welfare primarily to guarantee the presence of medical benefits for their children. This was a finding of the Children's Medicaid Program, a prepaid managed care demonstration in Suffolk County, New York (Davidson et al., 1987). Thus, providing the medical care eligibility separately from welfare would lead some AFDC mothers to seek work, reducing welfare caseloads. Those savings, in turn, could be used to raise the eligibility level for Medicaid so that more low-income children and others could qualify. Ironically, though, if Medicaid is separated from welfare programs, it may be bureaucratically more difficult to recapture savings in this way.

2. Remove key policy decisions from the states. Although no state established Medicaid eligibility at a level that approached the poverty line, it was clearly better to be poor in some states than in others. Two principal means are available to achieve greater levels of equity and adequacy. One would retain the present federal-state structure but reduce the degree of decision-making authority by setting higher federal standards. Regarding eligibility, the minimum income criteria could be set as a proportion of the poverty level. Then, residents of all states with incomes at, say, 80 percent of the poverty line would be eligible for Medicaid benefits. States could still be free to set the rate at a higher amount, but at least the lowest rate would be more nearly adequate.

The other method for increasing equity and adequacy would be for the federal government to set the criteria, thus removing decisions from the states altogether. This result could be accomplished if the federal government simply assumed total responsibility for Medicaid policy and administration. The state could retain a role through a contract with the federal government to operate the program, but fundamentally it would become a federal program. Another, more radical alternative would be to create a national health insurance program for which all Americans would be eligible. It could be financed through a combination of taxes and beneficiary contributions on a sliding scale so that lower-income people would contribute less (or nothing at all if their income were low enough) and higher-income people would contribute more. Everyone would have the same eligibility card and, to that extent at least, would be indistinguishable one from another.

3. Encourage more experimentation with comprehensive managed care and prepayment. This recommendation addresses the need to be more efficient in the delivery of services without having the state estab-

lish a set of arbitrary limits on benefits. Considerable attention in recent years has centered on the concepts of case management (in which access to care is channeled through a primary care physician who acts as gatekeeper to other services) and prepayment (in which the primary care provider—whether a physician or an organization that employs him— is at risk for the cost of the services used by his panel of patients.) Results from experiments to date are intriguing but inconclusive; while they may not warrant a rush to convert the entire American medical care system to prepayment, they do justify continued experimentation.

Of particular importance are the implementation issues. It is not enough simply to announce that, henceforth, all care is to be received through a case manager physician or that primary care physicians will be prepaid and at risk for the cost of services. Systems must be put in place to effect those changes so that managed care and prepayment have the best opportunity to demonstrate their potential value. Among these are computerized information systems that provide the data about utilization and expenditures which permit clinical and administrative managers to intervene if the patterns are less than recommended. In addition, once the data are present and indicate conditions that need improvement, processes of intervening with physician case managers and other care-givers to produce more satisfactory results must be developed and implemented. Since these are professional services, the process of effecting change can be a delicate one involving conversations and negotiations over a period of time with clinicians. The roles of the general manager, the medical director, and others must evolve. The point is that these methods do not just happen; they must be developed with care. They can be done well or poorly. And since national Medicaid policy involves thousands of sites and thousands of professionals, it is likely to work more smoothly in some instances than in others. It is critical that experiments be conducted systematically and their results broadly disseminated.

Notes

1. Other Title XIX recipients are children who do not fit into either the categorically needy or medically needy groups, but are eligible at state option (e.g., Ribicoff children).

2. Federal subsidy rates are higher for states with lower per capita incomes.

3. These coverage groups have changed somewhat since 1985, as noted in the text.

4. The income permitted for eligibility was limited by the 1967 amendments to 133$^{1}/_{3}$ percent of the maximum amount paid to a family of comparable size under Aid to Families with Dependent Children.

5. For a complete description of each of the annual reconciliation budgets and their AFDC and Medicaid provisions, see Hill (1984, 1987) and Fox (1984, 1986a, 1986b).

6. Two provisions of the original Title XIX required that a program operate identically throughout an entire state ("statewideness") and that similar people should be treated similarly no matter where they lived in the state or what their color or ethnic background were ("comparability"). From the beginning, however, the Secretary of the Department of Health and Human Services (originally, Health, Education and Welfare) has had the authority to waive provisions of the law under certain conditions.

7. In the low-benefit states (Tennessee and Texas), between 60 and 63 percent were uninsured; and in the high-benefit states, between 16 percent and 30 percent were uninsured.

8. The only exclusions were children under 18, or at a state's option, those under 21, 20, or 19; pregnant women; institutionalized persons; emergency services; family planning; and HMO enrollees who were categorically needy or, again at state option, those who were medically needy.

9. Eligibility in each state is based on a set of income and asset criteria as well as family composition. Each state establishes a need standard, which represents the official determination for that state of what a family of 4 needs to subsist (HCFA, 1983). It also sets a payment standard, which indicates the level below which it accepts a public obligation for a family. The payment standard is the de facto AFDC and Medicaid eligibility level. Finally, a state determines separately the maximum payment it will make to a family. Thus, it is possible for a state to declare a family eligible for AFDC and Medicaid and, yet, make no cash payments to that family because it already has more income than the maximal payment the state will make. For Medicaid, the major importance of the maximal payment is that eligibility under federally supported medically needy provisions cannot exceed $133^{1}/_{3}$ percent of the maximal payment for an AFDC family of similar size.

10. The statute defines case management as services that will assist persons in "gaining access to needed medical, social, educational, and other services" (U.S. Social Security Act, Section 1915 (g)(2)).

11. Even though the increase in poverty has leveled off since 1983, as many as 20.5 percent or 12.4 million related children under 18 lived in poverty in 1985 (Current Population Survey, 1986).

12. For more information regarding innovative models and EPSDT strategies, see the new American Academy of Pediatrics' EPSDT handbook (AAP, 1987).

13. Actually, the bases for selection of Medicaid policies and, more generally, welfare policies are complicated by a multiplicity of factors, and are beyond the scope of this paper (Davidson, 1985).

References

Aday, L.A., R. Anderson, and G. Fleming. 1980. *Health Care in the United States: Equitable for Whom?* Beverly Hills, Calif.: Sage Publications.

American Academy of Pediatrics. 1986. *Medicaid Policy Statement.* Elk Grove Village, Ill.

———. 1987. *Medicaid EPSDT Program: A Pediatrician's Handbook for Action.* Elk Grove Village, Ill.

Anderson, O. 1985. *Health Services in the United States: A Growth Enterprise since 1875*. Ann Arbor, Mich. Health Administration Press.

Congressional Research Services and Congressional Budget Office. 1985. *Children in Poverty*. Washington, D.C.: G.P.O.

Cromwell, J., et al. 1984. *The Evolution of State Medicaid Program Changes*. Final Report Prepared for the Office of the Assistant Secretary for Planning and Evaluation, Department of Health and Human Services under Contract No. 066A-83.

Current Population Survey. 1986. *Money Income and Poverty Status of Families and Persons in the United States, 1985*. Advance data from the March 1986 Current Population Survey. Washington, D.C.: G.P.O.

Davidson, S. 1983. Full and Limited Medicaid Participation among Pediatricians. *Pediatrics* 72(4):552–559.

Davidson, S., et al. 1985. Regional Differences in Medicaid: Their Origins and Effects. Unpublished paper.

———. 1987. *The Children's Medicaid Program: A Prepaid Managed Care Experiment*. Final report submitted to the Health Care Financing Administration.

Davis, K., and C. Shoen. 1978. *Health and the War on Poverty: A Ten-Year Appraisal*. Washington, D.C.: Brookings Institution.

Federal Register. 1984. *Final Rule of the Early and Periodic Screening, Diagnosis, and Treatment Program*. 42 CFR Parts 400 and 441. Vol. 49, No. 212. October 31.

Foltz, A. 1982. *An Ounce of Prevention: Child Health Policies Under Medicaid*. Cambridge, Mass.: MIT Press.

Fox, H. 1984. *Memorandum on New Mandatory and Optional Medicaid Provisions Regarding Eligibility and Benefits for Children and Pregnant Women*. Washington, D.C.: Fox Health Policy Consultants.

———. 1986a. *New Mandatory and Optional Medicaid Provisions Regarding Eligibility and Benefits for Children and Pregnant Women*. Washington, D.C.: Fox Health Policy Consultants.

———. 1986b. *1986 Legislative Amendments Affecting the Access to Care by Children and Pregnant Women*. Washington, D.C.: Fox Health Policy Consultants.

Fox, H., and R. Yoshpe. 1986. *Technology Dependent Childrens' Access to Medicaid Home Care Financing*. Washington, D.C.: Fox Health Policy Consultants.

General Accounting Office. 1985. *An Evaluation of the 1981 AFDC Changes: Final Report*. Washington, D.C.

Goggin, M.L. 1987. *Policy Design and the Politics of Implementation: The Case of Child Health Care in the American States*. Knoxville: University of Tennessee Press.

Health Care Financing Administration. 1983. *The Medicare and Medicaid Data Book, 1983*. Baltimore.

———. 1984, 1985. *Medicaid Services State by State*. Prepared by the Office of Intergovernmental Affairs. Baltimore.

———. 1986. Unpublished Tabulations on Medicaid Recipients and Expenditures. Baltimore.

Held, P., et al. 1982. *The Effect of Medicaid and Private Fees on Physician Participation in California's Medicaid Program, 1974–1978*. Working Paper 1306-02-04. Washington, D.C.: Urban Institute.

Hill, I. 1984. *Medicaid Eligibility: A Descriptive Report of OBRA, TEFRA, and DEFRA Provisions and State Responses*. Washington, D.C.: National Governors' Association.

———. 1987. *Broadening Medicaid Coverage of Pregnant Women and Children: State Policy Responses*. Washington, D.C.: National Governors' Association.

Holahan, J. 1982. *A Comparison of Medicaid and Medicare Physician Reimbursement Rates.* Grant Report to HCFA. Washington, D.C.: Urban Institute.

Institute of Medicine. 1985. *Preventing Low Birthweight.* Washington, D.C.: National Academy Press.

Intergovernmental Health Policy Project. 1986. *Major Changes in State Medicaid Programs and Indigent Care Programs, December 1985.* Washington, D.C.: George Washington University.

Law, S. 1974. *Blue Cross: What Went Wrong?* New Haven: Yale University Press.

Long, S., et al. 1986. Reimbursement and Access to Physicians' Services under Medicaid. *Journal of Health Economics* 5:235–251.

McManus, M. 1986. Medicaid Services and Delivery Settings for Maternal and Child Health. In R. Curtis and I. Hill (eds.), *Affording Access to Quality Care: Strategies for State Medicaid Cost Management,* pp. 95–125. Washington, D.C.: National Governors' Association and Center for Health Policy Research.

Margolis, L.H., and S.J. Meisels. 1987. Barriers to the Effectiveness of EPSDT for Children with Moderate and Severe Developmental Disabilities. *American Journal of Orthopsychiatry* 57(3):424–430.

Marmor, T., D. Wittman, and T. Heagy. 1983. The Politics of Medical Inflation. In T. Marmor (ed.), *Political Analysis and American Medical Care: Essays.* New York: Cambridge University Press.

Neuschler, E. 1986. Alternative Financing and Delivery Systems: Managed Health Care. In R. Curtis and I. Hill (eds.), *Affording Access to Quality Care: Strategies for State Medicaid Cost Management.* Washington, D.C.: National Governors' Association.

Newacheck, P., and N. Halfon. 1986. Ambulatory Care Services for Economically Disadvantaged Children. *Pediatrics* 78(5):813–819.

Rodgers, J. 1986. *Memorandum on a Methodology for Estimating the Impacts of Extending Medicaid Coverage to All Pregnant Women and Children with Incomes Below the Poverty Level.* Washington, D.C.: Congressional Budget Office.

Rosenbach, M. 1985. *Insurance Coverage and Ambulatory Medical Care of Low-income Children: United States, 1980.* National Medical Care Utilization and Expenditure Survey, Series C, Analytical Report No. 1, DHHS Publication No. 85-20401. Washington, D.C.: G.P.O.

Rosenbaum, S., and K. Johnson. 1985. *The Early and Periodic Screening, Diagnosis and Treatment Programs: Reconciling Child Health Goals with Medicaid Realities.* Washington, D.C.: Children's Defense Fund.

Rymer, M., et al. 1984. *Short-term Evaluation of Medicaid: Selected Issues.* Cambridge: Urban Systems Research and Engineering.

U.S. Congress. 1986. *Report of the Committee on the Omnibus Budget Reconciliation Act of 1986.* Report 99-727, July 31.

Wilson, R.W., and E.G. White. 1977. Changes in Morbidity, Disability and Utilization Differentials between the Poor and the Nonpoor: Data from the Health Interview Survey, 1964 and 1973. *Medical Care* 15:636–646.

7

Provider Payment and Children's Health Care

Constance M. Horgan, Sc.D., and Samuel S. Flint, Ph.D.

Ongoing changes in methods of paying American health care providers are profoundly altering the way medical care is organized and delivered. Fuchs (1985) argued that these changes represent the third revolution in health care finance since World War II, the first two being the spread of private insurance and the enactment of the public insurance programs of Medicare and Medicaid. Fuchs suggested that changes in payment methods may in fact be the most revolutionary change, since they are intended to alter fundamentally the organization and delivery of care, while public and private insurance programs sought only to increase access to the existing health care system.

Several broad, interrelated trends during the first half of the 1980s encouraged the use of alternative payment systems. Payers, particularly private employers, have attempted to exert greater control over the delivery of health care as the costs of their employees medical benefits have increased (Goldsmith 1984). The growing supply of providers has limited physicians' ability to resist this control. Table 7.1 illustrates that between 1976 and 1985, there was a sharp decline in the number of children per pediatrician and per "child health physician" (i.e., all pediatricians and 25 percent of family physicians and general practitioners). These data are consistent with the 1980 GMENAC (Graduate Medical Education National Advisory Committee) predictions of five to seven thousand excess pediatricians by 1990. Indeed, GMENAC projections may underestimate the oversupply, since rapidly growing managed care systems require 22 percent fewer primary care physicians for children than do traditional practice arrangements (Steinwachs et al., 1986).

Efforts to influence physicians' practices by payment incentives have been encouraged by evidence of substantial variations in medical practice. In one analysis of inpatient care in thirty communities between 1980 and 1982, pediatrics was shown to be among the most variable of all types of treatment. For example, there was a twentyfold difference in admission rates for pediatric gastroenteritis and differences of similar orders of magnitude for many other diagnostic groupings (Wennberg et al., 1984). To many observers, this suggests that professional norms are not in themselves sufficient to avoid substantial amounts of inappropriate

Table 7.1 The National Ratio of Children to Child Health Physicians

	Children under 18 (in Millions)	Pediatricians[1]	Children per Pediatrician	FPs/GPs (25% F.T.E.)	Children per Child Health Physician
1976	64.9	20,152	3,222	53,508	1,936
1982	62.4	27,776	2,245	59,680	1,461
1985	62.7	31,065	2,018	63,960	1,332
Percent change (1976–1985)	−3%	+54%	−37%	+20%	−31%

Source: AAP analysis of AMA Masterfile Data.

[1] "Self-defined" pediatricians (not fellows in AAP or board-certified/board eligible)

treatment. Innovative payment systems represent one method of addressing this problem.

This chapter describes the incentives in traditional and alternative payment systems with a particular emphasis on the consequences for children and for providers of services to children. In doing so, it follows the philosophy proposed by the Select Panel for the Promotion of Child Health (1981): that the design of alternative payment systems should be based on a "systematic assessment of the relationship between financing decisions and the availability, accessibility, appropriateness, quality, and cost of care."

It is necessary to examine the incentives created for children's medical care apart from those for other patients because pediatric health care needs are substantially different from the needs of adults. Hospitalization is a much rarer occurrence, and the constant process of growth and development requires an ambulatory orientation with a strong preventive component (Austin, 1984). Additionally, there is a greater need for providers to assume a strong "agency role" that is, to act on behalf of children. Children are often not able to identify their health needs or seek needed services. Parents and guardians can act as advocates for children; however, a strong agency role by the physician can complement the efforts of parents and may be essential if parents are not knowledgeable about child health needs or are not effective advocates.

The intent of this chapter is not to prescribe the single best payment system but rather to identify options, discuss trade-offs, and make recommendations as to how each payment system might be adapted to improve access to and quality of care for children in a cost-effective manner. This focus recognizes the fact that the American approach to health care is inherently pluralistic and that the providers of health care to children will continue to be compensated under a variety of systems. Any system can be made more responsive to children's health needs; we will assess which approaches look most promising.

Characteristics of Payment Systems

It is useful to examine four aspects of a payment system: the unit of payment, the method of setting the price, the level of payment, and amount of choice within the system. Under traditional systems the unit of payment is typically the procedure or service. Provider revenue thereby depends on the number of units and the unit price of procedure or service. To control costs under traditional systems, it is necessary to control either the volume or the price of the service or both. Alternative units of payment reflect higher levels of aggregation. Some systems pay by the case (e.g., payment for an entire hospital stay), by the episode (e.g., physician payment for the prenatal, delivery, and postpartum care associated with a pregnancy and delivery), or for an established time period (e.g., covering all services used by an individual for a year).

Under traditional payment systems, prices typically are either based on providers' costs or set according to the "prevailing" charge in a community. Under alternative systems, prices can be determined by a variety of methods. Some methods base payment on the complexity of the procedure. In others, prices are negotiated or competitively set through a bidding process (Dobson, 1987).

The generosity of the payment level, irrespective of the method of payment, has important implications for whether and how physicians participate in the program, which in turn affects beneficiary access and program costs (Sloan and Steinwald, 1978; Sloan et al., 1978; Hadley, 1979; Perloff et al., 1987). This is particularly true for providers who treat children. A survey of 800 pediatricians practicing in thirteen states found that a growing number are limiting their participation in the Medicaid program. Citing high collection costs, complex Medicaid regulations, slow receipt of payments from state Medicaid agencies, annoying retroactive claims denials, restrictive benefits packages, and low reimbursement levels, 26 percent of pediatricians in 1978 and 35 percent in 1985 had limited their treatment of Medicaid-insured children (Perloff et al., 1987). Low rates of physician participation in Medicaid have led to a greater reliance by beneficiaries on the more costly hospital outpatient departments, raising questions about both costs and accessibility of services to children from low-income families (Holohan, 1985).

In discussing a payment system, it is also critical to distinguish how provider groups are paid as opposed to how individual practitioners are compensated. Hornbrook (1985) used the term "method of payment" to refer to the first, "method of remuneration" to the second. For example, in an HMO, the physician may be remunerated on a fee-for-service, salary, or capitated basis. The economic incentives facing the physician under the three methods are quite different.

Payment systems also involve different degrees of choice for both beneficiaries and providers. Under traditional payment systems, the patient typically chooses a physician. In many alternative systems patient choice of physician is limited in some fashion. For example, members of HMOs are limited to using the providers participating in the particular plan to which they belong. This can limit access to subspecialists, such as pediatric surgeons and cardiologists who may be seen as expensive, exotic, and consequently not really necessary.

Payment systems cannot be viewed in isolation. Different methods of payment are often accompanied by different organizational arrangements or use of copayments. But any payment method can also be used in various organizational settings. For example, an HMO is a type of capitated payment system which can take many organizational forms, such as an independent practice association (IPA) or a prepaid group practice. Because other chapters focus on issues of organization and copayment, the major focus of this chapter is the method of payment. However, where there is an important interaction between organizational structure and method of remuneration, this will be mentioned.

Criteria for Evaluating a Payment System

A payment system must be evaluated in light of a variety of goals. First, the goal of *access* entails an assurance that an adequate supply of appropriate services are available and that providers have adequate incentives to serve all types of children, including those who may be less financially desirable, such as high cost patients. Second, the goal of *quality* requires that medical considerations not be compromised by the financial incentives of the payment system. Third, *costs* of medical care should be restrained by selecting the combination of setting, mix and amount of services which assures the most cost-effective care. Fourth, *equity* in the allocation of benefits across providers requires that certain types of providers do not unfairly gain or lose because of the method and level of provider payment. Fifth, the *administrative ease* with which a system can be operated reflects a trade-off between systems that are simple to administer but often unfair to individual providers and patients (because they do not take into account individual circumstances) and very detailed administratively complex systems that offer greater potential for equitable treatment.

Finally, financial *risk* to providers due to random variation in their case load needs to be minimized. Provider risk has two aspects: the unsystematic and the systematic effects of the payment system. Random variation in a provider's caseload is the cause of unsystematic risk. It occurs when a provider through the luck of the draw is faced with an unusual number of costly cases. Because of the law of large numbers, it is more problematic for small providers than large providers. Providers with smaller panels of patients face a higher risk that high cost patients will be disproportionately represented in their panel.

Systematic risk relates to provider equity and occurs when a provider typically has higher cost patients and the payment system does not compensate accordingly (McGuire et al., 1985). For example, children's hospitals may be underreimbursed under a prospective payment system because they must treat more resource-intensive patients who are referred to them by community hospitals throughout the region.

Some of these goals can best be met by encouraging providers to act as agent or advocate for children who are their patients. The extent to which a payment system furthers the societal goals depends in large part on how it effects this agency relationship. Under traditional payment systems, the provider and the patient share a mutual interest in the provision of more services—the provider for more revenue and the patient for more health care. This promotes access and, except in cases where patients may receive too much treatment, likely enhances quality of care. It provides no incentive, however, for providers to act as effective agents for society as a whole, which must bear the costs of increased health care use.

Under alternative payment systems, this shared interest is changed. Where the more services provided, the less net revenue is received by the provider (Ellis and McGuire, 1986). This threatens the agency role between provider and patient, while inducing providers to take into account broader social concerns for cost control. Designing or modifying either traditional or alternative payment systems involves a balancing of incentives, so that proper agency is encouraged, that is, so that providers appropriately balance the concerns of their patients and society as a whole.

Comparing Traditional and Alternative Payment Systems

Traditionally, physicians have been paid on a fee-for-service basis and hospitals through cost-based retrospective reimbursement. The principal mechanism for controlling costs and unnecessary utilization was cost sharing by the patient. Although cost sharing is still extensively used, there is a growing perception that to eliminate unnecessary care, without hindering access to needed services, financial incentives must be shifted to the provider (Lohr et al., 1987). Under alternative systems, providers are increasingly "at risk" (i.e., financially responsible) for the costs of the medical care of their patients.

A variety of alternative systems is growing rapidly. Most striking has been the emergence of prepaid health plans, often referred to as "health maintenance organizations" (HMOs). In 1975, 178 HMOs enrolled nearly 6 million individuals; by mid-1987 this had increased to 662 plans which enrolled 28.6 million individuals, or roughly 12 percent of the U.S. population (Interstudy, 1987). Medicaid enrollment in HMOs grew from under 200,000 in 1981 to 600,000 in 1986.

The shift in hospital payment to a per case, prospective system has been equally rapid. The first public sector price-per-case system for setting hospital rates was established in Maryland in 1976. Three years later the state of New Jersey began using Diagnosis Related Groups (DRGs) as a basis for establishing preset prices for hospital care. This type of payment mechanism is now being used by the Medicare program, more than a dozen state Medicaid programs, nine Blue Cross and Blue Shield Plans, and some commercial insurers (Hellinger, 1985; Matlin, 1985).

Although alternative payment systems appear to be the wave of the future, the majority of children still receive their ambulatory care from providers who are paid under traditional systems, though the nature of these payment systems are changing too. Traditional payment systems are increasingly adding incorporate utilization control techniques, such as preadmission review, second surgical opinions, concurrent and focused review (Dobson, 1987). By the early 1980s, virtually all major health insurers and many other health management companies were offering some of these options, frequently as components of broader managed care programs (Henderson and Wallack, 1987).

It is difficult to assess adequately these alternative payment systems because many of the changes are relatively recent and have a limited track record. Although more is known about HMOs, this knowledge is based on the experience of HMOs functioning in a relatively uncompetitive environment, a situation that is rapidly changing. Some of the discussion that follows is therefore necessarily speculative.

Traditional Systems

Traditional payment arrangements differ significantly for hospitals and physicians. There are many variations on cost-based hospital reimbursement; however, the essential ingredient of this payment method is that the hospital's payments are based on its actual costs of providing services (Foster, 1982).

Fee-for-service payment for physician services, in contrast, is based on the charges of physician's practicing in a community. Under the "usual, customary and reasonable" (UCR) procedure, payment is set as the lowest of (a) the physician's "usual" or median charge for that service, (b) the "customary" charge in the community, or (c) the "reasonable" charge if a particularly complex treatment is involved.

UCR encourages charge escalation by providers attempting to ensure larger future reimbursement, and there is also no incentive to decrease charges even if the cost of new treatment technologies is lower. It encourages the performance of procedures with high overhead and rewards the introduction of new and expensive technology (Dobson, 1987). This creates large differentials in fees between specialties (Hsiao et al., 1987) and leads to inadequate reimbursement for time-consuming procedures such as those performed by primary care providers (who deliver most medical services to children) (Select Panel for the Promotion of Child Health, 1981). UCR payment is subject to physician manipulation, such as increasing the quantity and complexity of services or billing separately for services previously bundled together (Langwell and Nelson, 1986). If patients pay a share of charges, these manipulations are passed on to the family in the form of higher out-of-pocket expenses.

Because traditional payment systems compensate providers on the basis of the number of units of service provided (i.e., procedures or days of care), there is an incentive for providers to increase the quantity of services and to offer more expensive services. These systems therefore lack incentives to provide services in a cost-effective manner.

These traditional systems are often defended because they create incentives to provide the most intensive services and at the highest possible quality, to the extent that quality is related to an absence of restraint on the use of resources. But traditional payment systems, embodying a "more is better" philosophy, result in care that is biased toward hospital-based, high-technology treatment by specialists. As discussed below, this approach is probably not in the best interests of most children.

Modified Fee-for-Service Payment: Hospital and Physician Prospective Payment Systems

Existing hospital prospective payment systems set charges either per day or per admission (Hellinger, 1985; Luft, 1985a; Matlin, 1985). Although these systems vary considerably in the detailed techniques used to set rates, all establish a fixed price per unit of service and thus give hospitals an incentive to restrain costs (Hsiao et al., 1986).

Per diem payments are not as widely used as per case payment; but have been adapted by some Medicaid programs, including those in California and Illinois. Per diem payment controls the price per day, but does not contain incentives to limit the volume of hospital days.

Indeed, if prospective rates are set low, hospitals can be expected to compensate by increasing utilization to maintain their revenues. Experience in New Jersey with prospective per diem payment, prior to the introduction of DRGs, found that it is associated with increased length-of-stays (Hsiao, 1986).

The remainder of this section focuses on the incentives created by paying hospitals per case. Because the hospital is at risk for costs that exceed these payments, per case payment creates financial incentives to curtail resource use by limiting intensity and duration of stay. There is no incentive, however, to control the number of admissions. The New Jersey experience with DRGs suggests that admissions are likely to increase (Hsiao et al., 1986). In recent years, though, there has been a significant decline in hospital admissions, particularly for children (Kozak et al., 1987; NCHS, 1987). To this point, this trend has offset any incentives created for increased admissions under per case payment.

Other incentives in per case payment are perhaps more worrisome. Incentives to minimize costs will encourage practices such as selective admissions, curtailment of needed treatment or "gaming" of the reimbursement system. These would have deleterious effects on access, quality, and cost-effective care.

Selective admission practices can occur when it is possible for a provider to identify before admission patients who are likely to be "winners" (i.e., cost less than the case payment) or losers (i.e., cost more than the case payment). The practice of selecting only low-cost patients ("skimming") might make it difficult for sicker children to find hospitals willing to admit them.

There is also concern that per case payment may lead to the premature discharge of costly patients or other forms of undertreatment. Indeed, outlier policies (paying expensive cases on the basis of costs) are frequently incorporated into payment systems to mitigate the financial risk associated with treatment of particularly costly patients. Even with such provisions, however, Medicare's prospective payment system has significantly increased the risks of premature discharge of patients (Bentkover et al., 1988). Finally, per case payments can be manipulated to increase hospital revenues. While this "gaming" of the system may not have deleterious effects on patients, it lessens the ability of the system to contain costs. Gaming may take many forms, such as reclassifying the patient into a higher paying case ("DRG creep"), splitting admissions (e.g., for bilateral procedures, such as hip replacement), and unnecessary transfers to more specialized facilities (Gertman and Lowenstein, 1984).

These issues are generic to prospective hospital payment and apply across all age groups. Some particular issues are of greater concern for pediatric hospitalization.

Pediatric hospital care tends to be more labor intensive than other hospital services. Children in general require more supervision than do adults and most hospitalization occurs at birth or in infancy. Children also tend to have different diagnoses from those of adults. Some pediatric conditions are congenital, resulting in death before adulthood, while other conditions are developmental and are associated with children of different ages (Payne and Restuccia, 1987).

Children pose significant problems for systems that pay hospitals on the basis of a patient's diagnosis. For a given diagnosis, pediatric hospitalization is characterized by a large number of both short and long hospital stays, so while on average stays are shorter than for adults, the variance in length of stay is greater (Kovar, 1978). Hospitals that have a high proportion of short stays relative to other institutions would gain financially and conversely hospitals with a high proportion of long stays would lose. Chronically ill and handicapped children tend to have repeated hospitalizations, which, depending on the diagnosis, may require more care as time progresses because of worsening of the condition or may require less care as development and treatment improve the condition (Payne and Restuccia, 1987).

Pediatric hospital care may be provided in specialized tertiary centers, including free-standing and university hospitals, as well as other types of hospitals. There is evidence that these tertiary centers treat a more severe case mix than do other hospitals, thus particular care must be given to developing a payment system that does not underpay these centers (NACHRI, 1985). These specialized tertiary centers are a component of a highly regionalized and differentiated system of care. The regionalization of services such as pediatric cardiac surgery, neonatal intensive care, and pediatric intensive care requires appropriate transfers to and from tertiary centers. It is thus important for a per case payment system to encourage appropriate transfers. If the per case payment is set too high, it encourages community hospitals to retain a patient when transfer up to a tertiary center might be more appropriate. If the payment is set too low, it may encourage the community hospital to transfer children solely for financial reasons (Payne and Restuccia, 1987).

Physician prospective payment systems shift the basis on which charges are calculated either by aggregating procedures into "cases" or episodes of care, or by resetting relative prices in terms of the complexity or time intensity required for the procedure. Paying for physician services on a per case basis has been of interest to policy makers since the early 1980s (Mitchell and Cromwell, 1984). This approach would shift the financial risk to the physician because the payment is fixed regardless of the intensity or actual cost of services to an individual patient. There is therefore an incentive to restrain resource use. It should also create incentives to provide care in less expensive settings. Children's health services can be provided in several sites of service delivery: hospital, emergency room, physician's office, outpatient departments, and free-standing clinics. In theory, per case payment should shift more costly outpatient hospital care to the physician's office. The major problem with a per case payment system is the difficulty in constructing an adequate classification system to reflect the great variation found in ambulatory claims (Lion et al., 1986). The amount of risk imposed on individual physicians may be excessive if the physician does not have a large enough volume of patients for the costs of high-cost patients to be offset by lower-cost patients (Ginsburg and Hackbarth, 1986). However, physician payment systems of this sort could be made more attractive by including some form of stop-loss limitations, analogous to an outlier policy for hospital prospective systems, that can mitigate the financial risk facing the physician.

Another problem with per case payment for physician services relates to who to pay when more than one physician is involved in treating the patient (Pauly and Langwell, 1986). Payment could be made to the primary physician, the hospital medical staff, or the child's family. Payment to the primary physician would place the person who initiates the course of treatment in a position to consider the costs of treatment options, but individual physicians would have limited ability to absorb the losses from high-cost cases, and this would discourage referrals to specialists. The hospital medical staff would be better able to pool financial risk, but could have difficulty in implementing a system of sharing costs and revenues among the staff. This approach would also be infeasible for care outside the hospital. Paying the family would enable the patient to exercise greater control, but would lead to selection of appropriate sites and types of care only if the parents are well informed. Risk pooling would be limited, leaving families liable for the financial consequences of unusually expensive illnesses.

These problems raise serious questions about the feasibility of per case payment for physician services. As yet, there are no operational systems that pay for care in this manner. Other alternatives to UCR methods, however, do exist and have been proven practical. Fee schedules of various types have been used for a number of years by private insurers and about half of the state Medicaid programs (Holahan, 1984). Under a fee schedule, a dollar value is set prospectively for specific services. This either represents the maximum allowable payment or is simply paid to all physicians. A fixed fee schedule is not subject to automatic increases if physicians increase their charges over time. It is therefore less inflationary than UCR payment systems.

Relative value scales (RVS), which rank the worth of all procedures relative to some standard, are frequently used as fee schedules. The first scale was the 1956 California RVS (CRVS), which used prevailing physician charges as the basis for determining relative value and is the basis for many current Medicaid fee schedules (Holahan, 1984).

It is argued that an RVS or any other comparable mechanism that sets fees on historical experience is inherently flawed because the market for physicians' services does not generate fair relative prices. Historically, medical procedures, particularly invasive procedures, are compensated at a rate substantially higher than patient evaluation and management, often termed "cognitive services." This is due in part to the historical willingness of third-party payers to fully insure procedural services and either exclude or only partially insure cognitive services. It is further alleged that this results in higher than necessary utilization of more costly (and some argue more risky to the patient) invasive procedures as providers seek to provide the most remunerative procedures (Matlin, 1986).

Efforts are currently under way to develop an alternative RVS methodology, the Resource-Based Relative Value Scale (RBRVS), which sets physician payments based on a broad definition of the costs to deliver medical care (Hsiao et al., 1987). These include estimates of the cost of physician time, service complexity, overhead or practice costs associated with delivery of each service, service-specific physician stress, and income foregone during specialty training (opportunity costs). Through estimates of these components derived through physician technical panels, field surveys, and statistical analyses, relative production costs for medical services are being determined. Preliminary findings indicate that payment for cognitive services would significantly increase relative to payment for procedural services (Matlin, 1986). For example, under charge based reimbursement, a heart catherization is reimbursed at 20 times the rate of a standard extended office visit. Using a relative value scale based on physicians' time spent on care, the differential between the two services is only one-third as large (Juba and Hadley, 1985).

An important aspect of child health care is health promotion and disease prevention. Fee schedules that undervalue cognitive services thus particularly hurt the quality of children's care (Select Panel on Child Health, 1981). Relative value scales based on physician time would correct this, but additional financial incentives to deliver preventive care could also be added to a RVS (Hadley et al., 1984).

There is ample evidence that generosity of payment affects providers willingness to treat patients or to provide particular services (Held and Holohan, 1985; Mauskoph et al., 1985; Perloff et al., 1987). Thus, changing relative fees in an RVS payment system can be used to encourage participation of certain types of providers or settings and to influence treatment decisions.

Capitated Systems

Capitation involves the payment of a fixed, prospectively determined rate for a specified range of services for a specified period of time, usually one year. Service use is restricted to participating providers. The unit of payment is much broader than in per case reimbursement and thereby results in a system that is somewhat less intrusive into medical practice (Ginsburg and Hackbarth, 1986). Under capitation, the incentive to provide less service involves two aspects: to reduce the intensity of service and to reduce the volume of care. There is also an incentive to shift from higher cost to lower cost services, in particular to substitute less costly ambulatory care for hospital care. Evidence suggests that HMOs are capable of making this substitution for enrollees of all ages (Luft, 1981).

Physician remuneration methods affect the size of cost savings. Physicians within capitated systems who are remunerated on a capitated basis have the strongest incentive to minimize costs (Welch, 1987), with physicians paid on a fee-for-service basis facing the weakest incentive for cost minimization. As of 1986, approximately 40 percent of all HMOs capitated their primary care physicians (Hillman, 1987).

When the provider is placed at financial risk there is an incentive not only to provide fewer services in the least costly manner but also to seek healthier enrollees. Many HMOs are aggressively marketing to healthy clients (Luft, 1985b). Although this selection should not adversely affect patients, it may actually increase the costs of health care for employees and public insurance programs. HMOs are generally paid based on the expected cost of an average beneficiary. If they only enroll the healthy, who would otherwise have spent little on health care, overall health care spending will increase (Schlesinger and Drumheller, 1988).

As with per case payment, there is concern that the financial incentives of capitated payment can result in reduced quality of care either through underutilization or inadequate referral to pediatric specialists and specialized pediatric hospitals. Capitated delivery systems may not have a large enough population of enrollees to justify the inclusion of both a specialist and a pediatric specialist within a particular field, thus the special competence required for children may not be available. The capability of serving children with special or unusual needs may be inadequate. Out-of-plan specialty care, including that in pediatric hospitals, may occur inappropriately late or not at all (Budetti, 1984).

Adapting Payment Systems for Children's Health Needs

The ultimate goal of a payment system is to obtain appropriate access to high-quality health care at the lowest possible cost in a manner that is fair to providers. This section focuses on how both traditional and alternative payment systems might be adapted to better achieve this goal for children. The incentives in both traditional and alternative payment systems can be structured to encourage providers to deliver desirable amounts and kinds of services, as well as ensuring that certain groups of children are not consistently viewed as financial "losers." The options discussed are not meant to be all inclusive and may be most effective if implemented in combination with one another.

Traditional Systems

Case management. Increasingly, traditional insurance systems are becoming more "managed," with an emphasis on control of hospital services. To limit "unnecessary" hospital stays, insurers are requiring: (1) mandatory second (and encouraging voluntary third) opinions for surgery, (2) prior authorization for certain types of hospital care, and (3) concurrent and retrospective utilization review (Dobson, 1987). Even though the main thrust of the "managed" approach has been to control utilization and expenditures, because it monitors treatment, it also has the potential to improve quality.

Catastrophic case management (or care coordination) is a type of managed care that is targeted to the small number of individuals who consume a large share of resources (Henderson and Wallack, 1987). These high-cost patients typically have experienced a major illness (e.g., low birth weight babies in need of neonatal intensive care; auto accident victims in need of high-cost inpatient care such as burn units); or patients who suffer from long-term chronic conditions (e.g., spina bifida). Although catastrophic case management programs contain mechanisms for limiting resource use, in theory their main objective is to mobilize and coordinate appropriate resources, which may not always be lower in cost. This may involve finding alternative settings and providers, arranging for the coverage of alternative services not offered under the patient's insurance plan, and facilitating communication among involved parties (Henderson and Wallack, 1987).

Case management also has potential for rationalizing the delivery of noncatastrophic care, but perhaps with less likelihood of cost savings. A demonstration to test the effects of case management on utilization and expenditures for Medicaid eligible children in Suffolk County, New York, was conducted between 1983 and 1985. Utilization of primary care was greater for the two types of case managed groups, compared with the regular Medicaid control group. The case-managed fee-for-service group had more primary care and an equal amount of subspecialty care as did the Medicaid enrollees while the case-managed capitated group had an equal amount of primary care and less subspecialty care. The conclusion was that offering a "medical home" (and guaranteed Medicaid eligibility for a minimum of one year) was desirable, though not cost reducing. Recipient utilization under the case-managed systems fit more closely the American Academy of Pediatrics' standards for preventive care (AAP, 1988).

Hybrid arrangements—PPOs. Preferred provider organizations (PPOs) are essentially a fee-for-service system with discounts. They contract with selected providers, hospitals and/or physicians, who agree to provide services at a discount. By minimizing patient cost sharing for these "preferred" providers, patients are encouraged to use these providers and costs will thereby be constrained (Luft, 1985a).

PPOs combine some of the limitations on choice of provider found in capitated systems with the fee-for-service payment mechanism. Most make extensive use of the utilization control mechanisms discussed above and in effect are a "managed" system. Thus although there is an incentive for the provider to increase the quantity of services while still providing them at the negotiated discount rate, the utilization controls curb this tendency. Patients have a limited choice of providers, which may compromise geographic access, but have the option to pursue out-of-plan treatment if they are willing to pay increased cost sharing (Gabel et al., 1986). These arrangements may discourage use of and referrals to higher-cost specialty providers and pediatric hospitals.

Because PPOs retain the essential ingredients of fee-for-service payment, they are less risky financially for the provider than prospective and capitated systems. PPOs can increase financial access to health care because there are minimal or no cost sharing provisions if "preferred providers" are used. This aspect can be particularly important for children whose health care needs requires a strong ambulatory orientation.

One apparent advantage to children insured by PPOs is full coverage of preventive care in most benefit plans. Approximately three-fourths of PPOs cover well-baby care and immunizations for infants during the first two years of life, and more than half insure well-child care into adulthood. The standard coverage of well-baby care during the first two years is particularly important since this period offers the greatest potential lifelong health benefits to children. Prenatal care is covered by 85 percent of PPOs (Logsdon et al., 1987). It is unclear, at this point, whether broader coverage is the result of cost savings produced by other aspects of the PPO, or coincidental, since PPOs have been most often adapted by large employers who already had generous health benefits.

Prospective Payment Systems

Change outlier policy. When Medicare adapted its hospital prospective payment system (which pays hospitals by the case based on the patient's diagnosis) children's specialty hospitals were explicitly exempted, out of a belief that the high variance in costs for children's' care within each diagnosis made this system inappropriate. As states and private insurers have adapted similar payment systems, however, much of children's hospital treatment has come to be paid on a per case basis. Methods must therefore be found to adapt this system to children's more variable costs.

Most per case hospital payment systems include some provision for exceptionally costly cases, often called "outliers." For these cases, an additional reimbursement is provided beyond the standard payment. The threshold at which a case becomes an outlier is an important determinant of the financial risk faced by the hospital. Modifying the outlier policy, by lowering the threshold or by paying for a higher proportion of costs beyond the threshold, is one way of reducing the risk that potentially high-cost children will have problems getting access to care or will be prematurely discharged. It should also provide greater equity for specialized tertiary children's hospitals, which treat a disproportionate number of high-cost pediatric cases.

Pediatric hospitalization is also characterized by a large number of short hospital stays. To keep the system cost-effective, it would be desirable to institute an outlier policy for particularly short lengths of stay to prevent windfall profits to hospitals treating these children. The savings could be used to finance more generous high-cost outlier provisions.

For similar reasons, a system that pays physicians by the case should also incorporate a fairly generous outlier policy. The greater number of physicians treating children—10 times as many as the number of hospitals—would, though, make such a system administratively complex. In fact, the burdens of administering outliers represents one of the most compelling arguments against adapting a per-case payment system for physician services.

All payers system for hospital care. Having all payers pay the same amount for the same service is intuitively appealing because it encourages more equitable treatment of patients. It also reduces the complexity and administrative difficulty for both providers and government regulations. In addition, all payer systems have also been successfully used to deal with the problem of uncompensated hospital care, i.e., hospital bad debt and charity care. By incorporating an adjustment into provider's rates to pay for care of the uninsured, bad debts are automatically reimbursed and shared among all payers in the state (Hsiao et al., 1986). This has particular relevance for children because some of the leading conditions associated with uncompensated care relate to pregnancy and neonatal morbidity (Singer et al., 1985).

Whether this indirect means of paying for the uninsured is the best way of dealing with the problem remains a matter of considerable debate. More direct approaches, such as the provision of public insurance for uninsured poor individuals by expansion of Medicaid or a program of national health insurance, are probably preferable but may not be politically feasible. On the other hand, no state has adopted an all-payers system since the early 1980s. To some extent, rate regulation under all-payers arrangements seems antithetical to the trend toward greater competition among providers, a trend often encouraged by policy makers. However, because both public and private insurers are increasingly paying hospitals based on patients' diagnosis, this common approach may facilitate future development of all-payers systems, particularly if interest in competition wanes.

Refine patient classification systems. Pediatric hospitalization differs from adult hospitalization in many respects. The classification system used to define the group into which a case falls can be adapted to reflect some of these differences. In particular refinements by age, diagnosis and procedure or treatment may result in a classification system which is a better predictor of resource use (Payne and Restuccia, 1987). Efforts are under way to adapt the DRG classification system for children's hospitalization along these lines (NACHRI, 1985).

One way to refine per case reimbursement is to better distinguish between acute and chronic care. Children who have multiple admissions for the same disease comprise a substantial proportion of pediatric hospitalizations (Zook et al., 1980). Appropriate treatment may change over time. Depending on the diagnosis, costs for care may decline because the patient outgrows the condition or costs may increase as the patient requires more intensive treatment (Payne and Restuccia, 1987). Per case hospital payment probably works best for the payment of single case episodes of acute care. Consideration should be given to reimbursing separately for the care of chronically ill or handicapped children (Payne and Restuccia, 1987).

Even with improvements in the classification system, the major concern related to per case payment remains: the incentives to minimize cost may result in various forms of undertreatment. Strong utilization review mechanisms external to the hospital should be implemented to ensure that adequate standards of quality are maintained.

Mixed system reimbursement. Ellis and McGuire (1986) suggested that a mixed system that combines cost-based and prospective reimbursement would mitigate the incentive to undersupply services inherent in prospective payment alone, as well as curb the incentive under cost-based reimbursement alone to oversupply services. A mixed system may have other advantages as well. Since the gain or loss per case is less under a mixed system, then the incentive to selectively admit profitable patients is moderated. A mixed system also narrows the differences in the prospective payment amount among categories, which reduces the incentive to game the system. Finally, a mixed system diminishes the financial risk faced by the hospital since part of the payment is based on the hospital's actual costs. It also lessens the need to strive for increased efficiency for these very same reasons.

These advantages come with liabilities. Partially paying for care based on costs reduces incentives for efficiency. It places more complex demands on those who administer the system—they must manage both a prospective payment system and determine what costs are reimbursable under the cost-based system. Whether these disadvantages outweigh the advantages cited above is unclear.

Capitated Systems

Chronically ill and handicapped children have average costs that are more than twice as great as those of nondisabled children (Fox et al., 1987). The incentive to minimize costs inherent in a capitated system may have particularly deleterious effects on these children to the extent that necessary services are underprovided (see Chapter 8). Establishing a higher capitation rate for chronically ill patients would increase the willingness of plans to enroll these children but not necessarily reduce the risk of inadequate care.

Others argue that developing a higher capitation rate for chronically ill children is poor public policy for two reasons. First, movement toward an individual experience-rated premium, whether for a capitated plan or traditional indemnity coverage, does violence to the socially desirable goal of health care risk sharing. If higher costs were financed through individual premiums, insurance would be beyond the financial means of families with the sickest children.

There are also questions about the quality of care received by high-cost children once enrolled in a plan. In theory, the incentives in a capitated system for continuity of care could particularly benefit the chronically ill or handicapped child. However, given the self-contained nature of capitated systems, consideration needs to be given to the possibility that the comprehensive needs of these children will not be provided within the plan. Supplemental payments could be used to support outside referral; however, if the bulk of treatment is provided externally, then the advantages of coordination of care inherent in a self-contained system are lost.

Summary and Recommendations

Changing from a traditional payment system to an alternative system that contains stronger incentives for provider efficiency does not by itself imply that children will be either more or less well off. It does, however, require that payment systems be designed recognizing the special needs of pediatric patients and the providers serving them. Both traditional and alternative systems can be better structured toward these ends, but all will require additional reform to do this.

To date the overwhelming preoccupation with payment system changes has been with their ability to contain costs. Attention should also focus on other aspects of adequate health care: access, quality, and health outcomes. Particular emphasis needs to be placed on quality, since it is more easily compromised under these alternative payment systems in which the provider is at financial risk for costs incurred in excess of a preestablished rate. In particular, payment systems should be modified to reduce undue financial risk to providers, restoring incentives for providers to act as reliable agents on behalf of their patients.

Most children are likely to fare quite well under the alternative payment systems which we have discussed, largely because most children are healthy with occasional acute health care needs. In particular, capitated systems seem desirable because they provide comprehensive ambulatory services, including preventive care, with minimal cost sharing and reduced the fragmentation of services. However, the desirability of capitated systems relates more to the payment mechanism than to organizational issues, because capitated systems typically cover comprehensive coverage ambulatory care.

New payment systems can be designed to enhance children's health in ways previously impossible. Recent evidence indicates that more generous coverage of preventive services and reduced cost sharing only slightly increase their use, and that preventive care remains below desirable levels (Lurie et al., 1987). Thus, patient incentives are not enough to ensure that children use preventive care adequately (McPhee and Schroeder, 1987). Incentives targeted to providers might prove more efficacious.

Payment systems must be structured to maintain adequate specialty care. If pediatric subspecialists or children's inpatient units are seen as an unnecessary level of care and referrals are stopped or slowed to the point where this care becomes economically unsustainable, the provision of specialized pediatric medical care will be jeopardized. Some children will require the sophisticated care provided in the specialty setting.

Given that all the alternative systems contain incentives to minimize the amount of care provided to varying degrees, special attention must be given to groups of children who are likely to be high-cost users. These include poor children, newborns, chronically ill, and the physically or mentally handicapped. The challenge of these alternative systems is to retain cost-minimizing incentives, while including incentives that assure that adequate access, continuity, and quality are not compromised, especially for these vulnerable groups.

References

Aaron, H. 1984. Prospective Payment: The Next Disappointment? *Health Affairs* 3:102–107.
American Academy of Pediatrics. 1988. *Children's Medicaid Program—Executive Summary*. Elk Grove Village, Ill.
American Association of Preferred Provider Organizations. 1987. *Directory of Operational PPOs*, 4th ed. Chicago.
American Hospital Association. 1986. *Cost and Compassion: Recommendations for Avoiding a Crisis in Care for the Medically Indigent*. Chicago.
Austin, G. 1984. Child Health-Care Financing and Competition. *New England Journal of Medicine* 311:1117–1120.
Austin, G. 1985. Consistent Care Leads to Payoff. *Business and Health* 2:10–14.
Brown, L. 1981. Competition and Health Cost Containment: Cautions and Conjectures. *Milbank Memorial Fund Quarterly* 59:145–189.
Bentkover, J., P. Caper, M. Schlesinger, and J. Suldan. 1988. Medicare's Payment of Hospital. In D. Blumenthal, M. Schlesinger, and P. Brown Drumheller (eds.), *Renewing the Promise: Medicare and Its Reform*, pp. 90–114. New York: Oxford University Press.
Budetti, P. (ed). 1984. *Capitation and Child Health Care*. Conference Proceedings, Institute for Health Policy Studies, University of California, San Francisco.
Butler, J. 1977. Financing Children's Health Care. In D. Mundel (ed.), *Developing a Better Health Care System for Children*, pp. 99–134. Cambridge, Mass.: Ballinger.
Butler, J., S. Rosenbaum, and J. Palfrey. 1987. Ensuring Access to Health Care for Children with Disabilities. *New England Journal of Medicine* 317:162–165.
Chafee, J. 1985. Ensuring the Health of Children. *Business and Health* 2:5–9.
Children's Medicaid Program (Brochure—undated), Suffolk County, Hauppauge, N.Y.
Cohen, J. 1986. Risk Pools for Chronically Ill Children. *Child Health Financing Report* 3:4. Elk Grove Village, Ill.: American Academy of Pediatrics.
Dobson, A. 1987. Physician Payment Reform: Prospects for the Future. *Business and Health* July:7–12.
Dutton, D. 1978. Explaining the Low Use of Health Services by the Poor: Costs, Attitudes, or Delivery Systems? *American Sociological Review* 43:348–368.
Egdahl, R., and C. Taft. 1986. Financial Incentives to Physicians. *New England Journal of Medicine* 315:59–61.

Ellis, R., and T. McGuire. 1986. Hospital Behavior under Prospective Reimbursement: Cost Sharing and Supply. *Journal of Health Economics* 5(2):129–151.
Ellwood, P., and B. Paul. 1986. But What about Quality? *Health Affairs* 5:135–140.
Flint, S. 1987. House Passes Medicaid Improvements. *Child Health Financing Report* 1:1.
Foltz, A. 1981. The Organization and Financing of Child Health Services: Options for Policy. In *Better Health for Our Children: A National Strategy*. Vol. 4, *Select Panel for the Promotion of Child Health*. DHHS Publication No. 79-55071. Washington, D.C.: G.P.O.
Foster, R. 1982. Cost-Based Reimbursement and Prospective Payment: Reassessing the Incentives. *Journal of Health Politics, Policy and Law* 7:407–420.
Fox, H., L. Neiswander, R. Yoshpe, and M. Anderson. 1987. Briefing Memoranda for Meeting on the Feasibility of High-Risk Pools to Provide Health Insurance Protection for Children with Special Health Needs. Mimeograph. Presented in Washington, D.C., December 14–15 at meeting sponsored by the American Academy of Pediatrics, Bureau of Maternal and Child Health, March of Dimes, and the National Association of Insurance Commissioners.
Frech, H. 1988. Introduction. In H. Frech (ed.), *Health Care in America: The Political Economy of Hospitals and Health Insurance*. San Francisco: Pacific Research Institute for Public Policy.
———. 1988. Preferred Provider Organizations and Health Care Competition. In H. Frech (ed.), *Health Care in America: The Political Economy of Hospitals and Health Insurance*. San Francisco: Pacific Research Institute for Public Policy.
Fuchs, V. 1985. *Paying the Piper, Calling the Tune: Implications of Changes in Reimbursement*. Working Paper No. 1605. Cambridge, Mass.: National Bureau of Economic Research.
Gabel, J., and M. Redisch. 1979. Alternative Payment Methods: Incentives, Efficiency, and National Health Insurance. *Milbank Memorial Fund Quarterly* 57:38–59.
Gabel, J., D. Ermann, T. Rice, and G. de Lissovoy. 1986. The Emergence and Future of Preferred Provider Organizations. *Journal of Health Politics, Policy, and Law* 11(2):305–322.
Gabel, J., and T. Rice. 1985. Reducing Public Expenditures for Physician Services: The Price of Paying Less. *Journal of Health Politics, Policy, and Law* 9:595–609.
Ginsburg, E., and M. Ostow. 1985. Organization and Financing of Medical Care: Resources. *Medical Care* 23:421–431.
Ginsburg, P., and G. Hackbarth. 1986. Alternative Delivery Systems and Medicare. *Health Affairs* 5:6–22.
Goldsmith, J. 1984. Death of a Paradigm: The Challenge of Competition. *Health Affairs* 3(3):5–19.
Hadley, J. 1979. Physician Participation in Medicaid: Evidence from California. *Health Services Research* 14:266–280.
Hadley, J., D. Juba, R. Berenson, and M. Sulvetta. 1984. *Final Report on Alternative Methods of Developing a Relative Value Scale of Physicians' Services*. Report to the Health Care Financing Administration. Washington, D.C.: Urban Institute.
Haggerty, R. 1985. Commentaries—The Rand Health Insurance Experiment for Children. *Pediatrics* 75:969–971.
Held, P., and J. Holohan. 1985. Containing Medicaid Costs in an Era of Growing Physician Supply. *Health Care Financing Review* 7:49–60.
Hellinger, F. 1985. Recent Evidence on Case-Based Systems for Setting Hospital Rates. *Inquiry* 22:78–91.
Henderson, M., and S. Wallack. 1987. Evaluating Case Management for Catastrophic Illness. *Business and Health* January:7–11.

Hillman, A. 1987. Financial Incentives for Physicians in HMOs. *New England Journal of Medicine* 317(27):1743–1748.
Holahan, J. 1984. Paying for Physician Services in State Medicaid Programs. *Health Care Financing Review* 5:99–110.
Horgan, C. 1985. *Prospective Payment and Psychiatric Care: Evidence from Research.* Waltham, Mass.: Bigel Institute for Health Policy, Brandeis University.
Hornbrook, M., and S. Berki. 1985. Practice Mode and Payment Method: Effects on Use, Costs, Quality, and Access. *Medical Care* 23:484–511.
Hsiao, W., P. Braun, E. Becker, and S. Thomas. 1987. The Resource-Based Relative Value Scale—Toward the Development of an Alternative Physician Payment System. *Journal of the American Medical Association* 258:799–802.
Hsiao, W., H. Sapolsky, D. Dunn, and S. Weiner. 1986. Lessons of the New Jersey DRG Payment System. *Health Affairs* 5:32–45.
Hsiao, W., and W. Stason. 1979. Toward Developing a Relative Value Scale for Medical and Surgical Procedures. *Health Care Financing Review* 1:23–27.
Hulka, B., and J. Wheat. 1985. Patterns of Utilization: The Patient Perspective. *Medical Care* 23:438–460.
Interstudy Edge, Fall 1987.
Juba, D., and J. Hadley. 1985. Relative Value Scales for Physicians' Services. *Health Care Financing Review* 6(4):93–102.
Kovar, M.G. 1978. Children and Youth: Health Status and Use of Health Services. *Health United States: 1978*. Washington, D.C.: DHEW, PHS.
Kozak, L., C. Norton, M. McManus, and E. McCarthy. 1987. Hospital Use Patterns for Children in the United States, 1983 and 1984. *Pediatrics* 80:481–490.
Langwell, K., and L. Nelson. 1986. Physician Payment Systems: A Review of History, Alternatives and Evidence. *Medical Care Review* 43:5–58.
Lion, J., M. Henderson, A. Bergman, and A. Malbon. 1986. The Second Generation of Ambulatory Visit Groups: How They Perform in a Hospital Based Specialty. Waltham, Mass.: Bigel Institute for Health Policy, Brandeis University.
Logsdon, D., M. Rosen, S. Thaddeus, and C. Lazaro. 1987. Coverage of Preventive Services by Preferred Provider Organizations. *Journal of Ambulatory Care Management* 10(2):25–35.
Lohr, K., R. Brook, C. Kamberg, et al. 1986. Use of Medical Care in the Rand Health Insurance Experiment. *Medical Care* 24 (Supplement).
Long, M., J. Dreachslin, and J. Fisher. 1986. Should Children's Hospitals Have Special Consideration in Reimbursement Policy? *Health Care Financing Review* 8:55–63.
Luft, H. 1981. *Health Maintenance Organizations: Dimensions of Performance.* New York: John Wiley and Sons.
———. 1985a. Competition and Regulation. *Medical Care* 23:383–400.
———. 1985b. HMOs: Friends or Foes? *Business and Health* December: 5–9.
Lurie, N., W. Manning, C. Peterson, G. Goldberg, C. Phelps, and L. Lillard. 1987. Preventive Care: Do We Practice What We Preach? *American Journal of Public Health* 77:801–804.
McGuire, T., C. Horgan, H. Goldman, and L. Saxe. 1985. Options for Including Psychiatric Hospitals and Exempt Units Under the Medicare Prospective Payment System. Working paper. Brandeis University.
McPhee, S., and S. Schroeder. 1987. Promoting Preventive Care: Changing Reimbursement Is Not Enough. *American Journal of Public Health* 77:780–781.
Matlin, N. 1985. Non-Medicare Insurers Moving to DRGs. *Child Health Financing Report* 2:3.
———. 1986. Pediatrics To Be Included in Harvard RVS Study. *Child Health Financing Report* 4:1.

Mechanic, D. 1985. Cost Containment and the Quality of Medical Care: Rationing Strategies in an Era of Constrained Resources. *Milbank Memorial Fund Quarterly* 63:453–475.

Mitchell, J. 1986. The Economic Motivation of Capitation. *Massachusetts Medicine* July/August: 46–48.

National Association of Children's Hospital and Related Institutions (NACHRI). 1985. Children's Hospital Case Mix Classification System Project, Phase I Report: Critique of DRGs Across Hospital Settings. March. Alexandria, Va.

———. 1985. Children's Hospital Case Mix Classification System Project, Phase II Report: Children's Diagnosis Related Groups. December. Alexandria, Va.

National Center for Health Statistics. 1987. 1986 Summary: National Hospital Discharge Survey. *Advance Data* 145. September 30.

Pauly, M. 1970. Efficiency, Incentives and Reimbursement for Health Care. *Inquiry* 7:114–131.

Pauly, M., and K. Langwell. 1986. Physician Payment Reform: Who Shall Be Paid? *Medical Care Review* 43:101–132.

Payne, S., and J. Restuccia. 1987. Policy Issues Related to Prospective Payment for Pediatric Hospitalization. *Health Care Financing Review* 9:71–81.

Perloff, J., P. Kletke, and K. Neckerman. 1987. *Medicaid and Pediatric Primary Care*. Baltimore: Johns Hopkins University Press.

Pratt, J., and R. Zeckhauser. 1985. Principals and Agents: An Overview. In J. Pratt and R. Zeckhauser (eds.), *Principals and Agents: The Structure of Business*, pp. 1–36. Boston: Harvard Business School Press.

Roper, W. 1987. Prescription for America's 'Morning After' Headache. *Health Week* December 23, p. 18.

Rymer, M., and G. Adler. 1987. Children and Medicaid: The Experience in Four States. *Health Care Financing Review* 9:1–20.

Schlesinger, M. 1986. On the Limits of Expanding Health Care Reform: Chronic Care in Prepaid Settings. *Milbank Memorial Fund Quarterly* 64(2):189–215.

Schlesinger, M., and P. Brown Drumheller, 1988. Medicare and Innovative Insurance Plans. In D. Blumenthal, M. Schlesinger, and P. Brown Drumheller (eds.), *Renewing the Promise: Medicare and Its Reform*, pp. 133–159. New York: Oxford University Press.

Schorr, L. 1983. Background and Highlights on the Report of the Select Panel. In R. Haskins (ed.), *Child Health Policy in an Age of Fiscal Austerity*. Norwood: ABLEX Publishing Corporation.

Select Panel for the Promotion of Child Health. 1981. *Better Health for Our Children: A National Strategy*. Report to DHHS Publication No. 77-55071. Washington, D.C.: G.P.O.

Showstack, J., B. Blumberg, J. Schwartz, and S. Schroeder. 1979. Fee-for-Service Physician Payment: Analysis of Current Methods and Their Development. *Inquiry* 16:230–246.

Steinwachs, D., J. Weiner, S. Shapiro, P. Batalden, K. Coltin, and F. Wasserman. 1986. A Comparison of the Requirements for Primary Care Physicians in HMOs with Projections Made by GMENAC. *New England Journal of Medicine* 314:217–222.

Valdez, R., R. Brook, W. Rogers, J. Ware, E. Keeler, C. Sherbourne, K. Lohr, G. Goldberg, P. Camp, and J. Newhouse. 1985. Consequences of Cost-Sharing for Children's Health. *Pediatrics* 75:952–968.

Vladeck, B. 1985. Reforming Medicare Provider Payment. *Journal of Health Politics, Policy, and Law* 10(3):513–531.

Welch, W.P. 1987. The New Structure of Independent Practice Associations. *Journal of Health Politics, Policy and Law* 12(4):723–740.

Wennberg, J. 1984. Dealing with Medical Practice Variations: A Proposal for Action. *Health Affairs* 3(2):6–32.

Wilensky, G., and L. Rossiter. 1986. Alternative Units of Payment for Physician Services: An Overview of the Issues. *Medical Care Review* 43:133–156.

Wyszewianski, L., J. Wheeler, and A. Donabedian. 1982. Market-Oriented Cost-Containment Strategies and Quality of Care. *Milbank Memorial Fund Quarterly* 60:518–550.

Zelten, R. 1981. Provider Reimbursement Alternatives and the Placement of Financial Risk: A Framework for Analysis. *Topics in Health Care Financing* 8:61–72.

Zook, C., S. Savickis, and F. Moore. 1980. Repeated Hospitalization for the Same Disease: A Multiplier of National Health Costs. *Milbank Memorial Fund Quarterly/Health and Society* 58:454–471.

III

Changes in the Organization of Service Providers and Their Effects on Children's Health Care

8

Private Medical Providers and Children's Health Care

Mark J. Schlesinger, Ph.D.

American medical care is rapidly changing. Physicians are joining organized systems of care, many with formal ties to hospitals and other institutions. Institutions themselves are becoming linked in multifacility systems. These emerging organizational forms compete with each other and with more traditional providers to attract increasingly price-conscious purchasers of services.

Many within the children's health care community welcome such changes, seeing in them opportunities for improving the delivery of services. Others simply acquiesce, believing change to be an unavoidable consequence of profligate spending on health care over the past two decades. But whether these changes are helpful or harmful to children is likely to have little effect on their spread.

Children who are most likely to be adversely affected by changes are in large measure those from low-income households. Less frequently insured, and without the financial resources to purchase medical care if not insured, these families have always been economically disenfranchised, with their concerns and needs being reflected only as an afterthought by most private providers. As will be discussed in this chapter, as medical providers have recently become more sensitive to large purchasers of care, they are now less responsive to the needs of the uninsured.

In addition, recent years have seen a growing "privatization" of health benefits. Increasingly, how and what health services are paid for has become a choice of private employers rather than of governmental officials. The extent to which health needs are met thus depends on successfully presenting those needs to corporate health benefits managers and within labor-management negotiations over fringe benefits. But no formal institutions, nor informal social compacts, exist to ensure that children's interests are effectively represented in these forums. Past experience suggests that all too frequently they will not be (Austin, 1984).

Although continuing change in the U.S. health care system seems inevitable, the consequences for children are not. It may be possible to insulate providers of children's health care from some of these ongoing trends. Alternatively, provider behavior can be adapted to better match children's health needs. For children who cannot be buffered from changes in these ways, we can develop compensatory policies to ensure that their health is protected.

Policies of these types must be carefully crafted. The emerging picture for children is complicated. Children will be affected differently by some ongoing changes than are their parents. The same institutional changes that may benefit some groups of children will work to the disadvantage of others. Public policy in this area must reflect these nuances. Because it is unrealistic to expect that an ongoing transformation of American medicine will be halted simply because it threatens the well-being of some children, remedial policies must also be compatible with existing trends within the health care system. The goal of this chapter is to identify policy responses to the changing market for private medical services that meet these criteria.

The Changing Organization of American Medicine and the Consequences for Children's Health Care

Organizational changes can alter the delivery of medical care in numerous ways, with varied consequences. In this chapter, the discussion will focus on the implications for the quality and accessibility of children's health care.[1] Accessibility is defined here in terms of three dimensions: *geographic,* based on the time necessary to obtain needed services, *financial,* based on the costs borne by the child's family in obtaining care, and *discretionary,* involving the willingness of providers to treat particular children. Three aspects of quality are also discussed: continuity of care, adequacy of treatment, and appropriate matching of needs to services.

Organizational changes will affect the accessibility and quality of care to varying degrees and in different ways for children with different needs and resources. For simplicity, the discussion that follows will be cast in terms of two conceptually useful stereotypes: "average" children and "high-risk" children. The latter are defined here as children with chronic illness or living in low-income families. These are often one and the same, since "children from disadvantaged backgrounds—lower-income (under $5000) and father-absent families—are between three and four times more likely to have limitations in their activity due to chronic conditions than children from more advantaged families" (Mundel, 1977, p. 11).

In this section we will explore the consequences for the adequacy and accessibility of care for these children caused by three significant trends in the organization of private medical providers: the growth of integrated ambulatory care (group practices and HMOs), the expansion of multifacility health care corporations, and the increase in price-based competition among private providers.

Integrated Ambulatory Practices

Children receive most of their health care in a physician's office (Starfield, 1980). Even for those from poor and near-poor households, the majority have a private physician as their regular source of care (Rosenbach, 1985). Consequently, changes in the structure of office practice can significantly affect services by altering the opportunities and incentives facing physicians. Over the past decade, several trends in practice arrangements have combined to increase the extent to which physicians' practices are integrated with one another, both physically and financially.

The decline of solo practice among U.S. physicians. Since World War II there has been a steady decrease in the proportion of physicians in independent, "solo" practice. Between 1950 and 1975, the number of physicians in group practice increased fivefold (Sorkin, 1977). In the late 1940s, 80 percent of pediatricians involved in direct patient care were in solo practice; by the early 1970s, this had declined to 45 percent (Starfield, 1980). Over the past decade, this trend has continued, particularly for pediatricians (Roghmann et al., 1984). According to surveys conducted by the American Medical Association (AMA), the proportion of all physicians in solo practice declined from 51 to 43 percent. The proportion of pediatricians in solo practice fell to 35 percent.[2] Pediatricians were especially likely to practice in small group settings (Wolinsky, 1982).

The continued shift into groups has been accompanied by two more recent, but equally important changes in physicians' practice arrangements. The first is the growth of prepaid group practices (PGPs). In these plans, providers are paid in advance for a year's worth of care. In 1974, 5 percent of all physicians, and 10 percent of those in group practice, were affiliated with prepaid plans (Feldstein, 1979; Reynold and Abram, 1983). By 1984, according to AMA surveys, more than 20 percent of all physicians cared for at least some patients through a prepaid group.[3] Again, this change has been even more pronounced among pediatricians. In 1984, more than 25 percent were affiliated with a prepaid group plan.

The second recent change in the organization of ambulatory practice has been the growth of independent practice associations (IPAs). The association is paid in advance to deliver care, but physicians remain in their individual offices and may be either paid on a fee-for-service basis, given an individual capitation payment, or reimbursed through a variety of other methods (Luft, 1981; Hillman, 1987). Virtually nonexistent 10 years ago, these have become the fastest growing form of prepaid plan. By mid-1987, half of all enrollees in prepaid plans were members of IPAs (Welch, 1987).

Physicians have thus increasingly become part of organized ambulatory practices. If current trends persist, by the mid-1990s there will be relatively few physicians in truly independent practice—one-third will be affiliated with prepaid groups, slightly more with independent practice associations, and perhaps another 15 percent members of fee-for-service groups. Solo practitioners, practicing under fee-for-service arrangements, will have become a disappearing breed. Though not all, indeed probably not even a majority, of patients will be cared for under prepaid arrangements, the vast majority of practitioners will to at least some extent operate under prepaid contracts.

The consequences of practice integration for children's health care. Although the solo practitioner has been romanticized in popular folklore and media, the integration of practice arrangements probably holds more promise than pitfalls for the average child's health care. Where there are problems, they are for particular groups of children whose health care needs are less compatible with the incentives created in various group settings. Integrated practices are thought to improve children's medical care in several ways. Group practices can more readily adopt various forms of utilization and peer review (Weber, 1975; Butler, 1977). In addition, integration creates linkages between primary care physicians and specialists that may facilitate continuity of care. This would be valuable for all children, but particularly for high-risk children (Starfield, 1980).

The evidence on the actual gains in continuity that occurs in practice is somewhat mixed. Compared to those treated by solo practitioners, patients treated in group practices have somewhat more continuity for serious illness (Richardson et al., 1976), but more so in fee-for-service groups than in prepaid plans (Scitovsky et al., 1979; Roghmann et al., 1984). These improvements, moreover, are somewhat deceptive, since they involve greater continuity with the overall group of providers but less with an individual physician (Mott et al., 1973; Roghmann et al., 1984). Some observers believe that the loss of individual continuity more than offsets the benefits of continuity with the group, leading to lower quality care for children (Austin, 1985).

Evidence comparing health outcomes of children in group and solo practices, however, more consistently and conclusively favors groups. Studies have found that outcomes of care for children (and at least in some cases pregnant women) are generally better in both fee-for-service and prepaid groups than in solo practices (Dutton and Silber, 1980; Osborn and Woolley, 1981; Wilner et al., 1981).

Whether prepayment enhances the benefits of group practice is less clear. It has been asserted that for children "the care provided, both preventive and corrective, is of generally higher quality in prepaid group practices than in other organizational arrangements" (Starfield, 1980, p. 75). Studies of prepaid groups (often termed health maintenance organizations or HMOs) found that enrolled children received more regular checkups, hearing tests, and eye exams than did comparable children in fee-for-service settings (Butler, 1977; Dutton, 1978; Ross and Duff, 1982), largely because HMOs offered care with minimal copayments (Luft, 1981). These findings were thought to be persuasive enough that in 1981 the Select Panel for the Promotion of Child Health specifically advocated enrolling low-income families in prepaid plans to improve access to services for their children. "The Panel recognizes that for the near future in most areas of the country, HMO's will not be the dominant mode of service delivery. But the promise of this service delivery mode at its best is substantial. . . . Where prepaid systems for providing cost effective comprehensive care to mothers and children are already in operation, such systems should be encouraged to add low-income families" (Select Panel, 1981, p. 242).

Not all the consequences of prepayment will necessarily be positive. Budgetary pressures in prepaid plans can encourage shorter contact between physician and patient. AMA data indicate that the average pediatrics or obstetrics visit is up to 50 percent shorter in prepaid groups than in a fee-for-service individual practice (Wolinsky and Marder, 1985). For patients with complex illnesses, this reduced contact may threaten quality of care.

The evidence on health outcomes for children in prepaid care is mixed. Studies indicate that enrollees in prepaid groups had better outcomes in some aspects of care, but that children in fee-for-service groups did better by other measures (Dutton and Silber, 1980; Luft, 1981). Both adults and children seem to be generally more satisfied with the care in fee-for-service groups and independent practices than in HMOs (Dutton and Silber, 1980; Luft, 1981; Ross, Mirowsky and Duff, 1982). In large part this is due to more limited contact between patient and physician (Mechanic, 1975).

Whatever the implications for the average child, prepayment portends some problems for high-risk children. Chronically ill children, for example, are not likely to fare well under prepaid care. An HMO has a financial incentive to treat illnesses to prevent future costs for the plan. Much of the costs of chronic illness, however, are borne by the child's family, not by health care providers (Salkever, 1985). As a result, physicians in prepaid plans have little financial incentive to treat chronic illness. Though economic incentives are certainly not the only factor that influence physicians' decisions, when financial incentives encourage undertreatment, they reinforce the inadequate professional norms and limited professional prestige from treating chronic illnesses (Sapolsky, 1977; Farrow et al., 1981). Fee-for-service reimbursement at least provides a financial incentive for continued treatment. In prepaid plans, in which providers must allocate a limited budget among various services and limited time for contact with patients, the chronically ill are likely to get short-changed (Schlesinger, 1986).

There has been relatively little experience with chronically ill children in prepaid settings, but it has not been especially promising. HMOs established in the early 1970s for Medicaid enrollees in California did treat some chronically ill children. Children's health care specialists in the state considered this care inadequate, even compared to the rather checkered record of the program as a whole (Smith, 1984). Subsequently, a number of the Medicaid programs that have used HMOs have explicitly exempted chronically ill children, leaving them a part of the fee-for-service system (Brazner and Gaylord, 1986).

The second problem facing high-risk children in prepaid plans is that they often come from homes in which the parents have limited education. Because HMOs often do not charge substantial copayments, they instead use various administrative restrictions and requirements to ration care (Luft, 1982b). As a result, some persistence and perseverance are required to work through the system and obtain needed care (Hetherington et al., 1975). Studies have found that less-educated enrollees in prepaid plans receive less preventive care (Freeborn et al., 1977; Shortell et al., 1977) and are apparently less satisfied with the care they receive (Pope et al., 1972; Hetherington et al., 1977).[4]

Whatever the impact of prepayment on access to services for those enrolled in the plan, recent research suggests that the expansion of HMOs may have a decidedly negative effect on access for uninsured children. According to AMA surveys, about 30 percent of all physician visits are not covered by insurance, and more so for pediatricians. When physicians join a prepaid group, however, they typically see only those enrolled in the plan.

Consequently, as more physicians join prepaid plans, fewer are available to treat uninsured patients. Data collected by the AMA reveal that physicians' participation in an HMO is associated with a significantly smaller proportion of uninsured patients in their practice, controlling statistically for various other aspects of their practice and the community in which they work (Blumenthal et al., 1987). Because children so often fall through the gaps in private insurance coverage (see Chapter 5), this has a particularly large impact on access to care for children. According to AMA statistics, in 1984 the average pediatrician affiliated with an HMO treated 25 percent uninsured patients, compared to more than 40 percent for nonaffiliated pediatricians.[5]

On balance, then, integration of physician practices probably does increase quality of medical care for children. Prepayment (associated with lower copayments) further enhances the accessibility of preventive services by reducing copayments, but these benefits may be outweighed by constraints on care for high-risk children. The spread of group practices may also limit access to physicians for children without insurance, exacerbating problems of financial access that have increased as the uninsured population has grown in recent years.

Changing Institutional Affiliations

Children are less likely than adults to require institutional care. Nonetheless, more than 2 million children are hospitalized each year, most in community hospitals, but about 20 percent in tertiary care children's hospitals. Several hundred thousand are residents of nursing homes, patients in long-term psychiatric hospitals, or residents of other long-term care facilities (Health Care Financing Administration, 1986; Millazo–Sayre et al., 1986). The accessibility and quality of care in these institutions have been significantly affected by ongoing changes in the hospital industry (Starkweather, 1971; Vladeck, 1981).

As physicians were joining organized systems of ambulatory care, health care institutions formed multifacility corporations. Virtually nonexistent until the mid-1960s, these corporations now control 35 percent of the short-term general hospital beds, almost half of the nursing homes, and one-third of the HMOs in this country (Schlesinger et al., 1986). To date, system affiliation has been less common among institutions specializing in the treatment of children. As of 1984, only a few children's' hospitals and 10 percent of the psychiatric facilities for children were affiliated with multihospital chains.

Specialty institutions, however, will increasingly be linked to multifacility corporations. Affiliation is in the interest of the hospital, because it creates a "feeder-network," facilitating transfers of patients to tertiary care facilities (McClure, 1985). Affiliation is also in the interests of the corporation, allowing it to diversify into less regulated aspects of health care. For example, most specialty hospitals, such as children's' hospitals and psychiatric facilities, are exempted from Medicare's prospective payment system. Partially as a result, multihospital systems have expanded their ownership of private psychiatric hospital beds (Wallace,

1987). It seems likely that they will seek ownership in institutions specializing in the care of children for similar reasons (Ermann and Gabel, 1984).

According to most current projections, multifacility corporations will continue to expand through "horizontal integration" (joint control of like facilities, such as a chain of hospitals) and "vertical integration" (shared control of institutions along the continuum of care, such as the joint ownership of an ambulatory care unit, a hospital, and a nursing home) (Brown, 1981). By the mid-1990s, such integrated corporations will likely control more than half the hospital beds in the country (Arthur Andersen and Co., 1984). Some observers make more extreme predictions, arguing that "by 1995 or sooner, the medical care system will be dominated by large vertically and horizontally integrated, closed panel organizations" (McClure, 1985, p. 45).

Institutional linkages can affect the delivery of health care in two different ways. On the one hand, they encourage the integration of interests of diverse providers. For example, physicians affiliated with an HMO that is owned by a multihospital system may be more likely to act in ways that promote the financial interests of affiliated hospitals than are physicians who simply have staff privileges at those institutions (Pauly, 1978). On the other hand, the emergence of multifacility systems is likely to disrupt the informal linkages that have traditionally existed among providers within a given region, linkages that are important for the care of children with multiple health problems (Starfield, 1980; Select Panel, 1981). Physicians in HMOs are likely to admit patients only to their affiliated hospitals, hospitals to discharge only to affiliated nursing homes. Thus, while systems consolidate health care facilities in some senses, they also fragment the health care system into a set of parallel tracks of care, tracks that patients may find quite difficult to cross. The greatest risks befall families who find themselves on the "wrong side" of these tracks.

Institutional affiliations and children's health care. The forces that encourage the growth of multifacility linkages are likely to fall short of creating a system of nation-wide megacorporations. There is no evidence that very large systems have any great economic advantages—in fact, large systems spend more in administrative costs than they save through large-scale purchasing of supplies and the like (Pattison and Katz, 1983; Renn et al., 1985). Under these circumstances, the future growth of systems will take the form largely of those integrated vertically and horizontally over several contiguous communities, rather than nation-wide systems.

These regional systems may have significant effects on the delivery of health care for children, some positive, others negative. Systemization will probably stabilize the financial condition of some facilities and thus preserve geographic access to care, but may also make it more likely that providers will discriminate against unprofitable patients. Systems should improve the quality of care for children living in communities with otherwise inadequate medical resources, but potentially reduce the quality of care for other children.

Multifacility systems are able to cross-subsidize facilities that are unprofitable because they are located in low-income communities or deliver services used disproportionately by unprofitable patients. There is some evidence, albeit anecdotal, that multihospital corporations are currently subsidizing some hospitals (McManus, 1985),[6] particularly tertiary care centers that bring prestige to the system (Feder and Hadley, 1987). "An impressive academic institution can serve as a "flagship" . . . to the extent that a flagship is seen as a kind of prestigious loss leader, there is greater incentive for the company to make decisions about the institution that are not based solely on profitability" (Egdahl, 1986, p. 21).

Younger patients will especially benefit from such cross-subsidization, because high-risk children receive much of their care from academic teaching hospitals (Select Panel, 1981). Children from low-income families particularly benefit from keeping local hospitals operating, since they are less able to travel long distances for care (Beauchesene and Mundel, 1977).

There are limits on the extent to which systems will cross-subsidize unprofitable facilities. They are less likely to affiliate with hospitals running a serious deficit (Feder and Hadley, 1987). Once affiliated, the shift of control from the locally elected board of trustees to the corporate central office may reduce the institutions' willingness to care for unprofitable patients.

> System-affiliated hospitals are said to "accept across the board the notion that the only health care they can provide in any significant way is that which returns them more revenue than their costs. Other care, whether needed or not, is relegated to some other providers or source" (Weinstein, 1984, p. 87).

Research suggests that hospitals affiliated with for-profit corporations, the fastest growing type of system, are indeed less likely to offer unprofitable services and more likely to discourage admissions by the uninsured than are other hospitals operating in the same community (Schlesinger et al., 1986a; Shortell et al., 1986).

The more care is vertically integrated—that is, the more ambulatory and institutional providers share common financial goals—the more difficult it will be for unprofitable patients to obtain access to care, since outpatient providers will become more sensitive to the costs of treating the uninsured if they're admitted to the hospital. Physicians who are paid through incentive payments from hospitals have been shown to treat a smaller proportion of uninsured patients. According to 1984 AMA survey data, 17 percent of the patients of physicians who were not paid through incentive payment arrangements were uninsured. This compared to 7 percent for physicians who received hospital-based incentive payments. This difference remains even after one controls for various characteristics of the physician's practice, the hospital and the community in which they are located (Blumenthal et al., 1987). These effects were more pronounced among physicians who treat children. The average pediatrician paid through hospital-based incentives had only 7 percent uninsured patients, compared to 37 percent for other pediatricians.[7]

Integration may affect quality of care in several ways. System membership encourages physicians to affiliate with hospitals in areas they would otherwise consider undesirable. The system becomes a network for professional contacts, making providers in other areas feel less isolated. By attracting better trained and qualified physicians, multifacility systems may thus improve the quality of care in rural and low-income regions (Treat, 1976; Townsend, 1983; Ermann and Gabel, 1984). In addition, interfacility linkages make patient transfers among institutions easier, creating the type of network of services often viewed as desirable for the effective care of children (Starfield, 1980).

It is also likely, however, that the growth of regional systems may reduce quality by partitioning the local health care system into a set of vertically integrated tracks of care. While system affiliation facilitates transfers among affiliated institutions, it may also encourage providers to view the system as self-contained, reducing their willingness to refer patients to unaffiliated providers. If these local integrated systems are too small to employ subspecialists, this inward orientation can hinder timely tertiary treatment. It may also cause providers to become less familiar with various health-related programs outside the system, including the Title V Crippled Children's Services (CCS), Medicaid's Early Periodic Screening, Detection and Treatment (EPSDT) program, and various child and maternal nutrition programs. While outside the boundaries of the traditional medical system, these other programs are important to the health and well-being of many children (Gephart et al., 1984).

Systems are sufficiently new that there have been no studies of their effects on patient referrals. A somewhat analogous situation exists within HMOs, which form a similarly self-contained system of care. Experience with these prepaid plans suggests that serious problems may exist for referrals to specialized or tertiary care providers. "Not all HMOs, IPAs and/or PPOs have a pediatric subspecialist on their panel of participating specialty or consulting physicians. Consequently, many general practitioners who belong to an HMO or PPO are finding they are no longer able to refer their patients to a pediatric subspecialist without the child's parents or their practice incurring a substantial financial loss" (Matlin, 1986, p. 3).

Past experience with HMOs in state's Medicaid programs also suggests that closed systems reduce referrals to health-related programs. From virtually every state that has required substantial enrollment by Medicaid beneficiaries in HMOs, including California, Arizona, and Wisconsin, have come reports of serious declines in referrals to EPSDT and CCS programs (Black, 1984; Clement, 1984; Brazner and Gaylord, 1986). In the first year of the Wisconsin program, for example, EPSDT screenings fell to one-third the level of the previous year (Brazner and Gaylord, 1986). This is problematic for several reasons. HMOs are unlikely to provide fully comparable services, so reduced referrals can hinder access for enrolled children. In addition, reduced referrals deprive these programs of revenues that may be needed to capture economies of scale. As programs shrink, they thus become less effective for children they continue to serve.

Increased Competition Based on Price

Over the past five years, the market for health care services has become more price-competitive. This reflects in part changing attitudes among purchasers, who have become more concerned with health care cost and who have sought to negotiate lower prices with providers (Goldsmith, 1984; Rice et al., 1985). In a period of declining rates of hospitalization and an increasing supply of physicians, health care has become a "buyers' market" in which providers are forced to reduce charges to attract patients.

The apparent oversupply of health care providers has its roots in several ongoing trends in the health care system. Over the past five years, hospitals have faced increased competition from newly emerging health care facilities (Goldsmith, 1984; Ermann and Gabel, 1985) as hospital occupancy rates have fallen dramatically (American Hospital Association, 1985). These free-standing facilities are expected to proliferate in the future, further increasing competitive pressures on hospitals (Arthur Andersen and Co, 1984). Beyond their mere numbers, many of these newly emerging organizations are more aggressive competitors than traditional health care providers have been. Recent research has found, for example, that for-profit health care facilities—the fastest growing form of ownership in the health care system—create stronger competitive pressures than do their private nonprofit counterparts (Schlesinger et al., 1986).

A second trend involves the growing supply of doctors. The number of physicians in this country rose 40 percent over the past decade, and the number of physicians per capita will grow by another 20 percent by the end of this century (McClure, 1985). Since the mid-1970s, more medical school graduates have specialized in primary care. Coupled with a slowing of the birth rate, this has led to sharp declines in the number of children per pediatrician in this country, which fell from 3355 in 1975 to a predicted 1500 in 1990.

Child health practitioners thus already face greater financial pressure than do most of their professional peers and the growing surplus of physicians who specialize in the care of children makes it "increasingly likely that competition for patients will increase" (Budetti, 1981, pp. 603–4). Since the late 1970s, general/family practitioners and pediatricians—who combined account for almost 90 percent of the physicians treating children (Baumann and Calkins, 1977)—have faced declining utilization and stable or falling real incomes (Table 8.1). Adjusting for inflation, all physicians' incomes in this country have declined since the mid-1970s, but the incomes of general practitioners have fallen 50 percent faster than that of the average physician, pediatricians 30 percent faster. This can be seen most dramatically among younger physicians. Between 1982 and 1984, the incomes of general practitioners and pediatricians under the age of 36 fell more than 20 percent, even before one takes inflation into account (Table 8.1).

As the number of practicing physicians continues to expand, hospitalization rates decline, and the price sensitivity of buyers increases,

Table 8.1 Growing Economic Pressures on Physicians Who Treat Children

	1978	1982	1984
Physicians of all ages			
Patient visits/week			
Family/general practice	180	161	143
Pediatrics	148	135	126
Mean income (thousands)			
Family/general practice	$55	$72	$71
Pediatrics	$51	$70	$75
Physicians less than 36 years old			
Patient visits/week			
Family/general practice		145	137
Pediatrics		127	122
Mean income (thousands)			
Family/general practice		$65	$57
Pediatrics		$59	$40

Sources: American Medical Association, Socioeconomic Monitoring System, 1983 and 1985.

competitive pressures on providers will grow as well. A panel of providers, administrators, and public officials predicted that "increased competition among health care providers appears to be a generally accepted trend of the future" (Arthur Andersen and Co., 1984, p. 6). This will inevitably affect both the accessibility and quality of children's health care.

The consequences of price-based competition for children's health care. Price-based competition in health care is something of a two-edged sword. It will enhance access to care for some children while inhibiting access for others. It will promote treatment of previously underserved groups, yet at the same time create the potential for overtreatment of other children. It will increase some aspects of quality, but lead to declines in other aspects, particularly those affected by disrupted patterns of referral and inappropriate patient transfers. We will consider each of these consequences in turn.

Growing competitive pressures will increase access for several sets of children. One group to benefit will be those enrolled in Medicaid. Historically, Medicaid programs in many states have paid providers at relatively low rates, discouraging provider participation (Health Care Financing Administration, 1986; Perloff et al., 1987). As price-based competition forces providers to deliver care more efficiently, they can more profitably treat patients even at low reimbursement rates and hence should be more receptive to Medicaid recipients (Schlesinger et al., 1986a).

A second group to benefit will be children who received inadequate care because their parents were unaware that they required treatment and health care providers lacked the outreach services to identify them. This should prove particularly important for prenatal care. Surveys suggest that lack of understanding on the part of pregnant women, particularly adolescents, is a major cause of inadequate prenatal care (General Accounting Office, 1989). Certainly one of the major differences between American and European health care systems is the lack of outreach programs in the United States that are designed to bring women into the health care system during pregnancy.

Declining utilization rates will undoubtedly motivate providers to seek additional patients. This is already reflected in efforts by health care providers to market their services—between 1984 and 1986 alone marketing expenditures increased fourfold (Health One Corporation, 1987). Physicians faced with increased competition expand their office hours, increasing access for children with working parents (American Medical Association, 1985). These same motivations should also encourage a growing array of outreach services and related activities aimed at attracting young patients.

Not all potential patients, though, will be pursued with equal vigor. In fact, some families will find it more difficult to obtain care for their children in a price-competitive market—particularly those without health insurance. Providers have traditionally treated the uninsured by cross-subsidizing this treatment using profits made from insured patients (Ohsfeldt, 1985). Children—particularly newborns—have been major recipients of this uncompensated care (Perrin, 1986). As competition drives down prices paid by the insured, the potential for cross-subsidization is limited. Studies have shown that where competition among providers is intense, they become less willing to offer services that are used by the poor and less likely to subsidize care for the uninsured (Luft et al., 1986; Schlesinger et al., 1986a; Shortell et al., 1986).

These cutbacks will disproportionately affect high-risk children from low-income families (Rosenbach, 1985). Access restrictions will be most pronounced among the most aggressively competitive facilities, such as those operated for profit. For-profit facilities have been shown to be less likely to locate in communities with relatively low income and limited insurance coverage, less likely to supply services that are inadequately reimbursed, and less likely to treat patients who require care at reduced charge (Schlesinger and Dorwart, 1984; McNerny and Gray, 1986; Schlesinger et al., 1986a; Sloan et al., 1986; Schlesinger et al., 1987; Shortell et al., 1987).

Providers' quest for additional patients can also create a peculiar paradox—services will be developed or expanded that will simultaneously address unmet needs yet at the same time create the potential for excessive treatment. This is well illustrated by the recent growth of mental health facilities providing services to children and adolescents.

Historically, children have often not received needed mental health care—studies suggest that about three-quarters of the mentally ill or emotionally disturbed children get inadequate services or no treatment at all (Office of Technology Assessment, 1986). But as competition among private psychiatric facilities has grown more intense, they have been driven to pursue new markets, including younger patients. The National Association of Private Psychiatric Hospitals estimated that admissions of adolescents to private facilities increased more than fourfold between 1980 and 1984. This willingness to treat younger patients has been welcomed by a number of observers, but it has also created concerns that the "wrong" children are being admitted to these facilities.

Private facilities are increasingly attracting patients through direct marketing. Children may thus be admitted without the acquiescence of a private practitioner and, in many states, without adequate legal safeguards (Warren and Staples, 1985). Too often admissions may involve "behavior problems" that are not in fact mental illness at all. These problems are often exacerbated by a hospitalization. Forty percent of postpsychiatric admissions for children and adolescents have been judged inappropriate (Knitzer, 1982). As the need to fill beds grows, providers will be under increased financial pressure to increase admissions. With weak professional norms and inadequate screening of admissions, competitive pressures may cause as much harm by encouraging inappropriate hospitalization as they bring benefits to children whose mental illnesses would previously have gone untreated.

Competition will also undoubtedly affect the quality of health services children receive. Although there is little definitive evidence, most observers anticipate that quality will decline in the face of price-based competition, that efforts to "cut out the fat" will inevitably take out meat and bone as well. As noted in Chapter 7, when institutional providers face cost-cutting pressures, they will eliminate some unnecessary days in the hospital but may also cause premature discharge of more serious cases.

Similar, though often less obvious problems may be created among ambulatory care providers. In a survey of health care professionals, half predicted that competition would significantly impair quality of care over the course of the next decade (Arthur Andersen and Co, 1984). With growing numbers of physicians and unfilled hospital beds, providers will become increasingly loathe to refer patients for fear of losing them as a source of revenue.

> Glut can seriously damage not only efficiency but also quality . . . providers stop referring patients to other specialists because they need the fee themselves. In cities where competition has begun to make the surplus obvious, even well-established physicians find noticeable holes in their schedules. Eminent specialists complain that 10 years ago physicians would call and say "I've got a tough one here. How soon can you see him?" Now they call up and say, "I've got a tough one here. What would you do if you saw a patient with symptoms X and Y and Z." They want a free consultation rather than sending the patient on to appropriate specialty care. (McClure, 1985, p. 44)

In areas in which competition is most intense, these effects are already being felt by providers specializing in the care of children. The states of California and Illinois have each introduced competitive bidding systems to reduce the cost of care for Medicaid enrollees. In each state, community hospitals have become less willing to refer many cases to children's hospitals but at the same time more eager to transfer very expensive cases (Hurd, 1984; Friedman, 1986).

These changes in transfer policies reflect a larger problem—a growing trend toward transferring patients for economic reasons. Such transfers increased as much as 300 percent in some cities during the early

1980s (Schiff et al., 1986). According to a recent survey conducted by the American Academy of Pediatrics, economic transfers are also becoming more common for children (Rosenbaum, 1985). Transfers threaten quality of care, because patients are often moved while in unstable condition (Schiff et al., 1986). Again, competition has induced a seemingly paradoxical problem—it inhibits some patient referrals that are desirable while encouraging others that are inappropriate or harmful.

The balance between gains in efficiency and cuts in quality will depend in large part on the ability of parents to determine when their children's health care has been inappropriately limited. The patient-provider relationship is increasingly assuming adversarial overtones as patients' trust in their physician's decisions has declined (Harvey and Shubat, 1986). Again, those patients who are best educated and who feel most comfortable challenging the decisions of health care professionals will be able to play this role most effectively. Children from other households will fare less well.

Policy Implications and Possible Responses

Integrated ambulatory practices, multifacility systems, and price-based competition will lead to some significant changes in children's health care. Some of these are favorable, some are not. Some changes will simultaneously benefit one group of children while putting others at increased risk. On balance, the status of the "average" child (Table 8.2) appears less problematic than the consequences for care of already high-risk children (Table 8.3).

Adverse effects will be particularly pronounced for children under two circumstances. First, the health care needs of some groups of children differ from those of the average patient. Organizational arrangements and system changes that may be beneficial for most individuals will not be for these children. For example, because for a given diagnosis, children have more variable lengths of stay in the hospital than do adults, they are more "risky" to treat under most systems of prospective payment (Restuccia and Payne, 1985; Essok-Vitale, 1986). Cost-conscious hospitals will therefore either avoid children or be under financial pressure to discharge prematurely those who turn out to be higher cost. Likewise, because maintaining the health of high-risk children requires a mix of medical and health-related services, they are more vulnerable to the problems that can develop if a vertically integrated system of care becomes too narrowly focused on medical services, disrupting patterns of referral to other sources of care.

Table 8.2 Summary of Expected Effects of Organizational Changes on the Health of the "Average" Child

Organizational Change	Nature of Effect	
	Positive	Negative
Integrated ambulatory practices		
Effects on access	Increased access to primary care due to low copayments	
Effects on quality	Increased peer review Some improved continuity	
Multifacility systems		
Effects on access	Subsidize tertiary-care facilities	
Effects on quality		Possibly reduce referrals to specialists
Price-based competition		
Effects on access	Increased access due to spread of freestanding providers Longer office hours by private practitioners	Reduced willingness to treat high-cost patients
Effects on quality	Greater direct patient admissions for previously untreated mental illness	Fewer referrals to specialists Excessive hospitalization for conditions with poorly defined professional norms for treatment Premature discharge of costly patients

The second source of problems emerges from incentives that affect the care of all patients, but from which children are less adequately buffered. Price-based competition will cut access for all the uninsured, not just children. Prepayment creates incentives for undertreatment for all enrollees with chronic illnesses or other conditions that have costs not borne fully by the medical system. Children are at greater risk under these circumstances, in part because they are less able to assess the care they receive. They are more likely to come from low-income households that have less capacity to voice complaints and concerns if treatment is inadequate.

Each of these problems requires a different approach to remedial public policies. Several alternative strategies are discussed in some detail below.

Addressing Children's Health Care Needs in a Changing Provider System

Three types of remedial public policies can protect children who are threatened by ongoing changes in American medicine. First, providers who treat children can be isolated from these system-wide changes. Second, ongoing organizational changes can be modified or converted to better meet the special needs of children. Third, children whose health care is most adversely affected by organizational changes could be com-

Table 8.3 Summary of Expected Effects of Organizational Changes on the Health of the "High-Risk" Child

Organizational Change	Nature of Effect	
	Positive	Negative
Integrated ambulatory practices		
Effects on access	Increased access to primary care due to low copayments	Fewer MDs willing to treat uninsured Administrative barriers hinder use by less-educated
Effects on quality	Increased peer review Some improved continuity	Undertreatment of chronic illness Reduced contact time for diagnosing and treating complex cases
Multifacility systems		
Effects on access	Subsidize tertiary-care facilities Subsidize "occasionally unprofitable" services and facilities	Facilities less willing to admit the uninsured
Effects on quality	Induce more qualified MDs to move to rural and low-income areas	Possibly reduce referrals to specialists Reduce referrals to EPSDT, CCS and health-related programs
Price-based competition		
Effects on access	Increased access due to spread of free-standing providers Longer office hours by private practitioners Improved access for Medicaid eligibles	Reduced willingness to treat high-cost patients Less willing to treat uninsured
Effects on quality		Fewer referrals to specialists Premature discharge of costly patients "Dumping" to public hospitals

pensated in various ways. Each of these strategies has been used, to some extent, in formulating children's health policy in the past. Each has advantages and disadvantages when applied to the problems looming in the future.

The isolation strategy. One means of minimizing undesirable effects on children is to keep them at arm's length from ongoing organizational changes. This was the approach adopted by the federal government when it exempted children's hospitals from Medicare's prospective payment system. Many European nations operate a maternal and child health system separate from their primary national health insurance or health service program. A similar approach could be used to address other ongoing organizational changes: for example, children's hospitals could be forbidden to join a multifacility system; HMOs could be required not to enroll any children with chronic illness. This isolation strategy, however, is effective only if it can in fact successfully insulate children from change. For a number of reasons, this may be neither desirable nor possible.

First, children can be isolated from the rest of the health care system only to the extent that providers can be induced to treat them differently from other patients. When children are treated by specialized providers, such as pediatricians or children's hospitals, these providers can be treated differently by those purchasing or regulating medical care. But often children are treated by providers who also treat adult patients (Baumann and Calkins, 1977; Starfield, 1980; Long et al., 1986). Only about half the physician visits for children under 15 are with pediatricians (Dept. of Health and Human Services, 1985). Practice patterns developed in treating older patients can easily "spillover" and alter treatment of children, even if this is not the intent of policy and even though no financial incentives directly affect children's health care. This has already happened for elder patients. For instance, when Medicare first began enrolling elders in HMOs, it paid the plans on the basis of costs like it did all other providers. Nonetheless, elders' hospitalization rates fell, commensurate with hospital rates for younger HMO enrollees whose care was prepaid (Weil, 1976). Physicians within the HMO didn't treat patients any differently as a result of their age or how care was being paid for.

Perhaps more important, promoting children's health requires an understanding and treatment of the problems of both children and their families. An isolation strategy is based on the notion of treating children differently from other patients. This necessarily makes it more difficult to develop systems of care that treat the family as a whole. For example, if Medicaid programs exempt children with chronic illness from mandatory enrollment in HMOs, they are faced with the dilemma of whether to exempt the whole family (and thus deny prepaid care to some family members who might benefit) or require that members of family receive care from different providers. Either option may have undesirable effects on the adequacy of children's health care (San Agustin et al., 1981).

The isolation strategy may also have unfortunate effects that are difficult to foresee. The exemptions built into Medicare's prospective payment system for hospitals are a good example. As noted earlier, by exempting specialty psychiatric hospitals, Medicare made these facilities relatively attractive to investors, because continued cost-based reimbursement seemed to them less risky than prospective payment. The resulting influx of private capital and expansion of capacity has created fears of excessive institutionalization, particularly for young patients. Thus, in attempting to insulate the mental health care system from the effects of prospective payment, Medicare inadvertently created a different set of problems.

Finally, the isolation strategy may be ineffective in the long run simply because it is politically unacceptable. Many of the organizational changes discussed in this chapter have been motivated by legitimate desires for reform of the American health care system. The increased acceptance of prospective payment, prepayment, and price-based competition are all products of a widespread belief that health care in this country has become too expensive. For an isolation strategy to be politically feasible, the case must be made that the potential dangers to children outweigh the advantages of greater efficiency in the delivery of health care. Although it is always difficult to predict the outcome of any political debate, it may well prove difficult to convince most policymakers that the dangers to children are sufficiently serious to merit totally abandoning these attempts at cost control.

The isolation strategy thus has a variety of liabilities. For these reasons, it does not seem a promising approach for coping with the changes affecting the health care of children.

The conversion strategy. A second approach involves designing policies that will adapt ongoing organizational changes to meet the special needs of younger patients. For example, because treating chronically ill children can become very expensive over the course of a year (Butler et al., 1985), these children may be undertreated in prepaid plans. One way to reduce or avoid this problem is to set a ceiling on the plan's liability for treating enrolled children. In fact, an experimental system of prepaid care for low-income residents of Monterey County, California, did just that. Plans were not financially responsible for any medical expenses over $15,000 per year for each enrollee; excess spending was paid by the Medi-Cal program. This ceiling seemed to improve the treatment of chronically ill children under the auspices of the prepaid plans (Smith, 1984).[8]

The conversion strategy may be politically more acceptable because it redirects, rather than directly opposes, organizational changes that have broad political support and considerable institutional momentum. This approach can be effective, though, only if ways can be devised to reshape the trends described above to create more appropriate incentives for children's care. This is not always the case. There are, for instance, no obvious ways to change the nature of competition among providers in ways that reduce problems of access to care by uninsured children. In general, a conversion strategy will be most effective when addressing problems stemming from organizational structure—which can be directly modified by policies that change the organizational arrangements—as opposed to less concrete changes in the goals or values of the organization. One would thus expect, for example, that this approach would be more effective in dealing with the emerging shortcomings of integrated ambulatory practices or multifacility systems than with providers' increased sensitivity to market pressures and other financial incentives.

The compensation strategy. The third approach to promoting children's health allows organizational trends to play themselves out, but compensates those children who are adversely affected. For example, if the families of high-risk children are less able to obtain care in prepaid settings, due either to providers' financial incentives or to administrative constraints, public initiatives could establish special outreach programs or patient advocates for these enrollees. Similarly, if uninsured children bear the brunt of problems in an increasingly competitive health care system, special insurance programs or risk-pooling arrangements could be created to specially compensate providers for the care of these patients.[9]

This approach is likely to generate the least political opposition, because it neither conflicts with popular reform movements nor requires that providers change their organizational arrangements. It too, however, has some serious limitations. Compensatory programs generally require governmental spending, and it may be difficult to sustain political support for these expenditures. History suggests that the absence of a strongly organized lobby for children's interests has led to unstable political support for spending programs targeted by age (Zigler and Muenchow, 1984).

In addition, compensatory programs can be effective only to the extent that they actually reach their target population. Often in the past, initially well-designed programs have been gutted by subsequent political and administrative constraints. Medicaid, a prototype compensatory federal program directed at low-income Americans, has been so constrained by budgetary pressures at state and federal levels that it currently serves less than two-thirds of those with incomes below the poverty line (Munnel, 1985). Similar constraints have hampered the EPSDT program (Rosenbaum and Johnson, 1986). Effective targeting can be particularly difficult if the appropriate target group changes over time. For example, as different forms of prospective payment are introduced, different sets of patients will become unprofitable for providers, and hence merit some compensatory action.[10]

Compensatory programs are most effective if they can be structured to encourage political support and reach their primary target group (Meyer and Lewin, 1986). Past experience suggests that the broader the group that benefits from the program, the more stable will be its base of political support, particularly if beneficiaries include middle-class voters (Marmor, 1973). Compensatory programs directed exclusively toward low-income high-risk children may therefore lack the necessary political base. In contrast, those aimed at chronically ill and developmentally impaired children may achieve broader and longer lasting political support, both because these illnesses potentially can affect any family and because there is a shared interest between chronically impaired children and older Americans with functional limitations.

Children and the General Course of Health Policy

Many of the shortcomings of emerging organizational changes for children's health care will also be problematic for other patients. The problems of funding care for the uninsured, of representing community interests in an industry of large corporate entities, and of defining the appropriate balance of monetary and nonmonetary incentives for health care providers are certainly not unique to children. That these inadequacies of our health care system are more widely experienced and acknowledged, though, does not make them necessarily easier to resolve. Indeed, in several ways their interaction with the special needs of children creates tremendous challenges for policy makers.

Ongoing organizational changes are altering our expectations of practitioners as well as the relationship between health care providers and those they serve. New organizations and payment systems are creating financial and institutional incentives that engender potential conflicts of interest of an unprecedented nature. Patients have become less willing to trust providers to act in their best interests (Schlesinger 1985; Blumenthal, 1986).The growth of a competitive ethic in health care likewise represents a change in the relationship between health care providers and the communities in which they practice (Weinstein, 1984; Schlesinger et al., 1986a). Many health care facilities have historically been guided by a sense of fiduciary responsibility to the community (Sigmond, 1985; Seay et al., 1986). As this informal contract erodes, government will likely be asked to define a new, formal relationship, one that clearly assigns both rights and responsibilities to health care providers.

Under these circumstances, it is natural to expect both patients and communities to take a more active role in health care decisions. This is already happening. A poll of physicians conducted in 1986 by the American Medical Association found that 76 percent of responding doctors felt that their patients had become more "knowledgeable about health" than three years previously and 63 percent believed their patients were more "demanding of their physician" (American Medical Association, 1986). It is thus natural for policy makers to build on this trend by seeking additional ways of empowering patients and community groups through additional education and information.

But these trends raise several important unasked questions: "Who speaks for children as patients?" and "How do we encourage better decision making on children's behalf?" The more one questions the legitimacy of decisions made by health professionals, the more one is forced to ask comparable questions of parents, advocacy groups, and other representatives of children's interests. These questions become particularly complicated for adolescents, who exist in a murky stage of quasi-independence in both legal and social senses.

A different type of challenge is created by the complex nature of ongoing organizational changes. In a real sense, the greatest problem created by prepaid plans, vertically integrated systems, or price-based competition is not that they lead to inadequate care for some patients. Any organizational arrangement or method of paying providers will create some incentives that we applaud, others that we abhor. The more fundamental issue is that ongoing organizational changes have created a health care system that embodies a mix of different organizational arrangements and payment systems. This diversity excites the advocates of competition, and certainly increases the choices open to the individual. But it creates a situation in which comprehensive health policy reforms may be very difficult to develop, and this is perhaps the most fundamental problem that these changes create for policy makers.

In contemporary American health care, prepayment and fee-for-service reimbursement exist side by side. Under growing competitive pressures, prepayment creates financial incentives for undertreatment, while fee-for-service reimbursement creates incentives for overutilization. For example, as discussed earlier, a mentally ill child enrolled in an HMO faces the risk of inadequate treatment, but the same child covered by fee-for-service insurance runs the risk of inappropriate and unnecessary hospitalization. If adequate safeguards are to be provided patients in this system, we must now simultaneously guard against too much care *and* too little care. System control of health care facilities creates a similar problem. As noted above, these interfacility ties both consolidate and fragment the local health system, linking more closely providers within each vertically integrated system of care, but attenuating contacts to providers affiliated with another system or with independent health-related programs. Each of these may lead to inadequate care for some patients, yet to develop a system that can simultaneously deal with too much and too little integration is a daunting task.

It is always difficult to muster political support in favor of any new program. When the problems of the health care system become seemingly self-contradictory and paradoxical, it may be virtually impossible to frame the relevant issues clearly enough to make comprehensive or even substantial reform possible at all. This complexity is exacerbated for children. Not only must policy makers cope with the complex and seemingly contradictory changes occurring in the health care system, but also they must differentiate those issues that are of greater concern or promise for children than for adults.

This complexity is likely to have one of two effects on policy making. Either it will lead to system-wide reform in an effort to simplify affairs, or it will render comprehensive reform impossible, locked in a stalemate of conflicting concerns. Policies addressing the special health needs of children may be easier to fashion and implement than those that deal with the more general shortcomings of the health care system. But partial and age-specific reforms will inevitably create tensions among age groups and demands for greater intergenerational equity.

These are issues with no easy solution. They portend a complicated future that is difficult to foretell accurately. It is clear, though, that advocates of reform to promote children's health must be sensitive to the growing complexity of the health care system. This change creates special challenges and opportunities for children, both of which must be vigorously addressed to ensure that all children have adequate access to health services of acceptable quality.

Notes

1. Organizational changes may also affect costs of care, both directly and indirectly. For example, if certain changes disrupt continuity of care, they could in-

crease costs by encouraging families to seek care in high-cost settings, such as hospital emergency departments (Austin, 1984). Though such cost-related effects are important, in the current political climate cost considerations get sufficient, perhaps excessive, attention. The discussion in the text will therefore focus on other, less publicized, implications of organizational change.

2. AMA statistics were obtained in part from annual reports entitled "Socioeconomic Characteristics of Medical Practice" (Reynolds and Abram, 1983; Reynolds and Duann, 1985). Unpublished data were obtained from the AMA's 1984 Socioeconomic Monitoring Survey, described in detail by White (1985). These statistics were calculated through the assistance of the staff at the AMA's Center for Health Policy Research.

3. This was 40 percent of all physicians in group practice. AMA surveys actually report the number of physicians who say they are affiliated with health maintenance organizations (HMOs). As discussed below in the text, however, a substantial number of these prepaid plans are so-called independent practice associations (IPAs), in which physicians are prepaid for patient care but continue to practice in free-standing offices. The statistics reported in the text are based on the responses to the AMA survey, adjusted assuming that the fraction of physicians in IPAs is proportional to the number of patients in those plans, as reported in the 1984 Interstudy census of HMOs (Interstudy, 1985).

4. These findings have to be interpreted with some caution, however, since less education is often associated with many other characteristics of the enrollee that might affect the quality of the care they receive or their own perceptions of treatment (Luft, 1981). Income is one of these. Studies find no relationship between family income and children's use of health services in HMOs (Colombo et al., 1969). Since children from poor families are more frequently sick, this equality may actually mask inadequate treatment for low-income children (Davis and Schoen, 1978), though comparisons of health outcomes by income in HMOs and other settings have been mixed (Dutton and Silber, 1980; Ware et al., 1986).

5. This difference was statistically significant at a 1 percent confidence level. Including both family/general practitioners and pediatricians together, the average proportion of uninsured patients was 18 percent for primary care physicians affiliated with a prepaid plan, 31 percent for other primary care practitioners.

6. Other studies have found, though, that systems tend to affiliate with hospitals that are located in areas with above average hospital profitability, per capita income, and prevalence of insurance (Mullner and Hadley, 1984).

7. For family/general practitioners and pediatricians combined, those with hospital-based incentives averaged 9 percent uninsured patients, others 29 percent. Both this difference and ones reported in the text are statistically significant at a 1 percent confidence level.

8. A similar case has been made for adapting the general principle of prepayment to meet the special needs of the elderly (Diamond et al., 1983) and the chronically mentally ill (Schlesinger, 1986a).

9. A number of states have already initiated programs for other groups likely to suffer under competition—those at high risk of illness and those unable to afford hospital insurance (Desonia and King, 1985).

10. If payments are based on the average cost of a patient in the facility, then providers have a financial incentive to avoid treating all patients with expensive diseases. If payment is based on average cost for a given diagnosis, then providers have an incentive to avoid the more severe cases in that diagnostic group (Jencks et al., 1984).

References

American Academy of Pediatrics. 1985. State and Local Governments Respond. *Child Health Financing Report* 2(3):1–3.
American Hospital Association. 1985. *Hospital Statistics.* Chicago.
American Medical Association. 1983. In R. Reynolds and J. Abram (eds.), *Socioeconomic Characteristics of Medical Practice.* Chicago.
———. 1985. In R. Reynolds and J. Abram (eds.), *Socioeconomic Characteristics of Medical Practice.* Chicago.
Arthur Anderson and Co. 1984. *Health Care in the 1990s: Trends and Strategies.* Chicago.
Austin, G. 1984. Child Health-Care Financing and Competition. *New England Journal of Medicine* 311:1117–1120.
———. 1985. Consistent Care Leads to Payoff. *Business and Health* 2:10–13.
Baumann, J., and D. Calkins. 1977. Providing Primary Care Practitioners for Children. In D. Mundel (ed.), *Developing a Better Health Care System for Children,* pp. 77–98. Cambridge, Mass.: Ballinger.
Beauchesne, D., and D. Mundel. 1977. Determinants of Utilization of Children's Health Services. In D. Mundel (ed.), *Developing a Better Health Care System for Children,* pp. 55–75. Cambridge, Mass.: Ballinger.
Black, R. 1984. Alternatives to Straight Capitation. Paper presented at conference on *Capitation and Child Health Services,* San Francisco, February 17, 1984. (Proceedings in Institute for Health Policy Studies Discussion Paper 84-4, University of California, San Francisco.)
Blumenthal, D. 1986. The Social Responsibility of Physicians in a Changing Health Care System. *Inquiry* 23:268–274.
Brazner, K., and C.L. Gaylord. 1986. *Medicaid, HMOs and Maternal and Child Health. An Assessment of Wisconsin's Mandatory HMO Enrollment Program for AFDC Families.* Madison, Wis.: Center for Public Representation.
Brown, M. 1981. Multihospital Systems: Trends, Issues and Prospects. In G. Bisbee (ed.), *Multihospital Systems: Policy Issues for the Future.* Chicago: Hospital Research and Educational Trust.
Budetti, P. 1981. The Impending Pediatric "Surplus": Causes, Implications, and Alternatives. *Pediatrics* 67:597–606.
Butler, J. 1977. Financing Children's Health Care. In D. Mundel (ed.), *Developing a Better Health Care System for Children,* pp. 99–134. Cambridge, Mass.: Ballinger.
Butler, J., P. Budetti, M. McManus, S. Stenmark, and P. Newacheck. 1985. Health Care Expenditures for Children with Chronic Illnesses. In N. Hobbs and J. Perrin (eds.), *Issues in the Care of Children with Chronic Illness,* pp. 827–863. San Francisco: Jossey-Bass.
Cauffman, J.G., M. Roemer, and C. Shultz. 1967. The Impact of Health Insurance Coverage on Health Care of School Children. *Public Health Reports* 82(4):323–328.
Clement, M. 1984. Capitation and California's Children's Services. Paper presented at conference on *Capitation and Child Health Services,* San Francisco, February 17, 1984. (Proceedings in Institute for Health Policy Studies Discussion Paper 84-4, University of California, San Francisco.)
Colombo, T., E. Saward, and M. Greenlick. 1969. The Integration of an OEO Health Program into a Prepaid Comprehensive Group Practice Plan. *American Journal of Public Health* 59:641–650.
Davis, K., and C. Schoen. 1978. *Health and the War on Poverty: A Ten-Year Appraisal.* Washington, D.C.: Brookings Institution.

Desonia, R., and K. King. 1985. *Programs of Assistance for the Medically Indigent.* Washington, D.C.: George Washington University, Intergovernmental Health Policy Project.

Diamond, L., L. Gruenberg, and R. Morris. 1983. Elder Care for the 1980s: Health and Social Service in One Prepaid Health Maintenance System. *Gerontologist* 28:143–154.

Dutton, D. 1976. A Causal Model of the Use of Health Services: The Role of the Delivery System. Unpublished doctoral dissertation, Massachusetts Institute of Technology, Cambridge, Mass.

———. 1978. Explaining the Low Use of Health Services by the Poor: Costs, Attitudes, or Delivery Systems? *American Sociological Review* 43:348–368.

Dutton, D. and R. Silber. 1980. Children's Health Outcomes in Six Different Ambulatory Care Delivery Systems. *Medical Care* 18:693–714.

Egdahl, R. 1986. The Involvement of For-Profit Hospital Chains with Teaching and Research Institutions. In R. Southby and W. Greenberg (eds.), *The For-Profit Hospital.* Columbus, Ohio: Battelle Press.

Ellis, R.P., and T.G. McGuire. 1986. Hospital Behavior under Prospective Reimbursement: Cost Sharing and Supply. *Journal of Health Economics* 5(2):129–151.

Ermann, D., and J. Gabel. 1984. Multihospital Systems: Issues and Empirical Findings. *Health Affairs* 3:50–64.

Farrow, F., et al. 1981. The Framework and Directions for Change. In J. Meltzer, F. Farrow, and H. Richman (eds.), *Policy in Long-Term Care,* pp. 1–37. Chicago: University of Chicago Press.

Feder, J., and J. Hadley. 1987. A Threat or a Promise: Acquisition of Teaching Hospitals by Investor-Owned Chains. *Journal of Health Politics, Policy, and Law* 12:325–342.

Feldstein, P. 1979. *Health Care Economics.* New York: John Wiley and Sons.

Freeborn, D., B. Franklin, and S. McLemore. 1977. Health Status, Socioeconomic Status, and Utilization of Outpatient Services for Members of a Prepaid Group Practice. *Medical Care* 15(2):115–128.

Friedman, E. 1986. The Health Lifeline: Out of the Reach of Women and Children? *Hospitals* 60:46–51.

Gabel, J., and D. Ermann. 1985. Preferred Provider Organizations: Performance, Problems and Promise. *Health Affairs* 4:24–40.

Ganelin, R. 1985. The Arizona Experience. Paper presented at conference on *Capitation and Child Health Services,* San Francisco, February 17, 1984. (Proceedings in Institute for Health Policy Studies Discussion Paper 84-4, University of California, San Francisco.)

Gaus, C. 1971. Who Enrolls in a Prepaid Group Practice: The Columbia Experience. *Johns Hopkins Medical Journal* 128:9–14.

General Accounting Office. 1987. *Prenatal Care: Medicaid Recipients and Uninsured Women Obtain Insufficient Care* GAO/HRD-87-137. Washington D.C.

Gephart, J., M. Egan, and V. Hutchins. 1984. Perspectives on Health of School-age Children: Expectations for the Future. *Journal of School Health* 54:11–17.

Goldsmith, J. 1984. Death of a Paradigm: The Challenge of Competition. *Health Affairs* 3(3):5–19.

Gray, B., and W. NcNernery. 1986. For-Profit Enterprise in Health Care. *New England Journal of Medicine* 314:1523–1528.

Harvey, L., and S. Shubat. 1986. *AMA Surveys of Physician and Public Opinion: 1986.* Chicago: American Medical Association.

Health One Corporation. 1987. *Serving Patients: Rededication to Basic Values* Minneapolis.

Held, P., and M. Pauly. 1983. Competition and Efficiency in the End Stage Renal Disease Program. *Journal of Health Economics* 2:95–118.

Hetherington, R., C. Hopkins, and M. Roemer. 1975. *Health Insurance Plans: Promise and Performance.* New York: Wiley-Interscience.

Hillman, Alan. 1987. Financial Incentives for Physicians in an HMO: Is There a Conflict of Interest? *New England Journal of Medicine* 317:1743–1748.

Hillman, D., and J. Christianson. 1984. Competitive Bidding as Cost Containment Strategy for Indigent Medical Care: The Implementation Experience in Arizona. *Journal of Health Politics, Policy, and Law* 9(Fall):427–452.

Hurd, R. 1984. Alternatives to Capitation. Paper presented at conference on *Capitation and Child Health Services,* San Francisco, February 17, 1984. (Proceedings in Institute for Health Policy Studies Discussion Paper 84–4, University of California, San Francisco.)

Interstudy. *National HMO Census 1985: Annual Report on the Growth of HMOs.* Excelsior, Minn.

Jencks, S.F., A. Dobson, P. Willis, and P.H. Feinstein. 1984. Evaluating and Improving the Measurement of Hospital Case Mix. *Health Care Financing Review* (Annual Supplement):1–11.

Johns, L., M. Anderson, and R. Derzon. 1985. Selective Contracting in California: Experience in the Second Year. *Inquiry* 22:336–347.

Long, M., J. Dreachslin, and J. Fisher. 1986. Should Children's Hospitals Have Special Consideration in Reimbursement Policy? *Health Care Financing Review* 8:55–63.

Luft, H. 1981. *Health Maintenance Organizations: Dimensions of Performance.* New York: John Wiley and Sons.

———. 1985. Competition and Regulation. *Medical Care* 23:383–400.

Luft, H., J. Robinson, D. Garnick, S. Maerki, and S. McPhee. 1986. The Role of Specialized Clinical Services in Competition among Hospitals. *Inquiry* 3:83–94.

McClure, W. 1985. Buying Right: The Consequences of Glut. *Business and Health* 2(9):43–46.

Marmor, T. 1973. *The Politics of Medicare.* Chicago: Aldine.

Marmor, T., M. Schlesinger, and R. Smithey. 1986. A New Look at Nonprofits: Health Care in a Competitive Age. *Yale Journal of Regulation* 3(13):313–349.

Matlin, N. 1986. HMOs, PPOs, and Pediatric Subspecialty Care. *Child Health Financing Report* 3(4):3.

Mechanic, D. 1975. The Organization of Medical Practice and Practice Orientations Among Physicians in Prepaid and Nonprepaid Primary Care Settings. *Medical Care* 13:189–204.

Milazzo-Sayre, L., P. Benson, M. Rosenstein, and R. Manderscheid. 1986. Use of Inpatient Psychiatric Services by Children and Youth Under Age 18: United States, 1980. National Institute of Mental Health Statistical Note No. 175. Rockville, Md.: National Institute of Mental Health.

Mott, F., J. Hastings, and A. Barclary. 1973. Prepaid Group Practice in Sault Ste. Marie, Ontario: Part II: Evidence From the Household Survey. *Medical Care* 11:173–188.

Mullner, R., and J. Hadley. 1984. Interstate Variation in the Growth of Chain-Operated Proprietary Hospitals, 1973–1982. *Inquiry* 21:144-151.

Mundel, D. 1977. Policy for Primary Medical Care for Children: A Framework for Basic Choices. In D. Mundel (ed.), *Developing a Better Health Care System for Children,* pp. 9–24. Cambridge, Mass.: Ballinger.

Munnel, A. 1985. Ensuring Entitlement to Health Care Services. *New England Economic Review* (Nov./Dec.):30–40.

Office of Technology Assessment, U.S. Congress. 1986. *Children's Mental Health: Problems and Services—A Background Paper,* OTA-BP-H-33. Washington D.C.: U.S. G.P.O.

Ohsfeldt, R. 1985. Uncompensated Medical Services Provided by Physicians and Hospitals. *Medical Care* 23(12):1338–1344.

Osborn, L.M., and F.R. Woolley. 1981. The Use of Groups in Well-Child Care. *Pediatrics* 67:701–707.

Pattison, R., and H. Katz. 1983. Investor-owned and Not-for-Profit Hospitals: A Comparison Based on California Data. *New England Journal of Medicine* 309:347–353.

Pauly, M.V. 1980. *Doctors and Their Workshops.* Chicago: University of Chicago Press.

Perloff, J., P. Kletke, and K. Neckerman. 1987. Physician's Decisions to Limit Medicaid Participation: Determinants and Policy Implications. *Journal of Health Politics, Policy, and Law* 12:221-235.

Perrin, J. 1986. High Technology and Uncompensated Hospital Care. In F.A. Sloan, J.F. Blumstein, and J.M. Perrin (eds.), *Uncompensated Hospital Care: Rights and Responsibilities,* pp. 54–71. Baltimore: Johns Hopkins University Press.

Pope, C., D. Freeborn, and M. Greenlick. 1972. Members' Evaluation of Their Experience in a Group Practice Prepayment Plan. Presented at American Public Health Association Annual Meeting, November.

Renn, S., C. Schramm, J. Watt, and R. Derzon. 1985. The Effects of Ownership and System Affiliation on the Economic Performance of Hospitals. *Inquiry* 22:219–236.

Reynolds, R., and J. Abram. 1983. *Socioeconomic Characteristics of Medical Practice.* Chicago: American Medical Association.

Reynolds, R., and D. Duann. 1985. *Socioeconomic Characteristics of Medical Practice.* Chicago: American Medical Association.

Rice, T., G. de Lissovoy, J. Gabel, and D. Ermann. 1985. The State of PPOs: A National Survey. *Health Affairs* 4(4):25–40.

Richardson, W., S. Shortell, and P. Diehr. 1976. Chapter I: Introduction to the Project, the Study, and the Enrollees. In *The Seattle Prepaid Health Care Project: Comparison of Health Services Delivery.* (pB 267488-SET). Springfield, Va.: National Technical Information Services.

Roghmann, K., R. Hoekelman, and T. McInerny. 1984. The Changing Pattern of Primary Pediatric Care: Update for One Community. *Pediatrics* 73:363–374.

Rosenbach, M. 1980. Insurance Coverage and Ambulatory Medical Care of Low-Income children, 1980. Series C, Analytical Report No. 1, *National Medical Care Utilization and Expenditure Survey.* Health Care Financing Administration. Washington, D.C.: G.P.O.

Rosenbaum, S. 1985. Testimony of the Children's Defense Fund Before the Subcommittee on Taxation and Debt Management of the Senate Finance Committee Regarding S. 367, the Child Health Incentive Reform Plan.

Rosenbaum, S., and K. Johnson. 1986. Providing Health Care for Low-Income Children: Reconciling Child Health Goals with Child Health Financing Realities. *Milbank Memorial Fund Quarterly* 64(3):442–478.

Ross, C., and R. Duff. 1982. Returning to the Doctor: The Effect of Client Characteristics, Type of Practice and Experiences With Care. *Journal of Health and Social Behavior* 23:11–31.

Ross, C., J. Mirowsky, and R. Duff. 1982. Physician Status Characteristics and Client Satisfaction in Two Types of Medical Practice. *Journal of Health and Social Behavior* 23:317–329.

Salkever, D. 1985. Parental Opportunity Costs and Other Economic Costs of Children's Disabling Conditions. In N. Hobbs and J. Perrin (eds.), *Issues in the Care of Children with Chronic Illness*, pp. 864–879. San Francisco: Jossey-Bass.

San Agustin, M., V. Sidel, D. Drosness, H. Kelman, H. Levine, and E. Stevens. 1981. A Controlled Clinical Trial of "Family Care" Compared with "Child-Only Care" in the Comprehensive Primary Care of Children. *Medical Care* 19(2):202–222.

Sapolosky, H. 1977. America's Socialized Medicine: The Allocation of Resources within the Veteran's Health Care System. *Public Policy* 25:359–82.

Schiff, R., D. Ansell, J. Schlosser, A. Idris, A. Morrison, and S. Whitman. 1986. Transfers to a Public Hospital: A Prospective Study of 467 Patients. *New England Journal of Medicine* 314:552–557.

Schlesinger, M. 1985. The Rise of Proprietary Health Care. *Business and Health* 2:7–12.

———. 1986. On the Limits of Expanding Health Care Reform: Chronic Care in Prepaid Setting. *Milbank Memorial Fund Quarterly* 64:189–215.

Schlesinger, M., J. Bentkover, D. Blumenthal, W. Custer, R. Musacchio, and J. Willer. 1986a. Multihospital Systems and Access to Health Care. In L. Rossiter, R. Scheffler, G. Wilensky and N. McCall (eds.), *Advances in Health Economics and Health Services Research*, Vol. 7. Greenwich, Conn.: JAI Press.

Schlesinger, M., D. Blumenthal, and E. Schlesinger. 1986b. Profit under Pressure: The Economic Performance of Investor-Owned and Nonprofit Health Maintenance Organizations. *Medical Care* 24:615–627.

Schlesinger, M., and R. Dorwart. 1984. Ownership and Mental-Health Services: A Reappraisal of the Shift toward Privately Owned Facilities. *New England Journal of Medicine* 311:959–965.

Schlesinger, M., T. Marmor, and R. Smithey. 1987. Nonprofit and For Profit Medical Care: Shifting Roles and Implications for Health Policy. *Journal of Health Politics, Policy, and Law* 12:427–457.

Schlesinger, M., and T. Wetle. 1986. Care of the Elder Veteran: New Directions for Change. *Health Affairs* 5:59–71.

Scitovsky, A., L. Benham, and N. McCall. 1979. Use of Physician Services under Two Prepaid Plans. *Medical Care* 17:441–460.

Seay, J., B. Vladeck, P. Kramer, D. Gould, and J. McCormack. 1986. Holding Fast to the Good: The Future of the Voluntary Hospital. *Inquiry* 23:253–260.

Select Committee on Children, Youth and Families. 1985. Emerging Trends in Mental Health Care for Adolescents. Hearing. Washington, D.C.: G.P.O.

Select Panel for the Promotion of Child Health. 1981. Better Health for Our Children: A National Strategy. DHHS Publication No. 77–55071. Washington, D.C.: G.P.O.

Shortell, S., E. Morrison, S. Hughes, and J. Coverdill. 1986. The Impact of Multi-Institutional Systems on Service Provision. In L. Rossiter, R. Scheffler, G. Wilensky, and N. McCall (eds.), *Advances in Health Economics and Health Services Research*, Vol. 7. Greenwich, Conn.: JAI Press.

Shortell, S., E. Morrison, S. Hughes, J. Coverdill, B. Friedman, and L. Berg. 1986. The Effects of Hospital Ownership on Nontraditional Services. *Health Affairs* 5:97–111.

Shortell, S., et al. 1977. The Relationships among Dimensions of Health Services in Two Provider Systems: A Causal Model Approach. *Journal of Health and Social Behavior* 18:139–159.

Sigmond, R. 1985. Re-Examining the Role of the Community Hospital in a Competitive Environment. The 1985 Michael M. Davis Lecture. Chicago: University of Chicago, Center for Health Administration Studies.

Sloan, F., J. Valvona, and R. Mullner. 1986. Identifying the Issues: A Statistical Profile. In F.A. Sloan, J.F. Blumstein, and J.M. Perrin (eds.), *Uncompensated Hospital Care: Rights and Responsibilities*, pp. 16–53. Baltimore: Johns Hopkins University Press.

Smith, E. 1984. Capitation and California's Children's Services. Paper presented at conference on *Capitation and Child Health Services*, San Francisco, February 17, 1984. (Proceedings in Institute for Health Policy Studies Discussion Paper 84-4, University of California, San Francisco.)

Sorkin, A. 1977. In P. Rohrbach (ed.), *Health Manpower: An Economic Perspective*. Lexington, Mass.: Lexington Books.

Starfield, B. 1980. Health Care Delivery System: Organization, Control, Costs, and Effectiveness. In S. Friedman and R. Hoekelman (eds.), *Behavioral Pediatrics Psychosocial Aspects of Child Health Care*. New York: McGraw Hill.

Starkweather D. 1971. Health Facility Mergers: Some Conceptualizations. *Medical Care* 9:468–478.

Starr, Paul. 1982 *The Social Transformation of American Medicine* New York: Basic Books.

Townsend, J. 1983. When Investor-Owned Corporations Buy Hospitals: Some Issues and Concerns. In B. Gray (ed.), *The New Health Care for Profit: Doctors and Hospitals in a Competitive Environment*. Washington, D.C.: National Academy Press.

Treat, T. 1976. The Performance of Merging Hospitals. *Medical Care* 14:199–209.

U.S. Department of Health and Human Services. 1980. *Health United States 1980*. DHHS Publication No. 81-1232. Washington, D.C.: G.P.O.

———. 1985. *Health United States, 1985*. DHHS Publication No. 85-1232. Washington, D.C.: G.P.O.

Vladeck, B. 1981. Multihospital Systems and the Public Interest. In G. Bisbee (ed.), *Multihospital Systems: Policy Issues for the Future*, pp. 63–75. Chicago: Hospital Research and Education Trust.

Wallace, C. 1987. Growth of Psychiatric Hospital Chains. *Modern Healthcare* 35: 8–11.

Ware, J., W. Rogers, A. Davies, G. Goldberg, R. Brook, E. Keeler, C. Sherbourne, P. Camp, and J. Newhouse. 1986. Comparison of Health Outcomes at a Health Maintenance Organization with Those of Fee-for-Service Care. *Lancet* 16:1017–1022.

Warren, C., and W. Staples. 1985. Mental Health: The Hidden System of Adolescent Social Control. Paper presented at conference: "Rethinking Child Welfare: International Perspectives," Minneapolis, June 17–21.

Weber, G. 1985. Alternatives to Straight Capitation. Paper presented at conference on *Capitation and Child Health Services*, San Francisco, February 17, 1984. (Proceedings in Institute for Health Policy Studies Discussion Paper 84-4, University of California, San Francisco.)

Weil, P. 1976. Comparative Costs to the Medicare Program of Seven Prepaid Group Practices and Controls. *Milbank Memorial Fund Quarterly* 54:339–360.

Weinstein, I. 1984. The Future of the MIO in a Price-Competitive, Price-Driven Market. *Topics in Health Care Financing* 11:84–92.

Welch, W. 1987. The New Structure of Independent Practice Associations. *Journal of Health Politics, Policy, and Law* 12(4):723-740.

Wilner, S., S. Schoenbaum, R. Monson, and R. Winickoff. 1981. A Comparison of the Quality of Maternity Care between a Health Maintenance Organization and Fee-For-Service Practices. *New England Journal of Medicine* 304:784–787.

Wolinsky, F. 1982. Why Physicians Choose Different Types of Practice Settings. *Health Services Research* 17:399–419.

Wolinsky, F., and W. Marder. 1985. *The Organization of Medical Practice and the Practice of Medicine* Ann Arbor, Mich.: Health Administration Press.

Zigler, E., and S. Muenchow. 1984. How to Influence Social Policy Affecting Children and Families. *American Psychologist* 39:415–420.

9

The Role of the Public Sector in Providing Children's Health Care

Lorraine V. Klerman, Dr.P.H., and Kyle L. Grazier, Dr.P.H., with Kathleen C. Thomas, B.A.

Health care provided through the public sector is of crucial importance to children in the United States. Although most infants, children, and adolescents receive their health care from physicians in private settings, those seen by providers in the public sector often have special problems, both medical and social. Many public providers have adapted their services to the needs of these populations. Thus, changes in financial or organizational arrangements which would reduce the number of such providers or the range of services that they offer can have disproportionately large effects on the health of children.[1]

A Definition of the Public Sector

A working definition of the public sector is made difficult by the complex relationships among the institutions that provide care and the public and private programs that finance it. In addition to those facilities that are owned and operated by governmental entities, many nongovernmental facilities, to receive government funding, must meet certain requirements that result in their acting in the public interest. Thus, the public sector can be defined as encompassing three broad categories of institutions. The first category includes those operated directly by governments. At the federal level, inpatient services are provided by armed services hospitals through the Department of Defense, by veterans' hospitals through the Veterans' Administration, and by Public Health Service and Indian Health Service hospitals through the Department of Health and Human Services. State and local governments (cities and counties) operate acute care facilities, as well as psychiatric, long-term care, and other specialized health care institutions. Outpatient services are often provided by these same facilities; in addition all freestanding health department clinics, school clinics supported by boards of education or health departments, many community mental health centers (CHMCs), and some community or migrant health centers (CHCs)[2] are operated as governmental agencies.

A second category of institutions sometimes included in the public sector are nongovernmental facilities that provide free or low-cost ser-

215

vices because of: (1) stipulations in their charters, as in some church-sponsored hospitals; (2) conditions of a grant, such as those in the Hill-Burton Act (Blumstein, 1986); (3) requirements to maintain their charitable, tax-exempt status under clause 501(c)(3) of the federal internal revenue code; and/or (4) substantial monetary subsidies from government sources. Using this definition, public providers would include all not-for-profit hospitals, virtually all CHCs, and school-based clinics operated by CHCs or other nongovernmental agencies, as well as women's centers and family planning clinics operated by Planned Parenthood and other nonprofit organizations and most CMHCs.

Finally, the most expansive use of the term "public provider" would include all individuals or institutions that obtain a substantial share of their reimbursements from governmental sources. Under this definition, physicians in private practice, investor-owned hospitals, and many for-profit health maintenance organizations (HMOs) would be included, because they receive substantial revenue from Medicaid or Medicare.

Despite the complexities of separating the public from the private sector, this chapter will focus on the first two definitions of public providers. These include inpatient and outpatient facilities owned and operated by federal, state, county, or local governments, plus those private not-for-profit 501(c)(3) organizations that have received or are receiving substantial public subsidies. Only facilities providing preventive services or acute care for physical conditions will be discussed, excluding those that primarily offer mental health or long-term care.

Statistics about the services received by children through the public sector are difficult to obtain. While some information is available about the number of public providers (Table 9.1) and the total number of

Table 9.1 Number of Public Providers

Type of Provider	Number of Facilities		Year
Hospitals*† (federal, state, and local)	1,784		1986
Local health departments*	2,925		1985
Community health centers	580		1986
Migrant health centers	123		1986
Family planning agencies	Agencies	Sites	
Health departments	1,419	2,928	1983
Hospitals	275	377	1983
Planned Parenthood	182	698	1983
Other (community health centers, women's health centers, and community action groups)	586	1,171	1983

Sources: American Hospital Association (1987); Health Resources and Services Administration (1987) (personal communication); Public Health Foundation (1987); and Torres and Forrest (1985).

*Not all of these provide medical care to children and women with fertility-related needs.

†Government-owned general and specialty hospitals.

patients they serve, these are infrequently analyzed by age group or type of service received. Data from a variety of sources suggest, however, that public agencies provide a significant amount of care for children, particularly those with limited incomes.

This is certainly true for inpatient hospital services. For example, 23 percent of all deliveries in 1986 were in government-operated facilities (American Hospital Association, 1986). But more than 35 percent of the hospital admissions for uninsured patients, primarily the poor and near poor, were to these same facilities (Committee on Implication of For-Profit Enterprise in Health Care, 1986).

A similar picture emerges for ambulatory care. Although most national surveys do not distinguish between public and private providers, the magnitude of the "other" category of care indirectly reflects the importance of publicly operated facilities for low-income families. ("Other" places of contact exclude telephone, office, or hospital contacts, but include CHCs, health department, school, and company clinics, and other nonprivate ambulatory care facilities.) Data from the NHIS for 1986 reveal that for all persons under 18 years of age such contacts represented 12.7 percent of all ambulatory care. They were 19.4 percent of all contacts for those with family incomes under $10,000. Hospital contacts in an emergency room, clinic, or doctor's office are also more important for the poor. They represented 13.2 percent of contacts for all persons under 18, but 24.8 percent for those with family incomes under $10,000 (National Center for Health Statistics, 1987).

The National Medical Care Utilization and Expenditure Survey (NMCUES) illustrated the importance of publicly operated clinics for both pregnant women and children. Children under 18 made significant use of these sites of care (Table 9.2). Low-income children, defined as those with incomes below 150 percent of the federal poverty level, were more likely to use health centers, emergency rooms, or hospital clinics than were nonpoor children (Rosenbach, 1985). More fragmentary data

Table 9.2 Percentage of Children with at Least One Visit, by Place of Visit

	Physician's Offices	Health Clinics*	Emergency Rooms	OPDs	Other**
All children	79.8%	19.5%	29.2%	16.3%	9.7%
Low-income children	67.8	28.7	35.2	24.8	10.1
Nonpoor children	83.7	16.5	27.2	13.5	9.6

Source: Rosenbach (1985).

Note: Since some children visited more than one place, the figures add up to more than 100 percent.

*Health clinics include CHCs and school clinics.

**Other includes laboratory and home visits, as well as visits to unspecified places.

are available for specific types of clinics and agencies. In 1984, 23 state health agencies (SHAs) provided physical assessments to 373,700 infants and 22 SHAs to 482,500 preschoolers (Public Health Foundation, 1987).

According to the federal Health Resources and Services Administration, more than 1.9 million persons under age 20 received medical services in 1986 in community health centers supported by federal funds appropriated under Section 330 of the Public Health Service Act. In addition, slightly more than 0.5 million were seen in Migrant Health Centers supported by section 229 funds. (The two figures can not be added, because some of the CHCs also receive funds as Migrant Health Centers [Private communication, Health Resources and Services Administration, 1987].) Surveys in 1983 and 1984 by the National Association of Community Health Centers found that more than 60 percent of all CHC users had family incomes below the federal poverty level, that almost 70 percent were members of minority groups, and that nearly half were uninsured (Rosenbaum, 1986).

The Quality of Services in the Public Sector

The quality of health care is traditionally measured in three ways: structure, process, and outcome (Donabedian, 1988). Remarkably few studies have assessed public providers along any of these three dimensions, and even fewer compared them with private providers. A number of studies have included structural analyses of public providers, including surveys of public providers of family planning, abortion, and other reproductive health services; surveys of state maternal and child health divisions and community/migrant health centers to determine the prenatal and delivery services that they provided (Alan Guttmacher Institute, 1987); and a study of the maternal and pediatric services provided by state maternal and child health divisions (Rosenbaum, Hughes, and Johnson, 1988). But none of these studies included a private comparison group. The Public Health Foundation formerly provided information on the types of services provided by state and local health agencies, but its recent reports are restricted to sources of funding.

The small number of studies that incorporate process or outcome measures suggest that public facilities offer a wider range of services (process) and achieve equal or better outcomes than do private ones, controlling for characteristics of the patient such as ability to pay. Many public facilities offer a variety of services in addition to medical care. These may include casework, nutritional supplementation and counseling, health education, transportation, on-site child care, and outreach. The funding organization often requires that such services be offered as a condition of a grant. For example, the federal Children's Bureau established standards for its Maternal and Infant Care (MIC) and Children and Youth (C&Y) projects, demonstration programs developed in the 1960s. Similarly, community and migrant health centers operate under service requirements established by the Health Services and Resources Administration, and family planning clinics that receive funding under Title X of the Public Health Service Act and adolescent pregnancy programs that receive funding under Title XX of that Act must also provide a specified group of services. State health departments usually establish guidelines for their own facilities or local facilities operated with state funds. Few studies, however, have actually examined these facilities to determine whether they are providing the services mandated by law and/or regulation.

Perhaps the most thorough attempt to compare providers in terms of services offered was commissioned by the Office of Economic Opportunity in the late 1960s in an attempt to determine the quality of care in neighborhood health centers (Morehead, Donaldson and Seravalli, 1971). The records of a sample of obstetric, pediatric, and adult medicine patients were abstracted and scored using a predetermined series of items. In obstetrics, the Children's Bureau MIC Projects scored highest, followed by medical school-affiliated outpatient departments, group practices, and neighborhood health centers. The range, however, was relatively narrow. In pediatrics, the Children's Bureau C&Y Projects again scored the highest, followed, at considerable distance, by health department well-baby clinics, community health centers, group practices, and medical school-affiliated outpatient departments. Reviews of the records of solo practitioners, mostly in rural areas, who cared for similar types of patients on a fee-for-service basis using public funds, revealed ratings considerably lower than those of any other type of provider.

Several studies of prenatal care also suggest that the services provided by public facilities result in better outcomes than those achieved by private providers. Buescher, Smith, Holliday, and Levine (1987) found a lower percentage of low-weight infants among Medicaid patients in the prenatal care program of a large county health department as compared to Medicaid patients served primarily by physicians in private practice. The difference was attributed to a case management approach and greater use of ancillary services such as follow-up, education, and linkage to other programs. An analysis of the National Survey of Family Growth, however, revealed a higher percentage of women with delayed prenatal care among patients of clinics than among those of private facilities, even controlling independently for age, insurance, and education (Fingerhut, Makuc and Kleinman, 1987). A study of sources of prescription contraceptives among young women initially suggested that those who obtained their first prescription method from a clinic were at higher risk of a pregnancy after 24 months than those who received it from a private physician. When socioeconomic status, race, and prior contraceptive use were considered, source became insignificant (Zelnik, Koenig and Kim, 1984).

The limited number and scope of these studies highlights the need for additional research. But they suggest that public providers are generally at least comparable to their private counterparts; their range of services and measured outcomes equal or exceed those from private providers, when the composition of the patient group is held constant.

A Brief History of the Financing and Organization of Children's Services

The current system of provision of care to children in the public sector has its roots in early American history, though it was significantly shaped by several of the Great Society initiatives of the 1960s.

In colonial America, almshouses provided care to the indigent, including those who were sick. Children were also housed in these facilities, because their parents were there, because they were orphans, or because no other facility would care for their conditions, including infectious diseases, epilepsy, blindness, and retardation. These almshouses, supported by city and county governments, became the first public hospitals and, in that capacity, continued to treat sick children and those physically, mentally, and educationally handicapped. Philadelphia General Hospital, for example, opened in 1732 as the Philadelphia almshouse.

In some areas, the sick poor were cared for through grants to voluntary hospitals instead of or in addition to services at governmental hospitals. By the early twentieth century, states and local governments had begun to reimburse voluntary hospitals on a per diem basis for the care of the indigent. This contractual agreement was very different from the public hospital's obligation to accept any patient who could not receive care elsewhere (Cone, 1979; Rosenberg, 1982; Stevens, 1982).

Public responsibility within the voluntary sector was emphasized in the Hospital Survey and Construction (Hill-Burton) Act, passed in 1946, which provided funds for the construction of hospitals and later health centers. Facilities built with these funds had the obligation to: (1) serve all persons residing in the facility's service area without discrimination (the community service assurance); and (2) provide a "reasonable volume of services" to persons unable to pay (the uncompensated acre assurance). Unfortunately these assurances were ignored until 1972 and definitive rules were published only in 1979 (Fiori, 1980). In 1986, 4,400 health facilities still had uncompensated services obligations, though the extent to which they are honored is a matter of continued debate (Blumstein, 1986; Dowell, 1987).

The differentiation of health services specifically for children began at the federal level in 1921 with the federal Maternity and Infancy (Sheppard-Towner) Act, a state-federal partnership to provide services to pregnant women and children. Although this act was allowed to die in 1929, its principles were incorporated into Title V of the Social Security Act in 1935. As a result of these two acts, all states developed maternal and child health divisions within their state health departments and many began to operate or finance specialized clinics for pregnant women, well infants and children, and "crippled children." Such services were provided directly by or, more often, through the support of, local health departments. In the 1960s, the Title V program was authorized to distribute grants to agencies and facilities that could demonstrate, in areas of high need, the provision of exemplary care to mothers and infants, the Maternity and Infant Care (MIC) projects, and to children and youth, the Children and Youth (C&Y) projects.

Beginning in 1965, neighborhood health centers were established by the Office of Economic Opportunity (OEO) in economically deprived areas. The Public Health Service began funding community health centers (CHCs) in 1968 and in 1973 absorbed the OEO centers, along with migrant and other specialized centers. From their inception, these centers were mandated to provide services to children and pregnant women either directly or by referral. It is estimated that more than 35 percent of CHC patients are children under 14 years of age and 30 percent are women of child-bearing age (Rosenbaum, 1986).

CHCs and similar centers were expected to receive a major portion of their funding from Medicaid. Medicaid funding, however, has not proven to be a particularly reliable financial base for these agencies. First, although the CHCs are located in poverty areas, not all of their patients are eligible for Medicaid. CHC patients include the working poor whose incomes are slightly above the poverty level and others categorically ineligible for Medicaid despite the fact that their incomes are below the poverty line. Second, in some states Medicaid reimbursement levels are often below costs and do not cover certain services, such as outreach programs or certain personnel, such as physician's associates. And, third, some states still do not cover services in freestanding clinics and thus the CHCs must be reimbursed through direct billing by eligible providers.

The Impact of Policy Changes since 1980

The deliberations of the Select Panel for the Promotion of Child Health at the turn of the decade (1981) reflected a belief that federal and state governments were prepared to continue and increase support for services that could improve child health. The election of a Republican president, however, brought to Washington radically different ideas about the appropriate role of government. Consequently, only a few of the recommendations of the Select Panel were implemented; primarily those providing greater discretion to states in their use of federal funds (Haskins, 1983).

Four major initiatives of the Reagan administration affected the public sector. These included reductions in eligibility for AFDC, which cut the number of families eligible for Medicaid and squeezed a major source of financing for many public agencies; the development of block grants, which changed the balance of federal responsibility between federal and state governments; reductions in appropriations for some public providers, directly through appropriations and indirectly through Medicaid-eligibility restrictions; and changes in reimbursement mechanisms that reduced the ability of providers to shift to the insured the costs of caring for the uninsured.

Uncertainty about the implications of these changes led to an early prediction that "on the one hand, states could develop innovative programs for delivery of services to the indigent and might correct many current inequities. On the other hand, the simultaneous reduction of federal direction and funding could worsen existing inequities among states and undercut much of the progress of recent years" (Budetti, Butler and McManus, 1982). Both forecasts proved correct.

State reaction to federal initiatives did have an important impact on the public sector. Several states used the discretion provided by the block grants to increase funds to some programs while decreasing to others. For example, under the Social Services Block Grant many states increased their spending on child and adult protective services and adoption/foster care while reducing day care and family planning. Services to handicapped children previously provided under Title V's Crippled Children's Service (CCS) programs were not affected, however, because of the political strength of the parents' constituency (General Accounting Office, 1984; Peterson, 1984). Other states obtained authorization to restrict Medicaid-eligible families to private sector organizations such as HMOs, further reducing sources of revenue available to public providers.

Federal funding reductions were also offset, to some extent, by increased state funding and increased revenue from other sources for public and private nonprofit agencies (Peterson, 1984; Salamon, 1984). Nevertheless, these reductions had a measurable impact on public providers of health care. This was particularly noticeable among hospitals, which were already experiencing a secular decline in utilization.

Hospital Inpatient Units

A study of hospitals in the nation's 46 largest cities found that several services of considerable importance to children were associated with hospital deficits. These included organized outpatient departments, family planning services, premature infant nurseries, neonatal intensive care units, genetic counseling, burn care units, and social work. Public hospitals comprised less than 2 percent of the hospitals with surpluses and almost one-fifth of those with deficits (Hadley, Mullner and Feder, 1982).

Uncompensated care, defined as charity care and bad debts, is a particular problem for public and not-for-profit hospitals. Community hospitals provided $6.2 billion in uncompensated care in 1982. More than one-third (34.6 percent) was provided by public hospitals. Certain types of cases were more likely to be classified as self-pay or no charge. These included several involving children: nonsurgical deliveries, newborns, and those who had surgery on the day they were admitted (Sloan, Valvona and Mullner, 1986). Perrin (1986) noted that cases requiring high technology care were often uncompensated. This was particularly true for three conditions often found among the young: neonatal intensive care and care for victims of motor vehicle accidents and blood-related cancers.

Increased deficits in public hospitals were also due in part to patient "dumping," as private facilities transferred patients without insurance coverage to public facilities. This threatened the health of the patients, many of whom were women and children, as well as the financial viability of public facilities (Reed, Cawley and Anderson, 1986; Schiff, et. al., 1986).

To stay financially sound, public hospitals rationed care by requiring payments for nonemergency patients, reducing the availability of outpatient services, and refusing transfers from not-for-profit hospitals that were based on inability to pay (Feder, Hadley and Mullner, 1984). By 1982, one out of every five public hospitals had adopted explicit limits on the amount of charity care that it would provide (Sloan, Valvona and Mullner, 1986).

Closures were another adaptation to financial and other problems, with those hospitals serving the poor being particularly vulnerable. Sager (1983) found that between 1937 and 1980 the proportion of short-term beds under nonfederal public control declined from one-third to one-seventh. The hospitals that closed were more likely to be located in minority neighborhoods, to serve above-average proportions of minority or Medicaid-funded patients, to be small, and not to have teaching programs. The hospitals that remained open were the more expensive, larger teaching institutions.

Between 1976 and 1980, 296 hospitals closed. Of the 226 community hospitals that closed, 16 percent were public; more than one-third, not-for-profit; and almost half, for profit (Mullner, Byre and Kubal, 1983). In contrast, of the 340 hospitals that closed between 1980 and 1985, almost one-third were governmentally operated. Again, smaller hospitals were more likely to close than larger ones (Mullner, 1986). Recent research indicates that public hospital closings significantly reduce access to care for uninsured patients (Thorpe and Brecher, 1987).

The reduction in public capacity to treat patients was in some cases masked by transfers of ownership. A 1986 GAO study of nine public hospitals that recently had been sold or leased revealed that despite specific or general provisions regarding the new operators' responsibilities for the care of the indigent, one hospital had clearly decreased admissions of the indigent and the costs of service to this group. The other hospitals did not maintain records of the indigent care provided and the local governments did not monitor compliance (Government Accounting Office, 1986).

Several data sets were examined by the authors to determine whether the problems faced by the public hospitals had affected their capacity to serve children and women with fertility-related needs. Between 1980 and 1986 the number of live births rose fairly steadily from 3.61 million to 3.73 million, an increase of 3.29 percent. In contrast, obstetric units in state and local government-owned hospitals decreased, as did the number of beds. At a time when the proportion of Americans living in poverty and without private health insurance was increasing (Chapter 5), this decline almost assuredly limited access to services.

Statistics for pediatric care follow a similar pattern. Between 1980 and 1986 the number of discharges from nonfederal, short-stay hospitals for children under 15 years (excluding newborn infants) dropped from 3,672 to 2,783, a decline of 24.21 percent (National Center for Health Statistics, 1982, 1987). The total number of pediatric beds decreased from 56,484 to 49,523, a decline of 12.32 percent. Pediatric units in state and local government-owned hospitals decreased, as did pediatric beds. The same was true for pediatric units and beds in the not-for-profit sector, although the decrease was not as marked. In contrast, the for-profit sector experienced an increase in pediatric units and in pediatric beds. The trends in pediatric intensive care units, neonatal intermediate care units, and neonatal intensive care units are shown in Table 9.3.

Table 9.3 Pediatric Facilities by Sponsorship, 1980–1986

Hospitals, Units, and Beds	1980	1981	1982	1983	1984	1985	1986	Change 1980–1986 #	Change 1980–1986 %
Total Nonfederal, Short-term General, and Other Special Hospitals									
Pediatrics (general)									
Hospitals									
Number	50	57	48	46	46	45	40	−10	−20.00
Beds	5,565	5,217	5,333	5,199	5,031	5,100	4,581	−984	−17.68
Units									
Number	2,715	2,678	2,722	2,713	2,673	2,631	2,562	−153	−5.64
Beds	50,919	50,387	50,141	49,018	47,662	45,289	44,942	−5977	−11.74
Total Pediatric Beds	**56,484**	**55,604**	**55,474**	**54,217**	**52,693**	**50,389**	**49,523**	**−6961**	**−12.32**
Pediatric intensive care									
Units	206	224	236	265	273	272	298	+92	+44.66
Beds	1,613	1,810	1,777	1,983	2,031	2,081	2,515	+902	+55.92
Neonatal intermediate care									
Units	138	172	188	234	255	280	323	+185	+134.06
Beds	1,680	2,117	2,326	2,783	3,107	3,260	3,715	+2035	+121.13
Neonatal intensive care									
Units	401	438	476	528	557	578	596	+195	+48.63
Beds	6,079	6,433	7,294	7,901	8,701	9,033	9,603	+3524	+57.77
State and Local Government									
Pediatrics (general)									
Hospitals									
Number	1	1	0	0	0	0	0	−1	−100
Beds	139	139	0	0	0	0	0	−139	−100
Units									
Number	657	637	629	618	588	575	548	−109	−16.59
Beds	10,917	10,820	10,751	10,157	9,693	8,838	8,706	−2211	−20.25
Total Pediatric Beds	**11,056**	**10,959**	**10,751**	**10,157**	**9,693**	**8,838**	**8,706**	**−2350**	**−21.26**

Table 9.3 (Continued)

Hospitals, Units, and Beds	1980	1981	1982	1983	1984	1985	1986	Change 1980–1986 #	Change 1980–1986 %
Pediatric intensive care									
Units	63	65	64	73	72	71	70	+7	+11.11
Beds	438	435	418	458	465	469	478	+40	+9.13
Neonatal intermediate care									
Units	39	46	47	57	57	55	76	+37	+94.87
Beds	500	718	784	887	928	832	1,245	+745	+149.00
Neonatal intensive care									
Units	95	191	111	117	120	116	113	+18	+18.95
Beds	1,474	1,570	1,800	1,842	2,017	1,918	2,013	+539	+36.57
Nongovernment Not-for-Profit									
Pediatrics (general)									
Hospitals									
Number	48	45	47	46	46	45	40	−8	−16.67
Beds	5,362	5,014	5,269	5,199	5,031	5,100	4,581	−781	−14.57
Units									
Number	1,904	1,896	1,925	1,920	1,907	1,893	1,826	−78	−4.10
Beds	37,888	37,617	37,305	36,640	35,598	34,258	33,601	−4287	−11.31
Total Pediatric Beds	**43,250**	**42,631**	**42,574**	**36,839**	**40,629**	**39,358**	**38,182**	**−5068**	**−11.72**
Pediatric intensive care									
Units	141	158	171	188	198	196	216	75	53.19
Beds	1,166	1,370	1,357	1,509	1,552	1,578	1,968	802	68.78

Neonatal intermediate care									
Units	95	122	138	173	192	214	225	130	136.84
Beds	1,146	1,356	1,510	1,873	2,099	2,316	2,278	1132	98.78
Neonatal intensive care									
Units	297	327	354	397	408	437	448	151	50.84
Beds	4,505	4,755	5,388	5,943	6,380	6,799	7,177	2672	59.31
Investor-owned (For Profit)									
Pediatrics									
Hospitals									
Number	1	1	1	0	0	0	0	−1	−100
Beds	64	64	64	0	0	0	0	−64	−100
Units									
Number	154	145	168	175	178	163	188	34	22.08
Beds	2,114	1,950	2,085	2,221	2,371	2,193	2,635	521	24.65
Total Pediatric Beds	**2,178**	**1,014**	**2,149**	**2,221**	**2,371**	**2,193**	**2,635**	**457**	**20.98**
Pediatric intensive care									
Units	2	1	1	4	3	5	12	10	500.00
Beds	9	5	2	16	14	34	72	63	700.00
Neonatal intermediate care									
Units	4	4	3	4	6	11	22	18	450.00
Beds	34	43	32	23	80	112	192	158	464.71
Neonatal intensive care									
Units	9	10	11	14	29	25	35	26	288.89
Beds	100	108	106	116	304	316	413	313	313.00

Sources: American Hospital Association, 1981 through 1987.

Taken together, these data suggest that the capacity to care for deliveries and for pediatric problems is shifting away from the public sector, which must admit all regardless of ability to pay, toward the not-for-profit and for-profit hospitals, which may not believe that they have such obligations.

Maternal and Child Health Services

Before the passage of the Omnibus Budget Reconciliation Act (OBRA) in 1981, Title V of the Social Security Act authorized the federal government to provide funds to states for support of programs in Maternal and Child Health (MCH) and Crippled Children's Services (CCS). These funds were distributed by formulas, after a certain amount had been set aside for use by the federal MCH agency for research, training and demonstration projects. The division of funds between MCH and CCS was established by the federal government. Each state was also required to have a Program of Projects. This was interpreted to mean at least one each of the following projects: MIC, C&Y, Neonatal Intensive Care, Dental Health, and Family Planning. The initiation of the block grant led to a significant redistribution of funds among public providers.

OBRA consolidated the following programs into the Maternal and Child Health Services (MCHS) Block Grant: MCH, CCS, lead-based paint poisoning prevention, Sudden Infant Death Syndrome (SIDS), adolescent pregnancy, genetic disease testing and counseling, hemophilia diagnostic and treatment centers, and Supplemental Security Income for Disabled Children (SSI-DC). In 1981 these 8 programs had received $455 million. In 1982 Congress appropriated $373.75 million for the MCHS Block Grant, an 18 percent reduction. Fortunately, funding for the Block Grant was increased by more than $1 million in 1983 through the emergency "Jobs Bill." In 1987 it received $478 million. It still, however, had not reached the 1970s levels in constant dollars.

The Children's Defense Fund (CDF) conducted a survey to determine the impact of OBRA on MCH programs in the states during 1982. Forty-nine states and the District of Columbia responded, and 47 reported cutbacks in their Title V programs through reductions in eligibility and/or health services. Forty-four reduced prenatal and delivery services for pregnant women and primary and preventive services for women of childbearing ages, infants, and children; 27 reduced their CCS program; and 37 reduced or eliminated services offered under the Program of Projects, most often C&Y projects (Rosenbaum and Weitz, undated).

A 1984 CDF publication, *American Children in Poverty,* reported the results of a ten-state study of MIC projects. About 90 percent had experienced a reduction or a freezing of funding levels (an actual decrease when inflation is considered). The agencies' ability to pay for hospitalization or transportation had been severely reduced and patients were being turned away. In some cases, services had been restricted to include only counseling, nutrition, and education, with patients directed to obtain their medical services from private physicians (Children's Defense Fund, 1984).

The GAO (1984) studied the impact of the MCHS Block Grant and the appropriations cuts in 13 states. Between 1981 and 1983 the CCS program was funded at the same or higher levels, with some changes in eligibility requirements and integration with the SSI-DC program; but state support for the Program of Projects and the other programs that had been brought into the grant were reduced. Fortunately, funding for the adolescent pregnancy, hemophilia, and genetic services programs continued from the federal set-aside fund.

In 1985 Kimmich reviewed several Urban Institute studies of the impact of the Reagan administration changes. Based on an 18-state study, she confirmed early findings that the states had not made major changes in their Title V program in the first post-OBRA year because of the presence of carry-over funds. By FY 1983, however, many states began to use their newfound freedom to reassess existing programs. As a result there were changes in both the geographic distribution of funds and in the distribution of funds across service categories. Changes included modifications of existing formulas for distribution to counties, providing funds to counties that had not previously received them, shifting funds to nonmetropolitan counties, and developing new methods of assessing need that were then reflected in the distribution of funds. Across service categories, the traditional MCH and CCS programs received equal or greater dollars in 1983 than in 1981. The smaller categorical programs that had been consolidated into the MCHS Block Grant tended to lose ground. These included programs for lead-based paint poisoning, adolescent pregnancy, and sudden infant death syndrome (Kimmich, 1985).

The data collected by the Public Health Foundation were examined to determine whether these programmatic changes affected the number of individuals receiving services from state and local health departments whose MCH and CCS programs were largely supported by Title V. Unfortunately, year-to-year changes in definitions of services and in the states reporting make national comparisons quite difficult. The users of health department services as a percentage of total births declined from 13.2 percent in 1981 to 9.5 percent in 1983 (Table 9.4). It is difficult to draw conclusions from these data, however, since several states with large numbers of births were excluded because they failed to report in one of the two years.

Table 9.4 Users of State Health Department Maternity Services and Live Births by Selected States, 1981 and 1984

State	Users of Maternity Services in 1981	Users of Maternity Services in 1984	Births in 1981	Births in 1984
Alabama	17,231	18,648	61,554	59,217
Arkansas	13,701	7,758	35,807	34,840
Colorado	4,236	2,857	52,103	54,364
Connecticut	570	4,500	39,919	42,220
Delaware	420	535	9,184	9,266
Florida	37,767	4,100	138,490	155,397
Georgia	17,680	25,396	89,943	92,013
Hawaii	252	176	18,214	18,707
Idaho	643	506	19,623	18,028
Indiana	2,708	4,234	84,645	80,084
Iowa	1,772	3,242	45,928	42,367
Kansas	1,210	1,350	41,246	40,010
Kentucky	14,550	11,570	57,243	53,290
Louisiana	21,816	23,208	82,234	81,472
Massachusetts	1,887	4,800	74,025	78,279
Michigan	2,000	1,909	140,693	136,076
Missouri	4,751	3,336	76,964	74,736
New Hampshire	425	689	13,517	14,250
New Jersey	9,718	10,633	96,651	101,334
New Mexico	4,226	2,780	28,262	27,373
North Carolina	26,685	25,544	83,774	86,042
Ohio	13,409	3,262	167,055	158,519
Oklahoma	14,974	3,482	53,668	54,477
Oregon	1,719	3,757	43,020	39,563
Pennsylvania	1,583	18,119	160,428	157,110
Rhode Island	1,030	2,703	12,448	12,659
Tennessee	4,900	12,058	67,081	65,006
Texas	45,066	3,962	281,651	299,025
Utah	3,657	642	41,343	38,299
Washington	19,375	923	69,714	68,927
West Virginia	1,445	3,729	27,842	24,585
Totals	291,406	210,408	2,214,271	2,217,535

Users of Services as a % of births in 1981 = 13.16%
Users of Services as a % of births in 1984 = 9.49%

Sources: Association of State and Territorial Health Officials (1983); Public Health Foundation (1987); National Center for Health Statistics (1983); and National Center for Health Statistics (1986).

Community and Migrant Health Centers

Before the Reagan years, the number of CHCs and the federal appropriations for their support had grown steadily since their inception in 1965. In the last pre-OBRA year, CHCs (exclusive of migrant health centers) received $322 million. The 1982 appropriation, however, was less than $300 million, a reduction of almost 13 percent in nominal dollars and of 18 percent adjusted for inflation. In 1983 Congress replaced the lost funds through the Jobs Bill appropriation and funds in nominal dollars continued to increase until Gramm-Rudman led to further reductions.

During 1982 the Administration defunded 239, or more than one-quarter, of the 827 operating CHCs (Sardell, 1983). The remaining ones were forced to reduce outreach and other community health services due to reductions in constant dollars in Medicaid and in the National Health Care Services Corps, which provided many health care professionals to the centers. The number of centers has grown slightly since 1982 but has not reached pre-OBRA levels.[3]

Despite the claims of CDF and others that the closing of the centers affected thousands of women and children (Rosenbaum and Weitz, undated), data collected by the Human Resources and Services Administration indicate that the fluctuations in funding levels was not accompanied by a decrease in the number of children served by CHCs and migrant health centers. These, in fact, increased between 1981 and 1986, perhaps as a result of uncompensated cases being refused care at other sites.

The National Association of Community Health Centers reports, however, that the increase in the number of patients has not been accompanied by an increase in overall revenues, since almost all the new patients have been uncompensated cases. The association also reported that the comprehensiveness of CHC programs has been reduced, with health education, mental health, nutrition, outreach, and transportation services being particularly vulnerable to cuts. These specialized services are particularly important for the increased numbers of Southeast Asians and Haitians who are enrolling. Waiting time for nonurgent cases may be as long as three weeks and waiting lists have been created for new registrants (Hawkins, personal communication).

Trends in the Health Care System: The Future of Public Providers of Services to Children

Several ongoing changes in the health care system are likely to limit further the ability of public facilities to provide adequate care to children.

Increases in Uncompensated Cases

One set of trends will reduce the number of paying patients that come to public facilities and increase the number of uninsured patients who seek care at such facilities. These trends include increased enrollment of Medicaid-eligible populations in managed care systems, reduction in the number of private facilities with Hill-Burton obligations to treat the indigent, and continued purchase of not-for-profit hospitals by private investors.

The trend toward managed care for Medicaid and other welfare patients could significantly reduce the number of patients with third-party coverage being served by the public sector. State welfare departments are increasingly enrolling Medicaid patients in Health Maintenance or Preferred Provider Organizations. This draws an important source of revenues away from public providers. There is nothing to prevent welfare departments from enrolling Medicaid eligibles in public sector institutions, such as hospital OPDS, health department clinics, and CHCs; and some do. Managed care systems, however, should be able to provide comprehensive services and twenty-four hour coverage. Although public hospitals can meet these standards, most CHCs and health department clinics cannot without developing new service networks.

Public providers have not been aggressive in developing the arrangements that would enable them to bid successfully for such managed care contracts. Where they have been included, public facilities ran the risk of being "squeezed" by rates negotiated with HMOs, or of receiving inadequate revenues as a result of unanticipated problems in the enrollment process (Brecher, 1984; Anderson and Fox, 1987).

At the same time, public facilities are likely to face a growing influx of uninsured patients. The Hill-Burton Act obligated the facilities built under its provisions to provide a "reasonable volume" of uncompensated care for twenty years only. Each year more hospitals reach this limit and no longer have this obligation. These hospitals may shift uncompensated cases to the public sector. In addition, as nonprofit hospitals are increasingly purchased by private investors or hospital chains, the number of uncompensated care cases admitted will be reduced, regardless of agreements to the contrary with city or county governments or Hill-Burton obligations (Government Accounting Office, 1986; Schlesinger, Bentkover, and Blumenthal, 1986; Lewin, Eckels and Miller, 1988). Almost invariably, these cases will be shifted to the public sector.

Decrease in Other Forms of Support

As the ratio of patients whose charges are covered by third parties to uncompensated cases declines, the public providers may become more dependent on grants and other forms of direct subsidy to maintain services. A second set of trends will affect public providers more directly through reductions in grant and other forms of direct support, expansion of the prospective payment system (DRGs) to all payors, and the shifting of funds to serve an increasing number of AIDS cases.

Health departments, CHCs, and family planning clinics are dependent on federal and state grants for support. Few experts expected these facilities to become entirely self-sufficient, although the advent of Medicaid and Medicare was anticipated to reduce greatly their dependence on grant support, particularly the CHCs. Data presented earlier indicated that federal support for these programs has not kept pace with inflation. Unless third-party payments increase markedly, these facilities will begin to shrink in number and in scope. Plans for containing the federal budget deficit may further threaten the fiscal stability of public institutions.

A second source of concern involves changes in reimbursement. In the past, public facilities, particularly inpatient services, have been able to cover some of the costs incurred by individuals who did not have third-party coverage and who could not pay out of pocket by cost-shifting, i.e., by increasing charges to those covered by third parties to include the costs of those who were not. The advent of Medicare's prospective payment system based on DRGs made this more difficult. As case-based systems of payment are expanded to include payors in addition to Medicare, cost-shifting from patient to patient or from payor to payor will become increasingly difficult. Hospitals will have to seek other sources of payment for uncompensated cases, particularly in those states without provisions for charity care in their rate-setting program.

Finally, the rising number of AIDS cases is increasing the burden carried by public providers. Roughly one-quarter of all AIDS patients are uninsured, and more than half are covered by Medicaid (Andrulis et al., 1987). By the early 1990s, the costs of caring for these patients alone will exceed $5 billion a year (Iglehart, Read and Wells, 1987). This is 15 percent of the current budget of all government-operated short-term general hospitals (American Hospital Association, 1987). But the burden on some public hospitals will be much worse, since the vast majority of AIDS cases are concentrated in the cities of a relatively small number of states (Andrulis et al., 1987).

Unless funding for AIDS specifically, or public providers generally, is increased substantially, personnel, space, and money currently used for other, less life-threatening conditions will be shifted to the care of AIDS patients. Children will be among those whose care will suffer.

Policy Options

Since 1980, public providers have been under growing budgetary pressures that have led to reductions in the availability of health services to poor and uninsured women and children. To date, these reductions have been fairly modest. But in the absence of changes in public policy, financial pressures will continue to grow and further cutbacks in the public sector are almost inevitable. Thus, it is timely and important to reconsider the historical role of public providers of children's health care.

Many policy analysts have examined the problems faced by providers, particularly hospitals, due to the growing volume of uncompensated care and a number of states have already taken action to try to ensure continued access to health services. But few analysts or state policy makers have thoroughly examined options for the public sector as a whole.

Three broad strategies appear available to policy makers: bring all individuals into the medical care system operated by the private sector and close all public sector facilities; bring most individuals into the medical care system operated by the private sector but maintain a few public facilities to care for those to whom the private sector will not or can not provide care; or allow individuals to choose between public or private facilities.

Complete Privatization

Theoretically it should be possible to develop a single private system of medical care that would serve both the poor and the nonpoor. Financing could be provided through either a universal or a national health insurance program or through a continuation of the current multiplan private insurance system, with governments subsidizing the premiums for those unable to pay their own. Given the increasing number of physicians, it might be possible to absorb into the private system all the individuals now being seen in public facilities, even those in rural and ghetto areas.

Practically, this option seems unlikely, primarily because of the absence of a national commitment to pay for universal health care coverage. Even if such a commitment did exist, it is unlikely that private providers would be unwilling to see all patients. Some of those covered by insurance would still be unprofitable to treat (because their care costs more than the reimbursement), with the specific financially undesirable groups depending on the type of prospective payment system. If providers are paid by the episode of care, unprofitable patients will be those with complex conditions that require extended care. If providers are paid a flat amount each year, the unprofitable patients will be those with chronic illnesses that require repeated treatment.

Private providers could be required to treat all patients who seek care. But this would be difficult to enforce and providers would almost inevitably provide lower quality care to patients whom they considered less desirable.

Nor is it clear that patients could be successfully channeled to private providers whom the patients judge ill-equipped to meet their needs. Experience suggests that forcing patients to seek care at facilities other than those they prefer is difficult, as demonstrated by the problems encountered by the Municipal Health Services Program (Ginzberg and Ostow, 1985).

A Limited Public Sector

Present trends could be allowed to continue unchecked, with consequent reductions in the capacity of public providers. Under this model, the private sector would be encouraged to draw into its fold as many as possible of the individuals who were previously served by the public sector. Attempts could be made to increase enrollment in private insurance through multiple employer trusts (Lewin and Lewin, 1984), regulations requiring coverage of dependents, and similar mechanisms. In addition, many if not all Medicaid recipients could be shifted into the private sector; with some expansion of Medicaid coverage to include the unemployed or the employed-uninsured.

In the absence of comprehensive health insurance enrollment, some patients would still lack the ability to pay for care and require access to public facilities. Others would be unprofitable for private providers to treat, even if they had health insurance. To serve both these groups, appropriations would continue to be essential for the support of public facilities. The scope of the public sector would be limited to the size required to treat those who were unable to obtain care elsewhere, primarily those with no form of third-party coverage.

Although somewhat more realistic than proposals that call for complete privatization, this approach has one very serious flaw. By strictly segregating the insured population in private facilities from the uninsured in public agencies, quality in public facilities would almost inevitably degrade over time. It would prove difficult to attract providers to work in public settings. The uninsured, disproportionately those with limited education and financial resources, would be relatively less capable of identifying and complaining about care of inadequate quality. They also would lack the political power to ensure that public agencies remained adequately funded. Indeed, it was exactly this set of concerns that led Congress to require that all HMOs that enrolled Medicare or Medicaid patients draw at least half of their members from those with private insurance (Brown, 1983).

A Balanced Dual System

A third possibility is to restore the fading vitality of the public sector. Public providers would care for: (1) those who had no choice, i.e., who could not pay out-of-pocket and did not have third-party coverage; (2) those who lived in areas not served by private providers, such as rural areas or inner-city ghettos; and (3) those who preferred public facilities. Public providers might be preferred because they offered services not usually available in the private sector, such as counseling, interpreters, nutritional education, child care, and transportation; or in the case of facilities such as CHCs, because they were more responsive to community problems. (CHC boards of directors usually include community representatives and their staff members and directors are more willing to accept responsibility for health-related community problems.) Part of the revised mission for the public sector would include active outreach efforts to bring into the system those who did not realize that they needed services, those who did not know where to locate services, and those who were unable to overcome the barriers that they perceived limited their access.

Under such a system the public providers would be partially supported by third-party payments, but would expect to receive a large portion of their income from governmental grants, pooling approaches, or other sources not based on fee-for-service. Since individuals with third-party coverage could receive care through either the public or the private system, public facilities would have more heterogeneous patient populations. Although most of those with third-party coverage would probably choose the private sector, the two systems would not be totally segregated. This should serve to maintain quality and to attract physicians and other health care providers.

This is the option preferred by the authors of this chapter. To achieve such a dual, nonsegregated system, it will be necessary to stabilize existing public providers and to expand their numbers and scope where necessary. Actions that would assist such a process include the development of a system for assessing and planning the services needed by children in each community. Market forces may limit duplication of services in the private sector, but without a well-developed planning function within the public sector, duplication could develop and has in the past. A state-level agency could be made responsible for assessing the need for public service facilities and allocating resources on this basis, even if facilities were actually operated by local government (Mullan, 1987). The state Title V agency might be assigned this task, if its staff and advisory group could be convinced to address the full range of maternal and child health needs, not just those traditionally funded or provided by Title V.

The role of this new agency would involve several tasks. The first would be the development of state regulations mandating that high-risk populations receive a certain package of benefits, such as nutrition, health education, and home visiting. States should be given the ability to circumvent current ERISA restrictions and require that all private insurers cover these benefits. Since such services have traditionally been offered almost exclusively in the public sector, this would disproportionately benefit public providers and might encourage more patients to seek care from them. Such requirements would also ensure that the public system had the fiscal capacity to provide the level of care needed by high-risk populations.

The second charge would be to establish or negotiate more appropriate provider payments. Reimbursement of public providers should be at a level higher than that of most private providers. This would recognize that the public providers' population is probably sicker and often needs more services. It would also recompense the public providers for a variety of nonreimbursable activities, such as casefinding and environmental advocacy. Medicare's prospective payment system already recognizes this need in its "disproportionate share" hospitals.

Finally, the coordinating agency should encourage welfare departments to contract with public providers for the care of Medicaid and other welfare-dependent populations. Many public providers do not have the capability to design managed care or capitation systems and thus the contracts are given to private sector providers, who in many cases can not provide as full a range of services as the public sector. If a policy decision was made to encourage the continued existence of public providers, welfare departments could provide technical assistance to such providers to assist them in developing managed care plans including comprehensive services and twenty-four hour coverage.

Even with these initiatives, public sector facilities might need increased subsidization. The distribution of these subsidies should be tied to the planning process described above. The subsidization could take the form of: (1) federal grants, through Title V for maternal and child health clinics operated by health departments, Title X for family planning facilities, and Sections 330 and 329 for community and migrant health centers; (2) direct state and local appropriations to support public facilities; and (3) indigent care pools with the funds coming from a surcharge on hospital revenues and/or from insurers.

Whether in the long run such a dual system would actually be more expensive than a single system or a segregated one is questionable. Such a system might, through more aggressive outreach, be able to provide more preventive care, to bring sick patients into care earlier, and treat them more successfully than the current system and thus, in the long run, prove less expensive.

Final Thoughts

The country is facing a crisis in regard to the provision of health care to the poor, many of whom are children. Reinhardt (1985) noted that:

> the currently emerging problems in American health care are not driven by a scarcity of resources, but by uncertainty over what constitutes a "just" distribution of plentiful resources among members of society. These problems are a product of the nation's soul. As a nation, we seem unable to decide whether access to acutely needed health care is a citizen's basic right, or whether there merely exists an unenforceable moral obligation on the part of providers to render such care. Indeed, we have not even been able to decide just what level of government should define whatever rights there might be to health care in America.

As a country we must first decide that health care for children is a right. Then we should move to develop an approach to implementing that commitment.

Notes

1. For purposes of brevity, this chapter will use the word "children" to refer to infants, children, and adolescents.
2. Unless Migrant Health Centers are specifically cited, the abbreviation CHC will be used to include both Community and Migrant Health Centers.
3. The Sardell figures, including her citation of a 25 percent funding cut, do not agree with the figures provided by the Health Resources and Services Administration even when the Migrant Health Centers are added to the CHCs, suggesting differences in definitions.

References

Alan Guttmacher Institute. 1987. *The Financing of Maternity Care in the United States*. New York.
American Hospital Association. 1981. *Hospital Statistics*. Chicago.
———. 1982. *Hospital Statistics*. Chicago.
———. 1983. *Hospital Statistics*. Chicago.
———. 1984. *Hospital Statistics*. Chicago.
———. 1985. *Hospital Statistics*. Chicago.
———. 1986. *Hospital Statistics*. Chicago.
———. 1987. *Hospital Statistics*. Chicago.
Anderson, M., and P. Fox. 1987. Lessons from Medicaid Managed Care. *Health Affairs* 6(1):71–86.
Andrulis, D., V.S. Beers, J.D. Bentley, and L.S. Gage. 1987. State Medicaid Policies and Hospital Care for AIDS Patients. *Health Affairs* 6(4):110–118.
Association of State and Territorial Health Officials. 1983. Selected Title V Maternal and Child Health Services 1981. Kensington, Md.

Aved, B.M., and V. Harp. 1983. Assessing the Impact of Copayment on Family Planning Services: A Preliminary Analysis in California. *American Journal of Public Health* 73:763–765.

Blumstein, J. 1986. Providing Hospital Care to Indigent Patients: Hill-Burton as a Case Study and a Paradigm. In F.A. Sloan, J.F. Blumstein, and J.M. Perrin (eds.), *Uncompensated Hospital Care: Rights and Responsibilities*, pp. 94–107. Baltimore: Johns Hopkins University Press.

Brecher, C. 1984. Medicaid Comes to Arizona: A First-Year Report on AHCCCS. *Journal of Health Politics, Policy, and Law* 9(3):411–425.

Brown, Lawrence D. 1983. *Politics and Health Care Organization HMOs as Federal Policy*. Washington, D.C.: Brookings Institution.

Buescher, P.A., C. Smith, A.L. Holliday, and R.H. Levine. 1987. Source of Prenatal Care and Infant Birthweight: The Case of a North Carolina County. *American Journal of Obstetrics and Gynecology* 156:204–210.

Budetti, P.P., J. Butler, and P. McManus. 1982. Federal Health Program Reforms: Implications for Child Health Care. *Milbank Memorial Fund Quarterly* 60:155–181.

Children's Defense Fund. 1984. *American Children in Poverty*. Washington, D.C.

Committee on Implication of For-Profit Enterprise in Health Care. 1986. *For-Profit Enterprise in Health Care*, ed. B. Gray. Washington, D.C.: National Academy Press.

Cone, T.E., Jr. 1979. *History of American Pediatrics*. Boston: Little, Brown.

Donabedian, A. 1988. The Quality of Care: How Can It be Assessed? *Journal of the American Medical Association* 260:1743–1748.

Dowell, M. 1987. Hill-Burton: The Unfulfilled Promise. *Journal of Health Politics, Policy, and Law* 12(1):153–176.

Feder, J., J. Hadley, and R.M. Mullner. 1984. Falling through the Cracks: Poverty, Insurance Coverage, and Hospitals' Care to the Poor, 1980 and 1982. *Health and Society* 62:544–566.

Fingerhut, L.A., D. Makuc, and J.C. Kleinman. 1987. Delayed Prenatal Care and Place of First Visit: Difference by Health Insurance and Education. *Family Planning Perspectives* 19:212–234.

Fiori, F.B. 1980. Bureau of Health Facilities Increasing Responsibilities in Assuring Medical Care for the Needy and Services without Discrimination. *Public Health Reports* 95:164–173.

General Accounting Office. 1984. *Maternal and Child Health Block Grant: Program Changes Emerging Under State Administration*. GAO/HRD-84-35. Washington, D.C.: G.P.O.

―――. 1986. *Public Hospitals: Sales Lead to Better Facilities but Increased Patient Costs*. GAO/HRD-86-60. Washington, D.C.: G.P.O.

―――. 1987. *Prenatal Care: Medicaid Recipients and Uninsured Women Obtain Insufficient Care*. GAO/HRD-87-137. Washington, D.C.: G.P.O.

Ginzburg, E., and M. Ostow. 1985. The Community Health Care Center: Current Status and Future Directions. *Journal of Health Politics, Policy, and Law* 10:283–298.

Gold, R.B., and J. Macias. 1986. Public Funding of Contraceptive, Sterilization and Abortion Services, 1985. *Family Planning Perspectives* 18:259–264.

Gold, R.B., and B. Nestor. 1985. Public Funding of Contraceptive, Sterilization and Abortion Services, 1983. *Family Planning Perspectives* 17:25–30.

Hadley, J., R. Mullner, and J. Feder. 1982. The Financially Distressed Hospital. *New England Journal of Medicine* 307:1283–1287.

Haskins, R. (ed.). 1983. *Child Health Policy in an Age of Fiscal Austerity: Critiques*

of the Select Panel Report. Norwood, N.J.: ABLEX Publishing Corporation.
Hughes, D., K. Johnson, S. Rosenbaum, J. Simons, and E. Butler. 1988. *The Health of America's Children.* Washington, D.C.: Children's Defense Fund.
Iglehart, J., J.L. Read, and J.A. Wells. 1987, Fall. The Socioeconomic Impact of AIDS on Health Care Systems. *Health Affairs* 6(3):137–147.
Kimmich, M.H. 1985. *America's Children: Who Cares?* Washington, D.C.: Urban Institute.
Kovar, M.G., and L.V. Klerman. 1984. Who Pays How Much for Prenatal Care? Paper presented at the annual meeting of the American Public Health Association.
Leibowitz, A., W.G. Manning, E.B. Keeler, N. Duan, et al. 1985. Effect of Cost-Sharing on the Use of Medical Services By Children: Interim Results from a Randomized Control Trial. *Pediatrics* 75:942–951.
Lewin, L.S., T.J. Eckels, and L.B. Miller. 1988. Setting the Record Straight: The Provision of Uncompensated Care by Not-for-Profit Hospitals. *New England Journal of Medicine* 318:1212–1215.
Lewin, M.E., and L.S. Lewin. 1984. Health Care for the Uninsured. *Business and Health* September:9–14.
Lohr, K., R.H. Brook, C.J. Kamberg, G.A. Goldberg, et al. 1986. Use of Medical Care in the Rand Health Insurance Experiment. *Medical Care* 24(Supplement).
Morehead, M.A., R.S. Donaldson, and M.R. Seravalli. 1971. Comparisons between OEO Neighborhood Health Centers and Other Health Care Providers of Ratings of the Quality of Health Care. *American Journal of Public Health* 61:1294–1306.
Mullan, F. 1987. Rethinking Public Ambulatory Care in America. *New England Journal of Medicine* 316:544–546.
Mullner, R. 1986. Hospital Closures, Mergers, and Consolidations. Paper presented at the Third Annual Meeting of the Association for Health Services Research.
Mullner, R., C.S. Byre, and J.D. Kubal. 1983. Hospital Closure in the United States, 1976–1980: A Descriptive Overview. *Health Services Research* 18:437–450.
National Center for Health Statistics. 1983. Advance Report of Final Natality Statistics, 1981. Monthly Vital Statistics Report 32: Supplement. DHHS Publication No. 84-1120. December 29. Hyattsville, Md.
———. 1986. Advance Report of Final Natality Statistics, 1984. Monthly Vital Statistics Report 32: Supplement. DHHS Publication No. 86-1120. July 18. Hyattsville, Md.
———. 1987. Advance Report of Final Natality Statistics, 1985. Monthly Vital Statistics Report 32: Supplement. DHHS Publication No. 87-1120. Hyattsville, Md.
———. 1987. 1986 Summary: National Hospital Discharge Survey. Advance Data from Vital and Health Statistics, No. 145. DHHS Publication No. 87-1250. September 30. Hyattsville, Md.
———. 1988. Births, Marriages, Divorces, and Deaths for 1987. Monthly Vital Statistics Report 36. DHHS Publication No. 88-1120. March 21. Hyattsville, Md.
National Center for Health Statistics (Dawson, D.A. and P.F. Adams). 1987. Current Estimates from the National Health Interview Survey, United States, 1986. Vital and Health Statistics, Series 10, No. 164. DHHS Publication No. 87-1592. October. Washington, D.C.: G.P.O.
National Center for Health Statistics (Haupt, B.J.). 1982. Utilization of Short-Stay Hospitals: Annual Summary. *Vital and Health Statistics, Series 13, No. 64.* (DHHS Pub. No. [PHS] 82-1725.) March. Washington, D.C.: G.P.O.
Nestor, B. 1982. Public Funding of Contraceptive Services, 1980–1982. *Family Planning Perspectives* 14:198–203.
Nestor, B., and R.B. Gold. 1984. Public Funding of Contraceptive, Sterilization and

Abortion Services, 1982. *Family Planning Perspectives* 16:128–133.
Perrin, J.M. 1986. High Technology and Uncompensated Hospital Care. In F.A. Sloan, J.F. Blumstein, and J.M. Perrin (eds.), *Uncompensated Hospital Care: Rights and Responsibilities.* Baltimore: Johns Hopkins University Press.
Peterson, G.E. 1984. Federalism and the States: An Experiment in Decentralization. In J.L. Palmer and I.V. Sawhill, (eds.), *The Reagan Record: An Assessment of America's Changing Domestic Priorities.* Cambridge, Mass.: Ballinger.
Public Health Foundation. 1987. *Public Health Agencies 1984.* Vol. 3, *Services for Mothers and Children.* Publication No. 97. Washington, D.C.
———. 1987. Public Health Agencies 1987. *Expenditures and Sources of Funds.* Publication No. 103. Washington, D.C.
Reed, W.G., K.A. Cawley, and R.J. Anderson. 1986. The Effect of a Public Hospital's Transfer Policy on Patient Care. *New England Journal of Medicine* 315:1428–1432.
Reinhardt, U. 1985. Hard Choices in Health Care: A Matter of Ethics. In *Health Care: How to Improve It and Pay for It.* Washington, D.C.: Center for National Policy.
Rogers, D.E., R.J. Blendon, and T.W. Moloney. 1982. Who Needs Medicaid? *New England Journal of Medicine* 307:13–18.
Rosenbach, M.L. 1985. Insurance Coverage and Ambulatory Medical Care of Low-Income Children: United States, 1980. *National Medical Care Utilization and Expenditure Survey,* Series C, Analytic Report No. 1. DHHS Publication No. 85-20401. September. Washington, D.C.: G.P.O.
Rosenbaum, S. 1986. *Community and Migrant Health Centers: Two Decades of Achievement.* Washington, D.C.: National Association of Community Health Centers.
Rosenbaum, S., D.C. Hughes, and K. Johnson. 1988. Maternal and Child Health Services for Medically Indigent Children and Pregnant Women. *Medical Care* 26:315–332.
Rosenbaum, S., and J. Weitz. 1983. *Children and Federal Health Care Cuts: A National Survey of the Impact of Federal Health Budget Reductions on State Maternal and Child Health Services during 1982.* Washington, D.C.: Children's Defense Fund.
Rosenberg, C.E. 1982. From Almshouse to Hospital: The Shaping of Philadelphia General Hospital. *Health and Society* 60:108–154.
Sager, A. 1983. Why Urban Voluntary Hospitals Close. *Health Services Research* 18:451–475.
Salamon, L.M. 1984. Nonprofit Organizations: The Lost Opportunity. In J.L. Palmer and I.V. Sawhill (eds.), *The Reagan Record: An Assessment of America's Changing Domestic Priorities.* Cambridge, Mass.: Ballinger.
Sardell, A. 1983. Neighborhood Health Centers and Community-Based Care: Federal Policy from 1965 to 1982. *Journal of Public Health Policy* 8:484–503.
Schiff, R.L., D.A. Ansell, J.E. Schlosser, A.H. Idris, A. Morrison, and S. Whitman. 1986. Transfers to a Public Hospital: A Prospective Study of 467 Patients. *New England Journal of Medicine* 314:552–557.
Schlesinger, M., J. Bentkover, D. Blumenthal, R. Musacchio, and J. Willer. 1987. The Privatization of Health Care and Physicians' Perceptions of Access to Hospital Services. *Milbank Memorial Fund Quarterly* 65:25–58.
Select Panel for the Promotion of Child Health. 1981. *Better Health for Our Children: A National Strategy.* DHHS Publication No. 79-55071. Washington, D.C.: G.P.O.
Sloan, F.A., J. Valvona, and R. Mullner. 1986. Identifying the Issues: A Statistical

Profile. In F.A. Sloan, J.F. Blumstein, and J.M. Perrin (eds.), *Uncompensated Hospital Care: Rights and Responsibilities.* Baltimore: Johns Hopkins University Press.

Stevens, R. 1982. "A Poor Support of Memory": Voluntary Hospitals and Government before the Depression. *Milbank Memorial Fund Quarterly* 60:551–564.

Thorpe, K., and C. Brecher. 1987. Improved Access to Care for the Uninsured Poor in Large Cities: Do Public Hospitals Make A Difference? *Journal of Health Politics, Policy, and Law* 12:313–324.

Torres, A. 1984. The Effects of Federal Funding Cuts on Family Planning Services, 1980–1983. *Family Planning Perspectives* 16:134–138.

Torres, A., and J.D. Forrest. 1985. Family Planning Clinic Services in the United States, 1981. *Family Planning Perspectives* 17:30–35.

Zelnik, M., M.A. Koenig, and Y.J. Kim. 1984. Sources of Prescription Contraceptives and Subsequent Pregnancy among Young Women. *Family Planning Perspectives* 16:6–13.

10

The Health Care Implications of Early Childhood Group Care Programs

Judith S. Palfrey, M.D., and Alix Handelsman, M.D.

The past 40 years have witnessed significant increases in the number of women in the work force and the number of children in group care (Table 10.1). In 1940, 14 million women (27 percent) were employed outside the home. By 1980, this number was nearly 45 million (51 percent). In 1950, 12 percent of married women with children under six were represented in the work force. This had increased to 45 percent by 1980 (U.S. Bureau of Census, 1983a).

These trends have led to the expansion of a variety of child care systems. It is becoming increasingly likely that children under the age of five will spend part or all of their day out of the home, in some sort of group setting. It is estimated that 85 percent of three to five-year-old children with employed mothers currently attend a formal group program (Marx, 1985). The new child care arrangements present both problems and new opportunities for the provision of various child development and health care services.

Types of Child Care Arrangement

Child group care situations are basically of four types (see Table 10.2). The first type is the academically-oriented nursery school designed for the social stimulation of young children. In general, the sessions in these nursery schools are limited to 3–4 hour blocks with relatively little emphasis on meals, naps, or toilet training. The children who attend these settings are primarily from the middle class and the decision to send them to the program is based upon the parents' desire for their children to have social interaction with peers and for them to receive educational experiences. It is estimated that approximately 34 percent of three to five-year-olds attend these types of programs (Galinsky, 1987).

The second type of group care is center-based, custodial daycare. Daycare arrangements vary considerably, but are characterized by flexible, often long hours, provision of meals, naps, and toilet training. Over the past decade, there has been an increasing tendency for traditional nursery schools to take on daycare functions, including meals and after

Table 10.1 Trends in Work Force Participation by Women (in millions)

Number of Women	1950	1960	1970	1980	1984
In the work force	17.7	22.5	31.2	44.9	49.2
In the work force with children 6–17	2.2	5.7	10.0	14.4	16.2
In the work force with children under 6	0.7	2.5	4.5	6.1	7.2

Source: Data from U.S. Bureau of Labor Statistics.

Table 10.2 Estimated Number of Children Aged 3–5 in Various Group Settings in the United States

Type of Setting	Number of Children
Nursery/preschools	4,900,000[1]
Center-based daycare	20,300,000[2]
Family daycare	6,000,000[1]
Headstart	400,000[1]

[1] Based on data regarding children 3 to 5 years of age published in Kamerman (1983).
[2] Bureau of Census (1983) (children under 5 years old).

school hours, and for daycare programs to include planned educational activities. The distinctions between nursery school and daycare arrangements have thus become less pronounced. Ten percent of children under five are currently thought to spend all or most of the day in formal daycare centers (U.S. Census Bureau, 1983).

The third type of program is family daycare, a formal or informal arrangement for the provision of child care for small numbers of children (generally fewer than six), in the home of the caring adult. These arrangements simulate the home environment, are flexible, and include meals, naps, and toilet training. Figures on how many children are in family daycare are difficult to obtain because much of the care is unregistered. Estimates on family daycare run from 8 percent to 20 percent of children under five.

Finally, since the mid-1960s, a special program of comprehensive services has been available to children at socioeconomic disadvantage through project Headstart. This program's major goal is the enhancement of poor children's health and development so that they will enter the public school system on an equal footing with other more economically fortunate youngsters. As a result of Headstart's commitment to health, health goals were clearly articulated from the program's inception, unlike the experience in most other child care settings. Headstart services are available to almost one-half million children.

Potential Health Problems

Within the daycare setting, several areas of potential difficulties exist. When young children are together, infectious disease can spread. There are potential psychosocial effects of group care for vulnerable young children. In addition, depending on the environmental situation within the daycare, the setting itself may include hazards. Finally, because child care means the children are away from their families for a substantial part of the day, children in daycare may not have access to some health and developmental services that are open only during weekdays.

Infectious Diseases

As younger and younger children enter group care, a number of infectious disease entities are becoming problematic. Being immunologically immature, they may be at higher risk of contracting illness or becoming chronic carriers of bacteria and viruses. Infectious agents that have caused the most difficulty in daycare settings have been gastroenteritis (salmonella, shigella, campylobacter, and giardia), upper respiratory illnesses, bacterial illness (including hemophilus influenza), hepatitis A (Loda, 1972; Williams, Huff and Bryan, 1975; Black et al., 1977; Ward et al., 1978; Storch et al., 1979; Pickering et al., 1981; Pickering and Woodward, 1982; Redmond and Pichichero, 1984) and a number of less serious but nonetheless irksome problems including lice, scabies, conjunctivitis, and impetigo.

Because of the rising number of children in daycare and the reports of sporadic disease outbreaks within child care programs, there has been systematic attention by the American Academy of Pediatrics (1986) and the Child Day Care Infectious Disease Study Group (1984) in determining the best preventive policies for stemming the spread of infectious illness within group care settings. What has become evident is that relatively simple hygienic measures can contain most of the transmission of illness (Black et al., 1981).[1]

Haskins and Koch (1986) examined daycare from the point of view of the costs associated with childhood illness in group daycare. Based on an analysis of the accumulated information on morbidity and mortality associated with attendance in daycare, they concluded that "respiratory conditions, with the exception of otitis media, are not a major problem among any group, that meningitis in the daycare situation is a threat primarily to children, and that children, staff, and household contacts are all at increased risk for both gastroenteritis and hepatitis A." They speculated that the increased dependence on daycare in the United States would soon lead to a measurable increase in the incidence of otitis media, because this has been the experience in Scandinavia.

To look at the financial implications of daycare-associated illness, Haskins and Koch (1986) created an index that included medical costs, missed work, and long term consequences (death and chronic disability). They found it particularly difficult to assign specific weights to these outcome parameters and concluded their analysis by stating that "illness of children in daycare as a policy problem is moderate and that there is no need for a clarion call against daycare or on behalf of major new federal and state regulations."

While large daycare centers are at the greatest risk for epidemics and the most vulnerable to the consequences of having to shut down operations, similar kinds of difficulties occur in family daycare. Family daycare presents somewhat greater challenges in the area of prevention as standard-setting for family daycare is less stringent and much more difficult to enforce. Since sporadic reports in the literature do suggest the risk of the spread of infectious disease is higher in family daycare than in the general population (Palfrey, Weitzman, Hostetter and Howes, 1980), this is an area worthy of health policy concern.

Because most of the group programs for children are designed for children over two years of age, experience remains limited for infants and young toddlers. Infant daycare is relatively new. Moreover, there is little experience with daycare either for premature infants or for chronically ill infants. Programs such as the Infant Health and Development Program are promoting daycare as an intervention for prematurely born children. As a result, there will be a substantial body of experience with the at-risk population within the next three to four years. These data should be monitored carefully.

A new concern about infectious disease in daycare is the rising number of children with AIDS and AIDS-related complex (ARC). The Centers for Disease Control (CDC) issued statements indicating that children with AIDS should attend community programs such as schools unless they demonstrate behavior which would place them or other children at risk (1985). Since young children bite and the potential for transmission through biting is suggested (though not well quantitated), states have varied in their recommendations about whether toddlers and preschoolers with known AIDS or ARC could attend group care with non-AIDS affected children.

Children with AIDS often face a difficult family situation, with one or both parents dying of the disease. As a result, the need for custodial daycare for the child is enormous. Specialized daycare facilities that combine social service, education, and health care are being developed across the country. How many of these will be needed and their societal costs are open to speculation. In light of predictions about the increases of virus transmission in the heterosexual population, it is possible that such centers may become a larger component of the national child care program.

Psychosocial Effects

As women have moved into the work force and found the need to make arrangements for the care of their young children, these arrangements have varied considerably in terms of the children's comfort, environmental stimulation, and safety. The full effects of these arrangements on children's psychosocial development are not well understood. Bronfenbrenner (1974) catalogued the questions that should be asked about the out-of-home arrangements for preschool children. These include (1) the importance of the maternal-child relationship in the first years of life, (2) the differences in half-time versus full-time care, (3) the importance of social class mix, (4) the differences between cooperative and regular nursery schools, (5) the father's ability to care for young children as effectively as the mother, (6) the importance of other adults besides the parents, (7) age desegregation, (8) the presence of children at the parent's work site, and (9) the importance of parents being at home when the child arrives back from daycare.

While most children seem to do very well within the daycare setting, some groups of children may not. Temperamentally vulnerable children may have their problems exacerbated. Other difficulties may arise for children who have eating or toileting problems. Moreover, the staff within a child care setting clearly cannot always handle the behaviorally difficult child. Higher staff to child ratios might be helpful in these situations, but this, of course, has financial implications.

Potential Hazards

In the past 2–3 years the issue of daycare has found a prominent spot in the national media because of multiple reports of sexual abuse within the daycare setting. Some experts prophesied that without proper staff to child ratios the kinds of negligence and abuse which had been seen in some nursing homes for the elderly would appear within the daycare setting (Martinez, 1987). While most workers in the field of child sexual abuse feel that these reports overemphasized the hazards and underplayed the important protective role of daycare for stressed families (reducing the threat of child abuse at home), the need for standardized employment practices and other safeguards was highlighted. To minimize these hazards, adequate staffing has been considered essential.

Tension has accompanied the call for more regulations, however. Higher standards were juxtaposed against cost and access to services.

Congress voted against the reinstitution of the Federal Interagency Day Care Regulations (FIDCR) in 1980 because it was argued that higher staff to child ratios would be so expensive that some families would be excluded from daycare and end up back on the welfare rolls (Martinez, 1987).

The tension around the enforcement of higher staffing requirements is also witnessed by the fact that even daycare proponents express fear about the increased costs, because it is clear that there are not enough dollars in the current system. As a result, the daycare community itself has been relatively quiet with regard to promoting standard setting.

In the absence of external or internal regulation, there has been considerable state-to-state variation in staff to child ratios, with some states having as low as a 1:8 ratio for children under age one (Martinez, 1987). Moreover, few states have standards for the training of directors and staff.

Alternatives to increased staffing include periodic inspections programs of parent and child education. Each of these, however, entails significant costs and may place an unreasonable burden on parents.

Potential hazards also exist in the physical environment of daycare settings. Unaware of physical dangers, small children are at risk for accidental injury when playing unsupervised or on poorly maintained or inadequately adapted equipment. Studies of accidents in daycare have established that the rate of such accidents is substantial (Aronson, 1983). Again, the most direct way of addressing this problem is to require higher ratios of staff to children; the most significant constraint involves the costs of these staff.

Lack of Access to Weekday Services

Another concern about children in group care is that there may be few opportunities for their parents to take them for routine health and dental care. The implication of this is that routine services may need to be open and available in evening and weekend times. Alternatively, some of these services might be provided through the center itself.

Perhaps of more concern than the provision of routine care is the provision of sick-child care. When children who are in daycare become ill, it is often difficult to provide them the kind of support that they require. Increasingly, decisions are being made to allow children who are sick to remain in daycare rather than to be sent home. In these cases, the parents' work is considered more important than the child's discomfort or even his health. One wonders why there has not been a stronger call for a "parents' labor law" that would allow parents of young children to use their own sick days for the care of their sick children. Young adults are the least likely in the labor force to require sick days for themselves. These days could be used for the care of sick children.

What would be the impact of such a policy? Emlen and Koren (1984) studied the number of days missed by working parents and found that men tended to miss an average of 8 days from work per year and women an average of 10 days per year. The difference was attributed to child sick days. If two days per year is a reliable estimate of the costs of more flexible parental leave, the change could be implemented without causing productivity to suffer.

Instead of such a solution, though, it is more commonly advocated that we establish yet another institution, the "sick child care center." These centers would be "hospitals" or "infirmaries" for children to attend when they have a cold or fever and cannot go to their regular daycare. Concerns have been raised about this kind of arrangement since children might be placed in a less than desirable situation at a time when they most need the comfort of familiar surroundings and people. Of all the arrangements for child care, the sick child care center seems to place adult values above concern with children's welfare. It reflects a disturbing tendency in American society of the 1980s to downplay or ignore the needs of children.

Targets of Opportunity

The group care setting also offers a number of targets of opportunity for creative programming that could improve the health of children. In this section, we will look at the opportunities for health care monitoring, the delivery of some health services, developmental assessment, training of staff, parent education, child education, and the integration of culturally different and handicapped children.

Health Care Monitoring

Child care programs are in a very good position to monitor the adequacy of children's health care. Child care programs can make a substantial difference in assuring that each child has a primary care provider. However, our experience in the Brookline Early Education Project (where 97 percent of families maintained a source of primary care) indicated that biannual checks were required to accomplish this level of primary care involvement (Hanson and Levine, 1980). With significant ongoing reductions in insurance and children's access to health services, child care programs may serve as an important safety net, making sure that if families lose insurance, someone is still providing health services for the child.

While monitoring the existence of a provider is simply clerical, monitoring the quality of health care is more complicated. A nurse responsible for several daycare centers can assess the number of visits, the consistency of the care, and the comprehensiveness of the health care services. In addition, she may check that screenings, immunizations, and physical examinations have been carried out. Monitoring systems are easiest to mount in large programs such as Headstart and nursery schools attached to public or private educational institutions. Table 10.3 documents the recent experience of the New England Headstart Program in carrying out health monitoring. The cost of this activity averaged $77 for each child. This is fairly small compared to the overall cost of daycare. Such programs can also be arranged by groups of smaller centers who obtain consultation from VNA, public health, or medical centers (Stifler, Bronson and Palfrey, 1980).

Screening

In some cases, early childhood programs themselves may sponsor health screenings. Others may simply ensure that screening has been performed elsewhere for the children within their programs. Again, the larger and more formal the program, the more likely that the service can or will be provided through the center itself.

Frankenburg (1974) outlined the criteria for relevant screening measures. These include prevalence, importance, cost effectiveness, and

Table 10.3 Health-Related Characteristics of Children in New England Regional Headstart, 1986–1987

Characteristic	N	%
Children who have completed medical screening including appropriate tests and physical examinations	17,383	96
Children receiving medical treatment	4,475	98
Children who have completed a professional dental examination during the operating period	17,104	95
Children receiving dental treatment	3,855	95
Children who have completed all immunizations required for their age before the start of operating period	16,716	86
Of those children who had not completed all immunizations required for their age before the start of operating period, the number who completed all required immunizations by the end of operating period	1,429	7
Children enrolled in Medicaid/EPSDT	13,087	67
Total professionally diagnosed for handicapping conditions	3,059	16

interventions available. The following are areas generally considered appropriate for screening. Many can be carried out under medical supervision by professionals and/or trained community volunteers.

1. Vision. Guidelines for screening the vision of young children have been published by the American Academy of Pediatrics (1986). Before age three it is not possible to measure visual acuity accurately, but physicians can look for structural anomalies, squint, and tumors. After age three, a number of procedures can be applied to measure acuity (Allen, 1957; Sheridan, 1970; Lippman, 1974).

2. Hearing. Periodic screening of children for hearing loss has been recommended by a series of international conferences (Joint Committee on Infant Hearing Screening, 1972). Frequent screening supplemented by otologic evaluations for children known to have fluctuating hearing is the most justifiable approach (Palfrey et al., 1980). Child care programs can be helpful in referring children for evaluation when they seem to be inattentive or unusually reticent in group activities.

Because otitis media is a major risk factor for hearing loss and because the incidence of otitis is on the rise in group care, early childhood programs should be particularly vigilant with regard to screening otitis prone youngsters. While the language consequences of otitis-associated hearing loss are currently the subject of hot debate, the theoretical risk is appreciable and justifies programmatic concerns and planning.

3. Lead intoxication. Poisoning from the ingestion of peeling lead paint and plaster has reached epidemic levels among low-income children (Centers for Disease Control, 1975; Piomelli et al., 1984; Schneider and Lavenhar, 1986). While the incidence of severe lead poisoning cases has dropped dramatically since the institution of screening, Needleman et al. (1979) showed that chronic or repeated ingestion of even small amounts of lead can cause long-term behavioral symptomatology. Screening for lead poisoning is simple and accurate and should be carried out on an annual or semiannual basis, especially in geographical areas of high prevalence. Daycare centers can serve as the site for such testing or can arrange for the transport of children to nearby clinics or public health stations.

4. Anemia. Between two and nine percent of preschool children suffer from iron deficiency anemia. Oski and co-workers documented the behavioral consequences of such anemia (Webb and Oski, 1973; Oski and Hinig, 1978). Because anemia is often a marker of nutritional deficit, screening for anemia can serve as a possible indicator of poor health status or of family needs for nutritional education and support (Folman, 1977). Screening for anemia is often carried out in conjunction with lead testing.

5. Sickle cell screening. Sickle cell anemia affects approximately 1 percent of the black population. Because sickle cell screening is extremely important in the first year of life, daycare centers serving infants should be particularly alert to the documentation of sickle cell status.

6. Dental screening. A preschool nutrition survey carried out in the 1970s indicated that the prevalence of caries was 2.6 to 3.8 per child throughout the United States (Folman, 1977). Many studies have indicated a higher prevalence of carious teeth among poor children and those attending Headstart centers than among middle-class children. Dental screening, health education and the provision of fluoride are the major factors in the prevention of caries. These three interventions can be carried out very effectively through daycare settings that arrange consultation with local dental and public health programs.

Immunizations

In addition to screening, preschool projects can monitor immunization status. Despite massive national efforts in recent years, many of the nation's children are still not adequately immunized. In fact, immunization rates among preschool children have declined in recent years (Hughes et al., 1988). Reasons for this include inadequate access to health care providers, family morbidity and noncompliance, as well as growing public apathy about the importance of childhood immunization.

Immunization levels have been maintained in most states through the public schools' entrance requirement for full immunization status. Increasingly, daycare and Headstart have played this monitoring role for young children, often through the licensing arm of the Office for Children, which ties the operating permit for the center or school to the reporting of immunizations. Hinman (1986) showed that immunization levels in children attending daycare are 8–15 percent higher (depending on the particular antigen) than in those who are not daycare attendees. Daycare and Headstart have played an important role in the introduction of the new Hib vaccine by requiring the vaccine for attendance.

Nutrition

Because children may be in group settings for one to two meals per day, there is a good opportunity to provide balanced nutrition under child care arrangements. This may be extremely important for the children of families of limited means and may contribute significantly to raising the children's nutritional status. The Headstart nutrition program has been particularly effective, maintaining adequate iron levels among a group of children traditionally known to be at risk for anemia.

Developmental Assessment

A function that daycare centers could fulfill but have largely left to others is that of developmental assessment. In group care there are ideal opportunities for documenting and following the progression of children's abilities in gross motor and fine motor skills, in perceptual abilities, in perceptual motor integration, and in language acquisition. There is no better place than the daycare setting to assess social integration, dependence, and independence.

If a group care setting has a systematic program of developmental assessment, it is most likely in the area of speech and language. The testing materials are relatively well developed and prescreening of children more or less straightforward. While the assessments may feasibly be carried out in a routine manner, language-based training for children may be less readily accessed. Linkage with school systems for this kind of intervention will be encouraged by the new early intervention requirements in P.L. 99-457.

Daycare placements are sometimes designated for children with particularly difficult home situations, sometimes even for the protection of the child. These centers should have the capability of following the children's cognitive and social development. Too often, however, the daycare center will lack the funding or will be forced to refer the children to another provider so that the assessment(s) can be billed under public or private insurance programs.

If developmental assessment is to be undertaken in daycare, one caveat must be raised. Developmental assessment requires sophistication on the part of the assessors in performing a differential diagnosis in the case of deviation from any standards. Too often in screening programs, simplistic explanations are accepted for children's deviations (—) "he's immature," "it's a bad family," "she's Spanish-speaking." When there are difficulties, it is only fair to the child and family to explore all possible explanations, including medical problems (thyroid, lead, anemia, hearing loss, chromosome abnormalities, etc.); developmental dysfunction, such as perceptual disability, motor incoordination, receptive or expressive language deficit, attentional problems, psychosocial explanations, including family discord, environmental deprivation, loss, abuse, and psychiatric pathology, including childhood depression and autism. One means of incorporating this broader expertise would be to establish an affiliation with a medical center, such as the model program currently in effect between the Tufts Daycare Center and the Children's Hospital Preschool Function Program. Such a program includes visits by Children's team members to daycare settings and daycare teachers come into the Children's Hospital with the child being evaluated. While this is an expensive model, it has been possible to negotiate insurance coverage for such extended evaluations.

Innovative training programs represent an alternative means of developing staff expertise. Staff training has been an important element of multidisciplinary programs such as Headstart, where nutritionists, dentists and physicians are actively involved in in-service training programs designed to bring a professional level of awareness to all staff members dealing with young children. While such training sessions require funding and preparation, in the long run they can lead to greater staff satisfaction, lower staff turnover rates, and better care for children.

Parent Education

One of the greatest health enhancing opportunities afforded by child care programs is parent education. Parents can learn from child care staff and consultants about their children and about their roles as the educators and care given for their children.

The task of parent education was a central one at the Brookline Early Education Project (Pierson, 1974), where the project was designed to support parents from three months prior to birth until school entry. This was done through home visiting in the infancy phase, diagnostic examinations, and "guided observations" in the toddler and preschool phase. Parent participation in the multidisciplinary diagnostic evaluations proved exceedingly valuable. Parents found that they learned to identify their children's developmental "readiness" points so that they were attuned to the children's needs and could respond appropriately to the child's call for a particular type of developmental or emotional attention.

The "guided observations" were particularly useful to parents. Standing behind a screen with a developmental psychologist, the parents had the opportunity to observe their children interacting with other children and with teachers. The "guiding" teacher would point out salient events and put the child's responses into perspective with regard to the child's age, developmental status and emotional responsiveness. Parents could then understand any reports they would be receiving from the child care workers.

Another more conventional form of parent education is parent groups and workshops. These can be a meaningful form of intervention but are often poorly attended. Caldwell (1987) suggested the importance of providing incentives such as food or prizes to encourage busy, working parents who want to spend what little free time they do have at home with their children. Obviously, any parent education does require time and that the parent be able to attend. Again, increasing flexibility in parental leave from work could make attendance more feasible.

Child's Education

Quality child care must include an educational component. More and more child care, daycare, nursery school and early education are becoming interchangeable, even synonymous terms. Nonetheless, with the low level of pay that most child care workers receive, some may not be qualified to prepare and carry out a curriculum.

A daycare curriculum can incorporate a number of subjects that can foster children's health and development. Young children can be taught social interaction skills, sharing, listening to others, and working together in twos and threes. Independence skills in dressing, toileting, and eating can also be fostered. Healthy habits such as tooth brushing, good nutrition, wearing seatbelts, and not talking to strangers can be emphasized as part of the curriculum for three- to five-year-olds.

Integration

Child group care provides a very important target of opportunity for the social integration of children of different cultural backgrounds. By bringing children of different ethnic and racial groups together on common ground, the youngsters can develop friendships free of the preconceived notions of their parents and other adults. By celebrating the important contributions of the various ethnic groups, the teachers can highlight and instill an appreciation of different talents and skills into the children. Having learned these things as young children, it is likely that these friendships and attitudes will carry through into later life.

There are also important opportunities in child care programs for the integration of children with disabilities. Young children expect little or nothing and thus accept variation and difference much better than older children. By getting to know about disability at a young age they may be able to develop lasting friendships which will get them (and their disabled friends) through the tough throes of the early school years. This target of opportunity has been one that Headstart has acknowledged and pursued through its requirement that 10 percent of the spaces in Headstart be reserved for young children with disabilities (Zigler and Valentine, 1979). While data remain to be analyzed on the effectiveness of this type of integration, the early reports suggest success in this venture.

What Do Other Countries Do?

In contrast to virtually all the European countries, the United States does not have a coherent or comprehensive policy regarding families and children. Unlike the situation in the United States, child care in Europe can be considered in the context of overall family policy (Robey, 1975). One hundred and seventeen countries (including all members of the European Economic Community) guarantee maternity leave, job protection while on leave, cash benefits to replace lost earnings, and/or cash benefit to supplement income and assist with the cost of raising children. In addition, national programs assure comprehensive health care for mothers and children. The motivation for providing public or publicly funded family programs in other countries varies (Hewlett, 1986). While some do so out of a "progressive" impulse and a commitment to equality between men and women, others feel that a child-oriented national program is an investment in their country's future.

Europe is experiencing the same increases in work force participation by women as the United States with the concomitant need for additional child care services. While most countries cannot fully meet the need, they have adopted universal availability of child care as a widely accepted policy goal with out-of-home care for young children often considered "essential for children and optimal development" (Kamerman, 1980a and 1980b). To provide this "essential" service, a number of models have emerged with varying degrees of coordination between health and child care providers. The experience of France, Sweden, and East Germany may suggest some potential policy directions for the United States.

France

France has one of the oldest public child care systems in the world. Started in the nineteenth century, the system now includes a wide range of programs with day nurseries for children from three months to six years, supplemental daycare centers for children under six whose parents work and family daycare centers. Interestingly, France now requires that anyone, even a relative, who cares for a child outside the child's own home be licensed. Much of the care is subsidized by municipal and national funds (with a sliding scale for parental payment ranging from $15 to $50/week). In 1980, the French government estimated that 35 percent of two-year-olds, 90 percent of three-year-olds, and 100 percent of four- to six-year-olds attended daycare or preschool (Kamerman, 1980b).

France also has had a comprehensive child health program since 1945. Children may receive care from a variety of providers, including the national "Service de Protection Maternelle et Infantile," company-run clinics, or private practitioners. The staff of the Service de Protection Maternelle et Infantile includes pediatricians, midwives, pediatric nurses, social workers, and psychologists. Care is free, but only about one-fourth of all well-child exams take place there. National health insurance reimburses parents for 80 percent of fee-for-service care, and many families have private insurance to cover the other 20 percent. Governmental guidelines are for nine exams in the first year, three exams in the second year, and two a year from ages two through six years.

France is one of many European countries that provides a cash benefit to families with children. Since 1973, pediatric exams at eight days, nine months, and two years have been a prerequisite for mothers to receive their child benefit allowance. Child health care is primarily linked to the social service system, rather than to daycare. However, admission to nursery and primary school is contingent upon completion of the compulsory immunization program (Drucquer, 1983) and as part of a recent emphasis on improving the quality of its extensive child care system, France is encouraging experimental programs which integrate daycare, preschools, and maternal and child health programs (Kamerman, 1980b).

Sweden

Swedish children start school at age seven, and approximately one-third attend some form of public child care before then. Another third of the under-seven-year-olds are cared for privately, usually by unlicensed daycare mothers. Parents pay for public facilities on a sliding scale ($16 to $122/month) and priority is given to single mothers and low-income families. Funding comes from the federal government (50 percent), municipal government (40 percent) and parental fees (10 percent) (Hewlett, 1986).

Sweden has a number of family policies including a national parent education curriculum, laws prohibiting corporal punishment by parents, and paid time off to help a child adjust to a new child care program. The Swedes are also experimenting with "sibling groups" (children of different ages) in daycare programs, and are leaders in "mainstreaming" children with physical and emotional handicaps into regular child care programs (Kamerman and Kahn, 1981).

The Swedish national health policy is implemented at the local level by county and municipal medical boards. There is a network of child health centers, as well as a strong school health program. Virtually all children are seen for health supervision in the first two years of life, as well as at the mandatory four-year-old examination.

Swedish children and their parents have an average of 11.8 contacts with health providers in the first year of life. This includes clinic visits with a doctor and a nurse and home visits by a nurse. There is also a formal attempt at integration of child care and health care centers at the local level (Kamerman and Kahn, 1981).

The mandatory four-year-old exam in Sweden is designed to detect health problems and treat them well before a child enters school. Dental caries and vision problems are the most common functionally significant problems picked up at this time (8.3 percent and 9.3 percent, respectively). Neurologic problems, speech disorders, and psychological problems are also found (Sjolin and Smedby, 1979). The importance of teamwork among professionals affiliated with different programs is emphasized. In model projects, nursery teachers meet regularly with physicians, nurses, social workers, and psychologists to discuss problems and integrate services (Kohler and Anderson, 1979).

Germany

In the German Democratic Republic, at least 60 percent of children between five months and three years are in daycare. Preference is given to the infants of single and working mothers. Centers are subsidized by the government and families pay about 50 cents per day. Ninety-two percent of three- to six-year-olds attend free, education-oriented kindergartens. In addition, there are low-cost after-school programs for the many children from families with two working parents (Greenberg, 1984).

The German health system's programs reflect a national child and family-oriented attitude. Prenatal care for pregnant women is universally available. Eighty percent of women have their first visit before the 16th week of pregnancy. This is attributed to widespread publicity about the importance of care during pregnancy, as well as the fact that working women are allowed paid time off to attend prenatal clinics. In addition, women are offered cash incentives for participation. If medical services are not available nearby, women are provided with transportation funds. Working women also receive two 45-minute work breaks to nurse their babies.

Child health care is given similar importance. Ninety-seven percent of infants participate in well-baby clinics, and 87 percent have their first visit by age three weeks. More than 90 percent of children are fully immunized by age three years. This high level of care is thought to be due to several factors, including societal emphasis on the importance of child health care, financial incentives for participation, and delivery of services at convenient times and locations (Greenberg, 1984). About 58 percent of children under age three years receive their exams and immunizations at their daycare centers, and 92 percent of children receive health maintenance exams and services in their preschools.

Daycare teachers play an important role in the health maintenance program. Regular, formal evaluations of each child's development become part of their record. Assessments include physical growth, gross and fine motor development, social skills, self-help skills, speech development, and teacher comments on behavior or parent-child interactions. Each center has one doctor who has the opportunity to develop an ongoing relationship with daycare staff (Greenberg, 1984).

The European-American Contrast

Under a range of political systems in Europe, comprehensive family support policies, maternity leave, cash benefits, health care, and low-cost child care have been established. By comparison with the United States, where daycare programs are still considered by some to "undermine" the family, European countries take child care for granted. There may be debates over whether care should be family-based or center-based or around the content of the center's curriculum, but not over the need for daycare or for government support of it.

A recurring international theme is that comprehensive, coordinated care for children should be a high priority. Medical services are free, sometimes mandatory, and often linked to other components of the social service "package" such as the cash child allowance. Many child care programs have an affiliated physician and all centers require up-to-date health supervision for their attendees. While the German Democratic Republic has developed the most sophisticated program of coordination between health care and group care programs, the other European countries are emphasizing integration of services, and are trying to increase communication between daycare and health care providers. Unfortunately, in the United States both systems are so fragmented that this sort of coordination can exist only in a haphazard, idiosyncratic fashion where individuals have an interest in seeing such programming happen.

Discussion

As with so many human services in the United States, group care for young children is provided through a wide variety of distinct organizations and programs. There is no system of care for young children and no means of assuring that those in need receive appropriate care. While Headstart has been shown to be an effective program, it reaches only one tenth of the children eligible for the health and developmental services which it can provide. Daycare spaces also are severely limited as are quality family daycare opportunities.

Much of the reason for the eclectic nature of group care for young children is that there is little or no formal planning at the federal level. While some state-level policy groups such as public health personnel or officials do consider concerns such as infectious disease and hygiene, few formal resources have been allocated to the venture of group care for children. Table 10.4 outlines the federal sources of funds for child care and indicates the variety of agencies through which they are available.

This semiplanned approach is in stark contrast to what happens in other countries where child care is considered a high priority and issues of access and quality are addressed systematically (U.S. Bureau of Census, 1983b). The lack of a child policy in this country may reflect either

Table 10.4 Federal Funding for Early Childhood Programs

Program	Annual Budget	Number of Children Served
HCEEP[a] (88 demonstration projects)	$5.70 million (FY 1986)	2,742
Headstart	$1.30 billion (FY 1987)	451,732
Title XX	$436 million[b] (FY 1985)	514,988
EPSDT[c]	N/A	2,248,429 (FY 1986)
IRS Child Care Tax Credit	$2.6 billion (FY 1984)	7,500,000 taxpayers
Child Care Food Program[d]	$486 million (FY 1986)	1,187,666

Source: Compiled from published and unpublished government data and telephone interviews.

[a] Handicapped Children's Early Education Program.

[b] Title XX is a social service block grant, which the states spend for a variety of programs such as protective services, care for the disabled, family planning, and adoption, as well as to subsidize daycare. They are no longer required to keep records breaking down the amount spent for the various programs. It is estimated that, collectively, the states spend about 18% of the $2.7 billion on daycare, but there is tremendous variation. Title XX funding for FY 1985 was only 72% of funding for 1981 in real dollars.

[c] Early Periodic Screening, Diagnosis, and Treatment. Funding comes from state Medicaid budgets. There is no breakdown of the amount spend on EPSDT.

[d] Pays for meals served to children in licensed group and family daycare.

ineffective social planning, the lack of a family-oriented program, or the low regard which children receive in the United States.

In the absence of a formal system, there are substantial gaps in our understanding of current child care use. This lack of knowledge makes it hard to plan for future needs. In addition, the pressures of business and labor leaders for productivity and increasing the work force often take precedence over the discussions about part-time work, job sharing, or "flex time" that might promote more effective child care arrangements. On-site daycare and health care services for young children are frequently discussed but usually rejected as "just not feasible."

Improvements in daycare thus must start with parents. More vocal advocacy for child care policy in this country is required if state and federal policies are to be changed. In addition, a "parents' labor law" might allow parents to use their own accrued sick time for child-oriented activities such as caring for a sick child at home, attending a performance or some other child-centered activity.

In tandem with the need for a child care policy, there is a major need for child care to be valued as a profession. There is a clear financial price for this, but until child care workers are afforded the proper training, salaries and respect that they deserve, it will be difficult for them to provide adequate services and impossible for them to fulfill the challenges that group care for young children raises.

There are significant opportunities for promoting health and development in group care. Recognition of these opportunities and capitalization of them may lead to major cost savings for children. Screenings and immunizations have clearly been demonstrated to be efficacious and the group care setting is one in which these can be monitored and sponsored. Moreover, developmental assessment is beginning to show promise and targeted interventions such as those offered in the Ypsilanti project and some of the Headstart projects are being heralded as major cost savers to society.

If additional monies become available for group care, they should be targeted to advocacy efforts for a family-centered policy, upgrading the training, staff ratios and professional status of group care workers, and promoting health screening and developmental assessment in group care. With this sort of financial investment, group care for children could evolve into a positive force in this country rather than a second-best situation for children whose mothers must work.

Notes

1. Aronson (1987) outlined the following measures which seem to be effective in infectious disease control in group care: (1) the assignment of soft, cuddly toys

to individual children wherever possible, (2) the sanitation of mouthed objects (with the use of one quarter cup of bleach diluted in one gallon of water), (3) the establishment of routines for hand washing for staff and children, (4) the establishment of routines for handling fecally contaminated materials, (5) the enforcement of mandatory immunization, (6) the establishment of reasonable and scientifically supported policies for excluding children with transmissible infection, (7) the arrangement for every daycare program to have easy access to health consultation, and (8) a yearly inspection of every daycare facility by a qualified sanitarian. Clearly, these practices are straightforward and do not particularly tax resources or personnel. However, the situations in which these measures are not followed can result in serious increases in illness throughout the daycare setting.

2. One of the newest challenges for daycare directors is obtaining insurance for their centers. Costs of liability insurance are becoming prohibitive for smaller operations. The absence of standards is felt to be one factor driving up the costs. The others include increasing numbers of claims and the awareness that daycare is now a social institution that must be dealt with on institutional rather than individual terms.

References

Allen, H.F. 1957. Testing Visual Acuity in Preschool Children: Norms, Variables and a New Picture Test. *Pediatrics* 19:1093–1100.

American Academy of Pediatrics. 1986. Report of the Committee on Infectious Diseases . 20th ed., pp. 54-61. Elk Grove Village, Ill.

American Academy of Pediatrics Committee on Practice and Ambulatory Medicine. 1986. Vision Screening and Eye Examination in Children. *Pediatrics* 77:918–919.

Aronson, S. 1983. Injuries in Child Care. *Young Children* 38:19–20.

Aronson, S.S. 1987. Maintaining Health in Child Care Settings. In N. Gunzenhauser and B.M. Caldwell (eds.), *Group Care for Young Children*. Lexington, Mass.: Lexington Books.

Black, R.E., A.C. Dykes, K.E. Anderson, et al. 1981. Handwashing to Prevent Diarrhea in Daycare Centers. *American Journal of Epidemiology* 113:445–451.

Black, R.E., A.C. Dykes, S.P. Sinclair, et al. 1977. Giardiasis in Daycare Centers: Evidence of Person-to-Person Transmission. *Pediatrics* 60:486–491.

Bronfenbrenner, U. 1974. Developmental Research, Public Policy and the Ecology of Childhood. *Child Development* 45:1–15.

Caldwell, B. 1987. Introduction. In N. Gunzenhauser and B.M. Caldwell (eds.), *Group Care for Young Children*. Lexington, Mass.: Lexington Books.

Center for Disease Control. 1975. *Increased Lead Absorption and Lead Poisoning in Young Children*. Washington, D.C.: DHEW, Public Health Service.

———. 1985. Education and Foster Care of Children Infected with Human T-lymphocyte Virus Type III/lymphadenopathy Associated Virus. *Morbidity and Mortality Weekly Reports* 34:517–521.

Child Day Care Infectious Disease Study Group. 1984. Public Health Considerations of Infectious Diseases in Child Daycare Centers. *Journal of Pediatrics* 105:683–701.

Drucquer, M. 1983. Child Health Services in France—Vive la difference. *British Medical Journal* 286:1529–1530.

Emlen, A.C., and P.E. Koren. 1984. *Hard to Find and Difficult to Manage: The Effects of Child Care on the Work Place.* Portland: Portland State University, Regional Institute for Human Services.

Folman, S.J. 1977. *Nutritional Disorders of Children: Prevention, Screening, Followup.* HSA Publication No. 77-5104. Washington, D.C.: DHEW.

Frankenburg, W.K. 1974. Selection of Diseases and Tests in Pediatric Screening. *Pediatrics* 54:612–616.

Galinsky, E. 1987. Contemporary Patterns of Child Care. In N. Gunzenhauser and B.M. Caldwell (eds.), *Group Care for Young Children.* Lexington, Mass.: Lexington Books.

Greenberg, R.A. 1984. Maternal and Child Health Services Policy in the German Democratic Republic. *Journal of Public Health Policy* 5:118–130.

Hanson, M.A., and M.D. Levine. 1980. Early School Health: An Analysis of Its Impact on Primary Care. *Journal of School Health* 50:577–580.

Haskins, R., and J. Kotch. 1986. Daycare and Illness: Evidence, Cost, and Public Policy. *Pediatrics* 77:951–982.

Hewlett, S.A. 1986. *A Lesser Life.* New York: William Morrow.

Hinman, A.R. 1986. Vaccine-Preventable Diseases and Child Daycare. *Review of Infectious Diseases* 8:573–583.

Hughes, D., K. Johnson, S. Rosenbaum, E. Butler, and J. Simmons. 1988. *The Health of America's Children.* Washington, D.C.: Children's Defense Fund.

Joint Committee on Infant Hearing Screening. 1972. Joint screening. *Journal of the American Speech and Hearing Association* 16:1160.

Kamerman, S.B. 1980a. Child Care and Family Benefits: Policies of Six Industrialized Countries. *Monthly Labor Review* November.

———. 1980b. *Parenting in an Unresponsive Society: Managing Work and Family.* New York: Free Press.

Kamerman, S.B., and A. Kahn (eds.). 1981. *Child Care, Family Benefits, and Working Parents: A Study in Comparative Policy.* New York: Columbia University Press.

Kaupas, V. 1974. Tuberculosis in a Family Daycare Home: Report of an Outbreak and Recommendation for Prevention. *Journal of the American Medical Association* 228:851:854.

Kohler, L., and I. Anderson. 1979. Case Report of a Swedish School Health Clinic. *Acta Paediatrica Scandinavia* 275(Supplement):51–58.

Lippman, O. 1974. *Directions for Use of the H.O.T.V. Test.* Forest Park, Ill.: GoodLite Company.

Load, F.A. 1972. Respiratory Disease in Group Daycare. *Pediatrics* 49:428–437.

Martinez, S. 1987. Child Care and Public Policy. In N. Gunzenhauser and B. M. Caldwell (eds.), *Group Care for Young Children.* Lexington, Mass.: Lexington Books.

Marx, F. 1985. Child Care. In H. McAdoo and T. M. J. Parham (eds.), *Services to Young Families.* Washington, D.C.: American Public Welfare Association.

Needleman, H.L., C. Gunnoe, A. Leviton, et al. 1979. Deficits in Psychologic and Classroom Performance of Children with Elevated Dentine Lead Levels. *New England Journal of Medicine* 300:659–665.

Oski, F.A., and A. S. Hinig. 1978. The Effects of Therapy on the Developmental Scores of Iron-Deficient Infants. *Journal of Pediatrics* 92:21–25.

Palfrey, J.S. 1987. Commentary on Interdisciplinary Group Care for Young Children. In N. Gunzenhauser and B. M. Caldwell (eds.), *Group Care for Young Children.* Lexington, Mass.: Lexington Books.

Palfrey, J., M. Hanson, et al. 1980. Selective Hearing Screening for Young Children. *Clinical Pediatrics* 19:473–477.

Palfrey, J. S., M. Weitzman, M. Hostetter, and L. Howes. 1980. The New Recruits: Spread of H. Flu Meningitis in a Family Daycare Setting. *Massachusetts Journal of Community Health* 1:3–6.

Pickering, L. K., D. G. Evans, H. L. DuPont, et al. 1981. Diarrhea Caused by Shigella, Rotavirus and Giardia in Daycare Centers: Prospective Study. *Journal of Pediatrics* 99:51–56.

Pickering, L. K., and W. E. Woodward. 1982. Diarrhea in Daycare Centers. *Pediatric Infectious Disease* 1:47–52.

Pierson, D. E. 1974. The Brookline Early Education Project: Model for a New Education Priority. *Childhood Education* 50:132–136.

Piomelli, S., J. F. Rosen, J. J. Chisolm, and J. W. Graef. 1984. Management of Childhood Lead Poisoning. *Journal of Pediatrics* 105:523–532.

Redmond, S. R., and M. E. Pichichero. 1984. Hemophilus Influenzae Type B Disease: An Epidemiologic Study with Special Reference to Daycare Centers. *Journal of the American Medical Association* 252:2581–2584.

Robey, P. 1975. *Day Care: Who Care?* New York: Basic Books.

Schneider, J. D., and M. A Lavenhar. 1986. Lead Poisoning: More than a Medical Problem. *Journal of the American Public Health Association* 76:242–244.

Sheridan, M. 1970. *Stycar Vision Test Manual,* 2d rev. ed. Windsor, Berks, England: NFER Publishing Co.

Sjolin, S., and B. Smedby. 1979. The State of Health of Swedish Children. *Acta Paediatrica Scandinavia* 275(Supplement):16–27.

Stifler, D., M. B. Bronson, and J. S. Palfrey. 1980. *Physician Training at Daycare Sites: A Pediatric-Consultative Model.* Boston: Children's Hospital, Community Services Program.

Storch, G., L. M. McFarland, K. Kelso, et al. 1979. Viral Hepatitis Associated with Daycare Centers. *Journal of the American Medical Association* 242:1515–1518.

U. S. Bureau of the Census. 1983a. Trends in Child Care Arrangements of Working Mothers. *Current Population Reports,* Series P-23, No. 129. Washington, D.C.: G.P.O.

———. 1983b. Child Care Arrangements of Working Mothers: June 1982. *Current Population Reports,* Series P-23, No. 129. Washington, D.C.: G.P.O.

U.S. Department of Health and Human Services. 1980. *Family Day Care in the United States: Site Case Studies.* DHHS (OHDS) Publication No. 80-30286. Washington, D.C.: G.P.O.

Ward, J. I., G. Gorman, C. Phillips, et al. 1978. Hemophilus Influenzae Type B Disease in Daycare Center. *Journal of Pediatrics* 92:713–717.

Webb, T. E., and F. A. Oski. 1973. Iron Deficiency Anemia and Scholastic Achievement in Young Adolescents. *Journal of Pediatrics* 82:827.

Williams, S. V., J. C. Huff, and J. A. Bryan. 1975. Hepatitis A and Facilities for Preschool Children. *Journal of Infectious Diseases* 131:491–495.

Zigler, E., and J. Valentine. 1979. *Project Headstart.* New York: Free Press.

11

Children's Health Care and the Schools

Deborah Klein Walker, Ed.D., John A. Butler, Ed.D., and Annette Bender, M.S.

To assess the changing status of children's health care in this country, it is important to examine not only changes in the health care system itself but also changes in other major service systems that provide care or family support. Public school programs play a growing role. Over the past fifty years, and particularly since 1965 when the War on Poverty began, they have enlarged their responsibility to include the health and well-being, as well as the education, of their students.

Ever since school nurses and physicians were introduced into schools in the early 1900s, the appropriate scope of school health programs has been discussed and debated. Most practitioners in the field refer to "school health" as encompassing three principal sets of activities: health education, health services, and environmental health (Office of Child Health Affairs, 1976; Igoe, 1980a; Gephart, Egan and Hutchins, 1984). These can serve not only the children but also the student's parents, the school staff, and the community at large. Other school activities are also sometimes considered part of a school health program, such as physical education, food services and pupil personnel services (Kolbe, 1985). In assessing the future role of two school-based health programs on the larger child health care delivery system, this chapter will, however, focus only on school health services and health education.

The Rationale for Locating Health Services and Health Education Activities in Schools

The arguments for basing health services and health promotion activities in the schools derive from the notion that there are situations when the market for children's health services fails to deliver services efficiently and equitably. Arguments for using schools as a base for health interventions can be grouped into five general categories.

First, schools can more efficiently deliver services because they enroll the school-age population. The school is the only national institutional base with a captive audience of all children aged 5 through 16 (the legal age at which youth can drop out of school) and a majority of youth from ages 16 to 18 (Hodgkinson, 1986).[1] Because of the concentration of children in schools, there are major potential economies of scale in delivering a wide range of preventive services, including screening for health conditions and health education, in addition to case identification, referral, and certain standardized forms of treatment. This is the classic rationale for most school-based health services and health promotion activities.

Second, schools can more effectively address some health needs of children and youth because they provide environments in which students feel comfortable. Schools are a better and less intimidating environment than physician offices or hospitals for offering health education and counseling. Care also is more accessible there for adolescents, who are often reticent to seek services in traditional primary care settings (Resnick, Blum and Hector, 1980). Peer culture—so often a negative influence on health behavior—can to some extent be shaped to become a positive influence in the context of the school (Blum, Pfuffinger and Donald, 1982). This rationale is used today by advocates of school-based clinics (Dryfoos, 1985; Korby, 1985).

Third, schools are a potential base for case coordination, case management, and advocacy for children who require multiple public and private sources of care (Wold, 1971; Walker and Jacobs, 1984). Because of their continued contact with children, school personnel are also in a better position than those in other public agencies to determine which children are not receiving adequate health care and which families are most in need of support services.

Fourth, because schools provide access to an entire age-specific population, they can collect data useful in estimating unmet needs and monitoring children's health status in a community as well as planning community-based health and health-related services (Walker, Richmond and Buka, 1984). More recently, schools have surveyed high school youth directly (Parcel, Nader and Meyer, 1977; Walker et al., 1982) to assess needs, plan services, and evaluate model interventions.

Finally, schools can more equitably make services available, because all children are entitled to a free public education. Where else can communities provide access to care for children of all income groups? Where else can the least advantaged as readily be identified and targeted with compensatory programs? Also, to the extent that adequate health and nutrition are prerequisite to equal educational opportunity, it becomes to some extent the obligation of schools to help ensure that students are healthy. This rationale has been used to justify the national school lunch and breakfast programs, and the provision by the schools of selected health services for children with disabilities or economically disadvantaged backgrounds.

Because it can be justified from so many different perspectives, most Americans have supported some form of school health program

(Lynch, 1977; Nader, 1978; Igoe, 1980a). Where there has been disagreement, it has been around the appropriate scope of the programs.

The Scope and Objectives of School Health Services

To fill all the roles identified above, school health services should be designed to address a wide range of problems common to the school age population. These include acute and chronic illnesses, health and developmental screening and assessment, behavioral and social problems, absenteeism, family crisis, child abuse, and neglect. In practice, school-based programs have developed around more limited packages of services. The evolution of school health services can be understood in terms of shifting support for two models or paradigms: the traditional health organizer model and the enriched nurse practitioner model (Office of Child Health Affairs, 1976; Walker and Guyer, 1980). Our discussion of each will be schematic, and does not do justice to subtleties of either approach, but does capture the most important aspects of the two models.

The Health Organizer Model

The traditional health organizer model has remained largely the same in intent and structure since the beginning of this century, when physicians and nurses were first employed in the schools. This model defines the role of the school conservatively, excluding direct medical service delivery, except perhaps involving disease prevention such as periodic immunization campaigns or screening programs. The school or school district is seen as an organizing link between the child in school and the community's health service resources. Within the school or district, a school nurse and/or aide, usually under the supervision of a very part-time physician, is charged with responsibility for seeing that every student has been immunized, screened, and referred to an appropriate provider if unmet needs are discovered. The nurse also maintains records and, in theory, monitors follow-up. In fact, the monitoring process usually is imperfect. Health education is a part of the traditional model, although the role and time of the school nurse usually is quite circumscribed.

The traditional model has two aims: to assure minimal public health protections by preventing contagion, and to provide the schools with protection against certain forms of legal liability that might result from playground injuries or inadequate physical examinations for varsity athletes. Most states have school health laws that focus on these rather narrow objectives, as reflected in states' medical requirements for school entry (Table 11.1).

Because the traditional model is rooted in a minimalist vision of the school's role, programs in this tradition have faced an uphill battle to capture adequate resources. Part of this battle involved other organized interest groups in health care. To a great extent, school health services have been able to develop in the United States only when they have not threatened or offended the interests of private office-based physicians. The alliance developed between the American Medical Association and the National Education Association in the late 1920s strongly discouraged the delivery of any treatment services within the schools. This agreement dictated how school services were run from the 1920s until the 1970s, when the efficacy of the traditional model was challenged for communities with large, low-income populations (Igoe, 1980a; Lynch, 1984).

It would be a mistake to criticize the health organizer model simply because it has historically lacked adequate financial or political support. In principle the model can be quite effective, especially where sufficient resources are available within the school for case identification, referral and health education, and where an adequate infrastructure of health service providers are financially and geographically accessible. At its most successful, this approach relies on energetic work by school nurses and related personnel to (a) provide case coordination for high-risk

Table 11.1 Number and Percentage of States with Specific Medical Requirements for School Entry

Requirement	N	(%)
Immunization		
DPT	50	(98)
Measles	50	(98)
Polio	49	(96)
Rubella	46	(90)
Mumps	28	(55)
Hearing test	22	(43)
Vision test	21	(41)
Physical exam	17	(33)
Tuberculosis test	8	(16)
Height/weight	5	(10)
Dental exam	5	(10)
Developmental evaluation	4	(8)
Speech test	4	(8)
Scoliosis evaluation	4	(8)

Source: Allensworth (1986).

children, linking parents, school, and health care providers; (b) join with teachers and psychologists within the school to offer screening and health education; and (c) write notices, phone parents, and make home visits with enough frequency to improve parent knowledge and involvement in the health care of their children. It also should be noted that the minimalist version of the program can sometimes produce powerful results without additional personnel or resources. One of the most remarkable recent school health accomplishments, implementation of the national measles inoculation campaign, was achieved largely by preventing children from entering school until their immunization records were complete (Bumpers, 1984).

The Nurse Practitioner Model

The nurse practitioner model is a more recent phenomenon, with origins in the early 1970s. This model differs from the health organizer model in that primary care is provided in the school in addition to the activities of the traditional model (Nader, 1978; Guyer and Walker, 1980; Meeker et al., 1986). Adolescent health care services based in high school clinics represent a much debated special case of this approach (Blum, Pfoffinger and Donald, 1982; Dryfous, 1985).

Nurse practitioners and aides in school-based clinics offer routine pediatric care, including diagnosis and treatment of common health problems. They depend on local physicians for consultation and referral as well as a hospital backup facility for inpatient care. In addition to hands-on medical care, the nurse practitioner often acts as part of a team including teachers, administrators, health aides, psychologists, social workers, and others to provide mental health services, health education, and case management.

In some communities, the nurse practitioner model has been funded and managed through the local public health department, renting or borrowing space from the school but not relying on the education system for funding or administration. In other communities it has been funded and managed by the school system. In still other cases, sponsorship is by a consortium of private medical providers.

The rationale for the nurse practitioner model has proven strongest where other sources of care are least available or accessible, such as in low-income rural and central city areas. There is little potential for conflict with private providers, who tend not to serve these children in these areas. School-based clinics in such areas, in effect, substitute for a neighborhood health center serving as a specialized primary care unit for school-aged children.

Expenditures for School Health Services

Funding sources for school health services include local school district revenues, local health department resources, state health department funds distributed to the local level, state education funds, federal funds and voluntary sector/private foundation funds. Local revenues are the primary source of funding in the majority of states (Gephart, Egan and Hutchins, 1984; Igoe, Nelson and Slaughter, 1984). Reports of the actual expenditures are extremely scarce, making estimates of total expenditures very difficult.

Table 11.2 presents the expenditures for 1975–76 (Vance and Munse, 1977) and for 1979–80 for public school health services (National Center for Educational Statistics, 1981), including the salaries for health personnel (physicians, nurses, and aides), supplies and other expenses. Total health service expenditures were about $380 million in 1975–76 and about $585 million in 1979–80. Since expenditure data from school systems has not been collected nationally since fiscal year 1980, an accurate report of current expenditures is not available. A rough estimate for fiscal year 1987 expenditures, based on a projected 7 percent increase in expenditures per year (NCES, 1986) and a constant proportion of health relative to other expenditures, would be about $940 million, or $13 per pupil. This estimate is well under 1 percent (0.34 percent) of the total school budget, projected to be $278.8 billion, in that school year (*Boston Globe*, 1986).

Expenditures varied greatly among states, which led to significant variation in the availability of health services, most notably school nurses. For example, in 1985–86, when the average pupil/nurse ration was 2473:1 for all districts; there was a range from 1156:3 for districts with enrollments up to 25,000 pupils to 4903:1 for districts with enrollments of 25,000 pupils or more (Education Research Service, 1986).

The costs associated with the nurse practitioner model are substantially higher than what is spent in a traditional school health program. In the recent school health demonstrations mounted by the Robert Wood Johnson Foundation (1985), the cost of replicating or continuing the programs was between $43 and $82 per year, per child in 1983, compared to expenditures of about $5 per pupil in districts with a health organizer model. While this looks expensive if the school system is paying, it is important to remember that it may be inexpensive compared to costs for comprehensive primary care in a medical setting.

Lessons Learned about School Health Services

What do we know about the success of school-based health programs? Though there is considerable variation among individual programs,

Table 11.2 Expenditures for Public School Health Services for 1975–1976 and Estimated Expenses for Fiscal 1980 (in thousands of dollars)

State	1975–76	1980
Alabama	841	1,220
Alaska	N/A	21,784*
Arizona	0	0
Arkansas	5,551*	3,268*
California	36,238	47,686
Colorado	7,928	45,897
Connecticut	7,985	21,600
Delaware	1,746	2,139
District of Columbia	45	116
Florida	N/A	0
Georgia	4,866*	36,852*
Hawaii	4,218	5,750
Idaho	582	692
Illinois	38,417	33,037
Indiana	6,233	8,654
Iowa	4,591	7,028
Kansas	2,732	3,786
Kentucky	754	943
Louisiana	1,998	6,262
Maine	1,423	1,934
Maryland	2,994	3,427
Massachusetts	20,418*	35,436*
Michigan	5,659	6,888
Minnesota	7,720	10,094
Mississippi	1,303	5,234
Missouri	6,226	10,784
Montana	1,784*	4,135*
Nebraska	1,602	2,171
Nevada	963	1,790
New Hampshire	2,177	3,050
New Jersey	33,399	47,074
New Mexico	2,179	4,194
New York	62,630	66,667
North Carolina	1,054	2,172
North Dakota	235	267
Ohio	10,045	23,372
Oklahoma	1,969	2,890
Oregon	2,184	4,214
Pennsylvania	38,046	43,966
Rhode Island	1,262	2,339
South Carolina	2,985	4,603
South Dakota	481	1,961
Tennessee	1,328	1,584
Texas	23,679	38,092
Utah	617	1,226
Vermont	1,102	1,773
Virginia	8,021	11,642
Washington	6,066	9,346
West Virginia	2,467	4,188

some general patterns emerge from their past performance. This evidence suggests that four general problems are generic to implementing any school health program.

First, as alluded to above, the school health program in many communities has developed in political equipoise with the primary care services of private office-based practitioners and health department clinics. Historically this has limited school-based services to prevention and screening, activities with a clear public health rationale and which generate business for private physicians rather than taking patients away. Direct service delivery in the school has generally been possible only when (a) there were no local practitioners threatened by this activity or (b) the services offered were not sufficiently lucrative or technically exacting to be of interest to the private practitioner. Many inner city or rural areas, lacking adequate primary care accessible to low-income children, are examples of the first category. Health counseling of adolescents is an example of the second type of service, since it is time-intensive and thus tends to be unprofitable under current insurance provisions.

In most U.S. communities there are an adequate number of health service providers outside the school. Overall, less than 10 percent of U.S. children and youth are reported by their parents to lack a regular source of medical care (Select Panel for the Promotion of Child Health, 1981). As the amount of time spent by primary care pediatricians and family practitioners to treat infectious disease has declined in recent years, there has been a commensurate increase in willingness to treat the "new morbidity"—i.e., problems of psychosocial, psychosomatic and familial origin, learning disabilities, behavioral matters, nutritional deficits or excesses, and so forth. There is thus a limited and shrinking opportunity for schools to directly provide services without competing with private providers.

This general pattern is illustrated by the experience of the individual communities that we studied as part of the Collaborative Study of Children with Special Needs (Palfrey, Singer, Walker and Butler, 1986). In Palo Alto, California, for example, there are many physicians in the community and a very high average family income. Not surprisingly, the school district no longer sees the need for a general school nursing program; instead it has limited its program to clerical services and intensive services for children with disabilities that require medical supervision. By contrast, Houston, Texas, known to have one of the least adequate community-based care networks for low-income children (as well as one of the most disadvantaged school populations and the least generous Medicaid programs in the country), has expanded its school nursing program so that it compensates in some degree for lack of community based care. Although it is still for the most part in the traditional mold, it offers a larger component of case advocacy, management, and prevention than many other systems. Houston also has employed nurse practitioners, one for each subdistrict, to meet the need for direct service and case management for severely handicapped students.

A second general problem relates to bureaucratic constraints and inertia. The interests of school administrators are not entirely congruent with those of health care providers. The principal's mission is to ensure that the school is a good learning environment for students and a good teaching environment for teachers. To the extent that health services facilitate this end—by controlling infectious disease, sending children home if they are sick, avoiding sports accidents, providing adequate nutrition, and maintaining student mental health—the principal usually favors them (Lynch, 1977; Guyer and Walker, 1981). However, to the extent that health-related activities must be traded off against educational activities, either competing for the same dollars or competing for time in the school day, they become secondary in importance or just a nuisance. With limited educational budgets, few health services will be given equal priority to basic instructional services or mandated educational programs. Even when the health department or Medicaid program has offered a generous subsidy and all the necessary personnel, school-based health programs have met resistance from school officials who fear lost control over student time.

The more ambitious the health care model, the more likely it is that such conflict will arise. The evidence from a number of communities suggests that the nurse practitioner model has been more successful in establishing new and independent sites of primary care than in coordinating with school authorities on day-to-day interventions with students (Nader, 1978; Meeker et al., 1986). Additional tensions have been created because the new model bifurcated responsibility for students, with schools giving the entire task of health over to the nurse practitioner and/or health aide, assuming that school personnel no longer need to be involved at all.

A third problem found in many districts with traditional programs is that school resources are being spent for purposes that are at best anachronistic and at worst wholly ineffective. For example, until very recently one major eastern city school system used a portion of the school health budget to check for flat feet and perform repeated screening procedures with no adequate follow-up. Even if such procedures had some justification years ago, they no longer represent cost-effective use of school health resources.

Old priorities often reflect ossified school health programs embedded in the least dynamic area of the school superintendency or local health department. School doctoring never has been a prestigious or lucrative area of health care practice, and often has failed to attract highly qualified and energetic physicians. School health also has been a low-status choice within the nursing profession, often caricatured as attracting persons more concerned about job security and summer vacations than the delivery of high quality health care. These stereotypes are changing, especially with the arrival of nurse practitioners in the schools, but the incentive and reward structure that created the old system cannot be changed overnight, at least not without substantial sums of new money.

A fourth and final problem concerns role definition of the school nurse (Igoe, 1980b) and other health care professionals in a setting where numerous other individuals are found with partially overlapping expertise (Wold, 1981). In recent years the schools have seen a proliferation of career categories, each with its own declared competency, its own professional guild, and its own reasons for interacting with children and parents. Professionals in school settings now include psychologists, career counselors, social workers, teaching specialists (e.g., for children with learning disabilities), special educators, occupational or physical therapists, case managers, nutritionists, and the like. Many of these persons are in each school for a larger part of the day than the school nurse, who usually rotates among several schools and perhaps other locations as well. Role differentiation becomes a problem under such circumstances. Who collects what information? Who controls student records? Who contacts the family? Who interacts with the school principal about problem cases?

The solution often sought, though seldom fully attained, has been the team approach (Guyer and Walker, 1980). The concept of teamwork is sound—indeed inevitable—but in practice it has proven somewhat elusive. School health personnel seldom have had the time or status to be selected for leadership roles in team diagnosis or case management. Given the number of children for whom they have nominal responsibility, it has been all they could do to communicate basic information to principals, classroom teachers, and parents. It is the perception of many that their time needs to be reallocated so that they can spend more time attending in depth to the needs of fewer students. School health laws and current policies, which require review of all students, make this difficult.

The history of school health programs suggests that school health services tend to be effective only under certain conditions. To implement useful and cost-effective services in the schools at least requires (a) sensitivity to the expectations of the larger community, particularly medical care practitioners; (b) an awareness of financial, organizational, and bureaucratic complexities within the public schools and public health agencies; (c) an understanding of the history, evolution, and constraints on rapid reform inherent in school nursing programs; and (d) the existence of supportive state school health codes. Reform therefore involves challenges in both defining goals and implementation practices.

School Health Education

Health education is obviously an important aspect of school-based health programs. The past ten years have seen growing interest in health education (Table 11.3). This has occurred for a number of reasons. Many of the health objectives that have been established as national goals can be effectively addressed through school health education. This has been reflected in reports by the American Public Health Association and the U.S. Surgeon General. The latter's *Report on Health Promotion and Disease Prevention* said, "Our children could benefit greatly from a basic understanding of the human body and its functioning, needs and potential—and from an understanding of what really is involved in health and disease" (p. 3). An emphasis on health education has been further stimulated by recent increased concern with AIDS and other sexually transmitted diseases among teenagers.

Although a comprehensive school health education policy has been defined by the National Professional School Health Organization (1984), health education programs in local schools share a number of the problems previously described for school-based health service programs. There is little agreement about the appropriate content of courses, tremendous interstate disparities in the amount of resources committed to these programs and limited professionalization of the educational curriculum. There are no standard texts used for health education; those that are used are limited and not uniform in coverage (Richmond and Kotelchuck, 1984). Even with existing mandates, school systems are free to choose what to teach and how to teach it since funds for enforcement, training and curriculum development is limited. In addition, most states do not have specific requirements for health education teachers.

Health education courses can cover a variety of topics, and there is considerable disparity in content from one state to another (Table 11.4). While 34 states, or 67 percent of those surveyed in the 1986 American School Health Association study, mandated courses in drugs, alcohol, and tobacco, only 6 states (12 percent) required courses in sex education. Studies suggest that parents and child health professionals believe that content should vary by grade level (Walker, Clark, Jacobs, and Gortmaker, 1981) with nutrition education appropriately studied at

Table 11.3 Estimated Number of Pupils Enrolled in Health and Physical Education Courses in 1972–1973 and 1982–1983 (in thousands)

Subject	1972–1973		1982–1983	
Health, grades 9–12	1,030	8.6	2,309	18.2
Health and safety	179	1.5	69	0.5
Health, personal and family living/sex education	109	0.9	39	0.3
First aid	111	0.9	61	0.5
Alcohol, drug and tobacco education	140	1.2	20	0.2
Environmental health	20	0.2	N/A	
Health and physical education, grade 9	1,734	14.5	2,949	23.2
Health and physical education, grade 10	2,423	20.2	2,254	17.8
Health and physical education, grade 11	1,508	12.6	1,330	10.5
Health and physical education, grade 12	1,155	9.6	939	7.4
Physical education (adapted)	2	0.0	40	1.6
Body dynamics/conditioning/postural apparatus	17	0.1	N/A	
Dance, rhythm and dramatic events	30	0.3	59	0.5
Modern dance/gymnastic	54	0.4	51	4.4
Individual and dual sports/aquatics/swimming	57	0.5	387	3.1
Team sports	54	0.4	637	17.4
Recreation/lifetime sports/hobbies	44	0.4	67	0.5
Leadership/school support	11	0.1	197	1.6
Human relations	31	0.3	41	0.3
Psychology	597	5.0	656	5.2
Sociology	582	4.9	1,602	12.7
Social problems/criminology	136	1.1	93	0.7
Intergroup relationships	54	0.5	63	0.5

Source: The 1973 data are from a survey of public schools with grade 7 or higher. The 1983 data come from another education study of selected schools which had a grade 12 and included private as well as public schools.

Note: To account for discrepancies between the 1973 and 1983 data in compiling the report on which this table is derived (National Center for Education Statistics, 1984), only public schools with grades 9–12 were included, resulting in a sample of 5,379 schools in 1973 and 835 in 1982. Because of the small numbers in the samples, the somewhat disparate bases from which the data were generated and changes in course names and labels from year to year, data in Table 12.3 should be interpreted with caution, as they give only a gross indicator of health education activities in high schools across the United States in the two time periods.

Table 11.4 Number and Percentage of States that Required Specific Health Education Topics

Topic	N	%
Drugs, alcohol, tobacco	34	(67)
Hygiene	19	(37)
Safety	17	(33)
Diseases	15	(29)
Nutrition	12	(24)
Mental health	10	(20)
Environment	10	(20)
Consumer health	10	(20)
Anatomy, physiology	9	(18)
CPR	9	(18)
Community health	9	(18)
First aid	8	(16)
Growth and development	8	(16)
Oral hygiene	7	(14)
Venereal disease	7	(14)
Sex education	6	(19)
Health careers	1	(2)

Source: Allensworth (1986).

the elementary school level, alcohol at the elementary or junior high school level, contraception and birth control at the junior high school level, marijuana and other drugs at the elementary or junior high school level, and venereal disease at the high school level. The resources devoted to these programs also varies greatly from one state to the next. This is reflected in state requirements for a minimal number of instructional hours for health education—there is as much as a fivefold difference between the lowest and highest requirements (Table 11.5).

These interstate disparities are exacerbated by inconsistent and incomplete requirements for training those who teach health education courses. According to a survey conducted by the American School Health Association in 1986, twenty-six states (51 percent of those polled) do not require prospective teachers of elementary education to take any courses in health education in order to meet the state certification requirement. For those who wished to specialize in health education, eleven states had certification requirements for elementary health education teachers and forty-five states for secondary teachers of health education. The report pointed out that while forty-five states required certification for health education teachers, many of these states accepted training in combined health and physical education to satisfy the coursework requirement, when, often, these teachers are prepared to teach physical education but lacking in preparation to teach health.

The federal government has supported health education through a variety of agencies and departments which vary in scope of program and funding. What federal coordination exists comes through the Office of Disease Prevention and Health Promotion in the Centers for Disease

Table 11.5 Average Number of Health Education Hours per Year by Grade Range in States with a Time Requirement

State	K–6	7–8	9–12	K–12
Alabama	LD[a]	LD	18.75	5.77
Arkansas	90.00[b]	18.50	18.75	57.08[b]
Delaware	—	30.00	18.75	10.38
District of Columbia	LD	45.00	18.75	12.69
Georgia	30.00	45.00	18.75	28.85
Hawaii	30.00	37.50	18.75	27.69
Idaho	90.00	—	18.75	54.23
Illinois	0	37.50	18.75	11.54
Indiana	26.14[b]	30.00	37.50	30.23[b]
Kentucky	18.00	18.00	18.75	18.23
Louisiana	77.14[b]	100.00[b]	15.00	61.53[a]
Minnesota	30.86	60.00	15.00	30.38
New Jersey	77.14[b]	100.00[b]	22.50[a]	63.85[b]
New York	—	37.50	18.75	11.54
North Carolina	—	—	37.50[b]	11.54[b]
North Dakota	30.86	18.00	7.50	21.69
Ohio	LD	24.00	15.00	8.31
Oregon	—	—	32.50	10.00
Pennsylvania	LD	15.00	15.00	6.92
Rhode Island	30.00	30.00	30.00	30.00
South Carolina	38.57	37.50	—	26.54
Tennessee	90.00	75.00	18.75	65.77
Texas	15.43	12.50	18.75	16.00
Utah	36.00	37.50	18.75	30.92
Virginia	—	—	16.50	5.08
West Virginia	50.57	45.00	33.75	44.54
Wisconsin	—	—	18.75	5.77
Total	760.71	903.50	540.25	706.92
M[c]	47.54	40.64	20.77	26.19
SD	26.49	24.19	7.18	19.14

Source: Allensworth (1986).

[a] LD = Number of hours is locally determined.
[b] Health Education requirement is combined with physical education.
[c] Mean is based on the states that reported a requirement.

Control (Gilbert, Davis and Damberg, 1985). The federal agencies that have sponsored major school-based health promotion activities include the Center for Disease Control, the National Heart, Lung and Blood Institute, National Cancer Institute, the Alcohol, Drug Abuse and Mental Health Administration, and the Office on Smoking and Health in the Department of Health and Human Services, as well as selected activities in the Department of Education, Agriculture and Transportation. Although models for doing health education research have been developed, studies supporting the efficacy of health education are not extensive (Stone, 1983). Until recently, what research there is tended to be disappointing in demonstrating that health education effects changes in health behaviors.

The most scientifically sound school health evaluation completed to date (Connell, Turner and Mason, 1985) produced more positive results than previous studies; health education courses increased pupil's knowledge on health topics and to a lesser extent, increased positive health attitudes and self-reporting of positive health behaviors. Not surprisingly, the study found that the most effective programs were comprehensive, had administrative support, adequate teacher preparation, and the largest degree of adherence to the prepared curriculum (Fors and Doster, 1985). This is consistent with the findings for the comprehensive Seaside Health Education program that began in Oregon and has now been disseminated through comprehensive training sessions to many other states (Drolet, 1982; Stevens, Davis and Gutting, undated).

The Impact on School Health of Changing Public Policies

In this section we will reflect on some of the changes in education, health and social policies that have affected the shape and substance of school health services over the past decade. These include declining enrollments and reduction in financial support for education, major federal education and social initiatives including the Great Society Programs of the mid-1960s, the Education for All Handicapped Children's Act in the 1970s, major changes in the structure and financing of the public health care system, through Title XIX (Medicaid) and Title V of the Social Security Act, and various national health demonstration programs.

Student Enrollment and Public Attitudes toward Education

One of the casualties of federal budget cutbacks over the past ten years has been good national data on school-based health services. Although rough estimates can be made about the total amount being spent on health services by local and state education agencies, very little can be said about how this money is allocated, how many persons it employs, and other basic facts.

Because enrollment has declined in recent years, one might hypothesize that ratios of school nurses to students have become more favorable. In fact, however, our findings from the five metropolitan school districts in the collaborative study of Children with Special Needs suggest the opposite—ratios have become less favorable as cuts made in education and health department budgets have disproportionately been borne by school nursing. As already mentioned in the prior section, some affluent districts have suspended the school health program altogether except for recordkeeping and services to selected groups of medically involved students. This move has been justified in part by increasingly favorable ratios of office-based physicians to children in the community, and in part because the changing profile of childhood morbidity has made infectious disease less common, undermining the traditional rationale for school-based services.

In central cities and rural areas, of course, there remains much for a school nurse to do by way of case-finding, referral, and routine consultation. Here too, however, the limited data available suggest that large-scale cutbacks in public school budgets have had very significant impact on the scope and quality of services (Igoe, 1984; Education Research Center, 1986). Services which were underfunded in the first place now are even further reduced.

School health services are uniquely vulnerable to cutbacks because they are interstitial, not a high priority for either schools or health departments except insofar as they must conform to state law and program guidelines. State laws by and large have remained minimal, meaning that the only infusions of new funds and personnel for school-based health services have come from major new federal and state programs, or else major privately funded demonstration programs.

Great Society Programs

Against this background, the role of federal initiatives—especially the Great Society programs and the Education for All Handicapped Children Act—has been critical in bolstering and redirecting school health.

The Great Society programs initiated in the mid-1960s introduced several transforming concepts to school-based health programs. In the education sector, Headstart and ESEA Title I (later to become Chapter I) embodied the philosophy that enriched health and nutrition services should be an integral part of compensatory education for the disadvantaged. This view resulted in the commitment of federal and state dollars for new activities in health screening and referral.

The fact that Headstart is a preschool program means that a significant proportion of the nation's low-income 4- and 5-year-olds have their health needs assessed before they ever get to school (Zigler and Valentine, 1979). The program also offers new opportunities for continuity of records and services between the preschool and school.

The influence of this philosophical approach peaked in the early 1970s. Federal money for Follow Through programs, the extension of Head Start into the elementary schools, provided money for health and social services for students from disadvantaged families. The Elementary and Secondary Education Act, under the auspices of compensatory education programs, funded core health personnel in schools serving low-income populations. Funding for these health-related activities, however, has been reduced in recent years.

Two Great Society health programs also have been very influential over the past 20 years in shaping and partially supporting school health programs. These are the Community Health Center (CHC) program and Medicaid. In the late 1960s and early 1970s, the CHC program established, under federal support in many medically deprived central cities and rural areas, a new infrastructure of community-based primary care units. Many of these units still exist today, although funding and target populations are somewhat more diverse and the federal support reduced. Some CHCs reached out to schools, reinforcing, or in a few instances directly providing, school health services. They also performed many of the functions of referral and treatment that would have been provided by private practitioners if a sufficient number of physicians had been located in the community. A major health care financing reform from the late 1960s was the passage of Title XIX (Medicaid) and the Social Security Act.

Although the potential for Medicaid to have a major impact on the schools is available, particularly through the Early and Periodic Screening, Diagnosis and Treatment program (EPSDT), it has not to date significantly enhanced the delivery of school-based health services (Children's Defense Fund, 1977; Meisels, 1984). Some of the reasons for this are discussed below.

The Education for All Handicapped Children Act (EHA)

The advent of P.L. 94-142 (the Education for All Handicapped Children Act, or EHA) was among the most significant transforming influences on school health programs in the past decade. This federal legislation, passed by Congress in 1975 and implemented in 1977, created a major new entitlement for handicapped children and their parents (Singer and Butler, 1987). It was radical in several ways.

First, it requires that every child with a handicap—including a very wide range of disabling conditions—be provided a free appropriate education by the public schools. The majority of special education students are classified as learning disabled or speech impaired, but many of the rest have severe physical and mental disabilities and chronic conditions which might have kept them out of school altogether in the past. Second, EHA includes an elaborate set of due process guarantees for parents, requiring an active school-system search for disabled children, an individualized assessment and educational plan for each, parental involvement in the placement process, and administrative or legal recourse for parents in the event they wish to contest their child's placement and educational program. Third, it mandates that disabled children be served in a "least restrictive environment," which has resulted in the mainstreaming of many children who previously would have been found at home or in specialized care settings. Finally, although explicit reference to health services is limited, EHA implies that the schools have a new and enlarged role in soliciting adequate medical judgment and information, involving health care personnel in individualized program meetings, and prescribing and providing selected forms of health treatment (e.g., supervising catheterization, prescribing physical therapy) (Walker and Jacobs, 1984; Palfrey et al., 1987; Singer and Butler, 1987).

In analyzing the impact of EHA on school health services, a careful distinction must be drawn between its impact in traditional school health personnel and programs, and its impact in terms of new services made available in the school setting. By and large the additional health-related services mandated by EHA, rather than transforming the traditional school health model, have simply been superimposed on it. School nurses responsible for services to the general school population have been stretched so thin that they and their supervisors have not assumed new responsibilities. School districts have simply paid the new excess costs for selected services (usually for the most part nursing care of physically handicapped and/or chronically ill children). In some instances, however, new nurse practitioners have been employed with wider responsibilities for the entire special education population.

The main positive impacts of EHA on health services have been, first, to engage the health care community more fully in the process of school-based diagnosis and educational programing; second, to unify further the education and health sectors in a new shared mission to treat learning disabilities and other high prevalence conditions comprising the "new morbidity"; and third, to provide added incentive for the employment of nurse practitioner and new personnel other than traditional school health nurses. For purposes of training and certification, the EHA also has resulted in a broadening of requisite competencies even for traditional school nursing roles (Smith and Goodwin, 1982).

Changes in the schools in turn have begun to influence the entire pediatric practice community, requiring that they become familiar with the process of special education diagnosis, placement, and the "related services" received by their patients. Some sense of this change is reflected in schools' employment of health professionals. Between school year 1976–77 and 1983–84 the number of occupational and physical therapists employed by U.S. public schools grew from 1,905 to 5,091; the number of psychological and diagnostic staff from 17,731 to 20,659, the number of speech pathologists and audiologists from 11,502 to 20,946

(United States Department of Education, 1980, 1985). Growth would have been even greater had more trained professionals been available.

Physicians' involvement in special education programs has not been measured nationally. In our own five-site study we discovered only a moderate degree of physician involvement (Palfrey, Sarro, Singer and Wenger, 1987). Only 30 percent of special education students were reported to have been referred to physicians by the school, and only 10 percent had a physician who actually came to the school to participate in an interdisciplinary conference. Among particular subgroups, such as the physically handicapped, recurrent contact between doctors and the schools was, however, quite common.

Our data further suggest a bimodal pattern of involvement with special education programs among community-based pediatricians and family practitioners. A limited number of these doctors, often the leadership of the local chapters of medical societies like the Academy of Pediatrics, are intimately familiar with EHA and have extensive contact with school authorities. Some even allocate a day each week to the school program. However, the vast majority of office-based physicians remain largely uninvolved, transmitting materials to the schools when requested to do so but otherwise not communicating with school personnel and not having any real comprehension of the school-based program. For example, among children with speech impairments and learning disabilities in our five study sites, we discovered that around 40 percent have physicians who were completely unaware that their patient was classified as handicapped by the schools or was receiving special education services. The lesson is that, despite good will and positive rhetoric surrounding interpenetration of the health care system and the schools, there remains insufficient incentive for real exchange between these two service sectors, especially when a student does not present a severe chronic illness or other medically complex problem.

EHA occasioned a serious and sometimes painful reconsideration of school nursing priorities in many school districts. The public schools have experienced a sizable increase in the numbers of seriously disabled students who attend school. There has also been a general move toward placement of disabled children in mainstream classrooms, even among students who fifteen years ago would have been found in substantially separate settings or at home (Singer, Butler, Palfrey and Walker, 1986; Singer and Butler, 1987). Some of these children have extensive and recurrent medical care needs during the school day (e.g., respirator care, tracheal suctioning, catheterization) (Palfrey et al., 1987). Who is to provide such services? In many districts nurses are still operating under the traditional model and by law cannot provide any but preventive services at school. Likewise, they probably do not have the time to provide such care and still accomplish all of their routine, legally mandated tasks for the general school population. The mainstreaming movement has further complicated matters by dispersing medically needy children to numerous community schools rather than concentrating them in central locations. How does this issue resolve itself?

In general what has often happened is that the schools have invested in a small second tier of nurses or nurse practitioners to meet specific health objectives for a subset of the special education population (Palfrey et al., 1987; U.S. Congress, Office of Technology Assessment, 1987; Walker, 1989). This initiative usually has occurred at school system expense rather than health department expense, because it derives from federal educational requirements. Although no national data exist to confirm the point, it is our hypothesis that supplemental nursing budgets for physically handicapped and chronically ill students have been funded by school districts even where health departments contribute and control the rest of the school health budget. Health departments typically are very reluctant to cede control over maternal and child health monies or reallocate them according to new school system priorities unless they can first fulfill the basic public health functions of the traditional maternal and child health programs.

A primary component of the EHA involves the "related services" section which states that medically necessary services be provided to keep children in school (Walker and Jacobs, 1984). These services, like the others mandated by EHA, must be provided in the "least restrictive setting," which is interpreted to mean that most treatment is given by the health professional in the school attended by the child. Treatment is generally in the fields of speech, occupational, and physical therapy and psychological counselling.

Different localities have dealt with the need to incorporate more skilled health personnel into the educational environment in different ways. Some school systems have directly hired the appropriate personnel, under the supervision of the special education director, while others have contracted for services with outside health agencies. Some states are attempting to coordinate these services across the entire state (e.g., in Connecticut and Michigan), while most leave the responsibility in the local school districts. However such services are provided, the local school district remains, by law, responsible for assuring appropriate and adequate service. This decentralized responsibility may not be especially effective.

Originally, the schools were required to finance these related services entirely from their own budgets. To ease the burden on school budgets, laws have been passed in several states, including Massachusetts, to allow schools to seek third party reimbursement. Private health insurance, health maintenance organizations, and Medicaid are all potential sources of funds. Since health insurers have been hesitant to accept schools as certified providers of care, schools trying to obtain outside sources of payment for service have tended to contract with intermediary health agencies. A recent 1986 study in Massachusetts (Bender, 1986) suggested that there is wide disparity in quality control over services— particularly where the services were contracted from an outside agency. No special education director interviewed in the study had clear requirements or guidelines for the services provided. Overall, larger school systems with capability of third-party billing have more readily used these options than smaller and more rural systems.

Of all payers, Medicaid is most likely to cover these outpatient services because of its relatively comprehensive coverage. Cooperation between Medicaid and the schools, though, varies greatly from state to state. Cooperation has been hindered by a lack of clear national standards for either interagency arrangements or for the services being purchased.

National Vaccination Campaigns

Sometimes schools can have a positive effect on child health simply by exercising a gatekeeping function. Such has been the case in the implementation of recent national vaccination campaigns, as already mentioned. In 1977, the Center for Disease Control of the Federal Department of Health and Human Services launched a campaign to immunize the nation's children against measles. At that time approximately 40 percent of all children under 15 (20 million) had not been totally vaccinated. Because of this national effort, there was a dramatic decrease from 1975–1982 in reported cases of rubella, measles, mumps, and diphtheria (Bumpers, 1984). One reason for this dramatic success was the willingness of states and local school districts to cooperate by insisting that youngsters be vaccinated as a precondition for school enrollment.

Vaccination campaigns probably have not done much to change the scope or configuration of school health services except perhaps to improve and streamline record keeping, but these campaigns have significantly affected child health and health risk subsequent to childhood. As such they are an instance of schools being used efficiently to attain a major national health objective.

National Health Demonstration Programs

Health demonstration programs in schools have been designed with the expectations that they will model exemplary practices that, if successful, can be replicated elsewhere. In the recent past, large scale demonstrations have generally focused on three issues: (1) innovative ways of delivery school health services, mainly using the nurse practitioner model (Nader, 1978; Meeker et al., 1986), (2) innovative health promotion activities, mainly using health education curricula and materials (Stone, 1983; Connell et al., 1985, Gilbert et al., 1985), and (3) demonstrations funded jointly by the Office of Special Education in the Department of Education (1985) and the Bureau of Maternal and Child Health in the Department of Health and Human Services to show model practices of service delivery to students with disabilities.

It is beyond the scope of this chapter to summarize all that has been learned from the various demonstrations during the past decade or all the ways that they have influenced the scope and quality of child health, school health services, and the larger delivery system. We will venture three generalizations, however, focusing on these categories of demonstration rather than individual projects.

First, as long as there is an external source of funding, whether it be a private philanthropy or public program, it is possible to institute the nurse practitioner model and substantially improve access to health services for low-income children. However, schools are not likely to pick up the bill for such services when the demonstration ends (meaning that unless there is some prospect of continuity of support from Medicaid or another public source the program will die). The demonstrations have also raised questions about appropriate target populations. While the school is a good delivery site for children, it is a less effective site for addressing the whole family's health needs. The demonstration projects also showed that it is more feasible to serve all children in a given school than to try to serve only low-income children. This is not only because of complexities in determining eligibility on an individual basis but also because of the organizational problems presented by trying to introduce a service for only some students without creating stigma or any perception of unfairness among those not deemed eligible. This has proven an obstacle to effective collaboration between health and education sectors, since Medicaid administrators have not been willing to target reimbursement to entire schools in low-income neighborhoods.[2]

Second, health education works—for a while. Positive effects have been measured in the short-term for improved knowledge and attitudes, and occasionally, for some behaviors. However, evidence remains equivocal regarding long-term effects, especially in the behavior change area. A second issue surrounding health education is that the comprehensive programs which are most effective in evaluation studies cannot be shoehorned into most school curricula without incurring the disapprobation of educators, because of the time they require. Teachers, even though they would heartily agree about the primary importance of heath education in a young person's life, especially an adolescent's, also see health-related instruction as a secondary objective for the schools.

Third, appropriate community-based, family centered services for seriously disabled children which bridge the health and education worlds are difficult to implement without adequate resources. One key is the willingness of an agency to pay a full-time case coordinator/manager for the child and family. Even in this case however, several other conditions must be met for a program to be effective: the manager must have equal legitimacy (i.e., be bureaucratically accountable) in more than one service sector; he or she must be politically astute enough to know how to gain and maintain access to services in the child's behalf; and the manager must use a record system mutually acceptable to all parties. Usually this means that case management or coordination simply costs too much. A least-cost solution to case management that has sometimes proven successful is the use of parent aides and volunteers, who can act in informal networks.

However, even this solution is not totally viable, because school districts under severe budget constraints have tended to cut first from their payrolls exactly those "lower-level" personnel who perform a boundary-spanning function, most notably classroom aides, social work aides and health aides. In case management and family support for children with disabilities, these cuts are apt to be pound foolish and penny wise. Clearly there is no one best solution to the complex issue of how to span agency boundaries for children with disabilities, while providing a program resistant to budget curtailing.

The Future: School-based Health Care

Bringing together the resources and goals of schools which are autonomous, available to everyone, and locally controlled, and health providers, who are largely funded by a private system with little local control, is a major challenge. In anticipating the future of school health services, one could easily predict more of the same. Certainly the priorities of school administrators and superintendents are not likely to undergo any radical reformation, and fundamental issues of health financing and case coordination will not go away. However, some ongoing developments in the U.S. health care system may have significant implications for the future of school health programs. Without making any claim to having a crystal ball, we anticipate that three sets of trends will be particularly important; the first affecting the need for school-based services, the second the availability of health care providers willing to work in and with the schools, the third broader societal attitudes about the appropriateness of school-based programs.

The prevalence of children needing school-based health programs is likely to be altered by several ongoing changes in the health care system. The first is the growth of prepaid provider organizations such as HMOs. Prepaid benefit packages for children are likely to be quite broad, encompassing many forms of prevention and routine primary care as well as the forms of secondary and tertiary care normally covered at present by most health insurance plans. Hence, those who qualify for a major family health plan linked to a large health care provider are likely to have comprehensive child health benefits including preventive and primary care with modest copayment. This would further reduce the need, at least among children with a fully employed parent, for a full-scale primary health care program in the schools.

Prepayment, however, also creates a tendency to skim or seek only the most desirable patients (see Chapter 8). In the case of children, this would be most likely to affect chronically ill or disabled children, those at high risk for disability, and those from low-income families. Children in these categories would fall through the cracks or become a residual group referred increasingly, for all elements of care, to community hospitals and major teaching hospitals. This group is likely to become larger if Medicaid and private insurers increasingly restrict coverage to save costs.

This group of children comprises many of the same ones who are identified as handicapped in school programs or else are eligible for compensatory education under ESEA Chapter I. It is thus possible that schools will be turned to, more than before, to support health care for these students as well as their schooling, particularly if the educators are able to strike a bargain with teaching hospitals, health maintenance organizations, special insurance pools, or other agencies that finance the care for these children. For example, Freedman and colleagues (1988) suggested using schools as a basis for enrolling children and families in health insurance schemes.

The second significant ongoing trend involves the supply of physicians available and willing to work in schools. If the ratio of child health providers to children continues to increase, there will be a greater probability that some primary care physicians will spend time in school settings. The simple picture of supply and demand, however, is confounded with at least two other factors—the changing profile of pediatric practice and the changing ratio of male to female pediatricians. It seems reasonable to expect that further changes in the epidemiology of childhood disorders and corresponding shifts in the content of pediatric practice will drive primary care physicians toward at least partial involvement with schools, because treatment of psychosocial and familiar concerns will continue to gain saliency over traditional treatment of infectious disease and schools are where many "new morbidity" problems are seen. If, as is projected, in ten years more women than men will be practicing pediatrics, pediatric involvement with schools could be further increased. Women may be more willing—or more often required—to accept part-time and flex-time arrangements that would be consonant with school-based activities.[3]

Public willingness to support school-based services may increase as the ratio of children to elderly citizens continues to fall and concern about national productivity leads to a new public motivation to ensure that each child maximizes his or her potential. On the other hand, it may turn out that, as an increasingly smaller proportion of families have children of school age, taxpayer willingness to support new initiatives in the schools will further decline. A third possibility is that these two trends will cancel out each other, so the propensity to spend on health services in school settings will remain unchanged.

Apart from these general attitudes toward school-based services, at least some communities have become willing to organize such primary health care units in their high schools. Although the development is far from becoming a national movement, it is being given further impetus by widespread publicity surrounding several programs which claim to have succeeded in reducing adolescent pregnancy rates. The Robert Wood Johnson Foundation is investing $16.5 million in a national demonstration program, and there has been nascent Congressional interest in the possibility of some kind of federal support.

This trend has been encouraged by growing concerns about teenage pregnancies and will likely be further reinforced by the spectre of AIDS. If the public acceptance of school-based adolescent clinics continues to expand, this will further consolidate the nurse practitioner model, even in communities where access to care outside schools is adequate. Again, however, the lesson of past demonstration programs must be remembered: unless some agency is willing to pick up the bill for services after a demonstration ends, even the most successful programs will dry up.

These same trends present opportunities for policy makers to improve the quality of school-based health services. To increase the institutional support for school-based practitioners, it would be useful to establish closer affiliation between the school and organized community providers, such as HMOs. Prepaid plans already have a financial incentive to establish linkages as long as a sufficient number of the children enrolled in their plan are at a single school, so the cost of establishing a program is offset by potential savings to the HMO. More often, few children from any HMO will be enrolled at a particular school. Under these circumstances, it may be desirable for policy makers to require HMOs to establish such affiliations (e.g., "adopt a school") as a condition of either licensure or participation in the Medicaid program.

Similarly, it would be desirable for policy makers to further encourage private practitioners to become involved in school-based programs, since this would bolster those programs and likely improve continuity of care and effective sharing of records for individual children. Some form of public service requirement could, for example, be added to government guaranteed loans for medical students who specialize in pediatrics. Alternatively, this too could be made a requirement of licensure.

Finally, to take full advantage of current community support for school-based health services, it is essential that a continued source of funding be available for programs that move beyond the demonstration stage. Since the greatest potential and greatest need for these services is concentrated in low-income communities, Medicaid seems the most appropriate source for that financing. To facilitate this funding, states should increase the ease with which school-based clinics can qualify as Medicaid-eligible providers. Resources could be further freed by allowing students at schools in low-income communities to qualify as "presumptively eligible," without requiring a means test for each individual school.

In many ways, schools have become vehicles for addressing larger social issues that involve the health needs of children. Major barriers to accomplishing this include the lack of financing, the bureaucratic limitations of educational institutions, the philosophic differences in approaches between the health and education systems, and the lack of commitment on the part of the larger society to solve child health problems.

The future viability and quality of school-based health services and health education thus depends on the availability of money, the role schools are given with respect to larger social issues, the supply of pediatricians and other health professionals, and the existence of clear school health mandates at the state and federal levels. But it will also require a basic commitment by society to ensure children's health. As Lynch stated: "School health is the occupational health service for children. We don't ask the physicians in the community if we can have an occupational health program in the factory. We expect that there is a responsibility at all levels to have such a program" (Gephart, Egan and Hutchins, 1984, p. 11).

Only if we are willing to meet this responsibility directly will the potential of schools to meet children's health needs be fully realized.

Notes

1. Public schools enroll the vast majority (about 90 percent) of all children in schools (National Center for Health Statistics, 1979).
2. School-based targeting was permitted under the compensatory education reimbursement formula for ESEA Chapter I.
3. A feminist critique of this same scenario might be less positive, seeing it as yet another way in which women entering a profession could be shunted to its less prestigious and less remunerative sectors. It would, however, lead one to the same conclusion—that pediatricians will be increasingly found in school settings.

References

Allensworth, D.D. 1986. *School Health in America,* 4th ed. Kent, Ohio: American School Health Association.

Bender, A. 1986. *Third Party Reimbursement for Related Medical Services under Chapter 766.* Paper for applied research tutorial, Department of Health Policy and Management, Harvard School of Public Health, Boston.

Blum, R.W., K. Pfaffinger, and W.B. Donald. 1982. A School-Based Comprehensive Health Clinic for Adolescents. *Journal of School Health* 52:486–490.

Boston Globe. 1986. Educating Pupil to Cost $4,263 This Year. August 29, p. 18.

Bumpers, D. 1984. Preventive Health Care for Children. *American Psychologist* 39:896–899.

Children's Defense Fund. 1977. *EPSDT: Does It Spell Health Care for Poor Children?* Washington, D.C.

Comprehensive School Health Education. 1984. *Journal of School Health* 55:312–315.

Connell, D.B., R.R. Turner, and E.F. Mason. 1985. Summary of the Findings of the School Health Education Evaluation: Health Promotion Effectiveness, Implementation, and Costs. *Journal of School Health* 55:316–323.

DeAngelis, C. 1981. The Robert Wood Johnson Foundation National School Health Program: A Presentation and Progress Report. *Clinical Pediatrics* 20:344–348.

Drolet, J. 1982. *Evaluation of the Impact of the Seaside Health Education Conferences and the Nutrition Education Training Programs in the Oregon School Systems.* Unpublished Doctoral Dissertation, University of Oregon.

Dryfoos, J. 1985. School-Based Health Clinics: A New Approach to Preventing Adolescent Pregnancy? *Family Planning Perspectives* 17:70–75.

Education Research Service. 1986. *Report of School Nurse Services.* Arlington, Va.

Fors, S.W., and M.E. Doster. 1985. Implications of Results: Factors for Success. *Journal of School Health* 55:332–334.

Freedman, S.A., B.R. Klepper, R.P. Duncan, and S.P. Bell. 1988. Coverage of the Uninsured and Underinsured: A Proposal for School Enrollment-Based Family Health Insurance. *New England Journal of Medicine* 318:843–847.

Gephart, J., M.C. Egan, and V.L. Hutchins. 1984. Perspectives on Health of School-Age Children: Expectations for the Future. *Journal of School Health* 54:11–17.

Gertler, D.B., and L.A. Barker. 1973. *Patterns of Course Offerings and Enrollments in Public Secondary Schools: 1970–71.* Washington, D.C.: National Center for Education Statistics, DHEW.

Gilbert, G.G., R.L. Davis, and C.L. Damberg. 1985. Current Federal Activities in School Health Education. *Public Health Reports* 100:499–507.

Grant, W.V., and A.R. Munse. 1977. *Statistics of State School Systems: 1975–76.* Washington, D.C.: National Center for Health Statistics.

Guyer, B., and D.K. Walker. 1980. *Summary Report: School Health Services in Flint Elementary Schools.* Boston: Community Child Health Studies, Harvard School of Public Health.

Hodgkinson, H.L. 1986. What's Ahead for Education. *Principal* 65:6–11.

Igoe, J.B. 1980a. Changing Patterns in School Health and School Nursing. *Nursing Outlook* 28:486–492.

———. 1980b. What Is School Nursing? A Plea for More Standardized Roles. *American Journal of Maternal Child Nursing* 5:307–311.

Igoe, J. B., N. Nelson, and E.L. Slaughter. 1984. *Report of a National Survey of School Nurse Supervisors.* Denver: School of Nursing, University of Colorado Health Sciences.

Kirby, D. 1985. *School-Based Health Clinics: An Emerging Approach to Improving Adolescent Health and Addressing Teenage Pregnancy.* Washington, D.C.: Center for Population Options.

Kolbe, L.J. 1985. *Indicators for Planning and Monitoring School Health Programs.* Paper presented at the Symposium on Indicators of Health Promotive Behavior, University of California, Los Angeles, November.

Lynch, A. 1977. Evaluating School Health Programs. In A. Levin (ed.), Health Services: The Local Perspective. *Proceedings of the Academy of Political Science* 32:89–105.

———. 1982. Organizational and Legislative Issues Related to Health Care of School-Age Youth. In J.C. Swart, J.B. Igoe, and J. Gephart (eds.), *Health of School-Age Children: Expectations for the Future.* Washington, D.C.: Division of Maternal and Child Health, Bureau of Health Care Delivery and Assistance, DHHS.

Meeker, R.J., C. DeAngelis, B. Berman, H.E. Freeman, and D. Oda. 1986. *Image: Journal of Nursing Scholarship* 18:86–91.

Meisels, S.J. 1984. Prediction, Prevention and Developmental Screening in the EPSDT Program. In H.W. Stevenson and A.E. Siegel (eds.), *Child Development Research and Social Policy.* Chicago: University of Chicago Press.

Nader, P.R. (ed.). 1978. *Options for School Health: Meeting Community Needs.* Germantown, Md.: Aspen Publications.

National Center for Education Statistics. 1979. *The Condition of Education.* Washington, D.C.: U.S. Department of Education.

———. 1981. *Revenues and Expenditures for Public Elementary and Secondary Education: FY 1980.* Washington, D.C.: U.S. Department of Education.

———. 1984. *A Trend Study of High School Offerings and Enrollments: 1972–73 and 1981–82.* Washington, D.C.: U.S. Department of Education.

———. 1986. Personal communication.

Office of Child Health Affairs, Department of Health, Education and Welfare. 1976. *School Health: Working Paper.* Washington, D.C.

Palfrey, J.S., L. Diprete, J.D. Singer, and M. Wenger. 1987. Physician Familiarity with the Educational Programs of Their Special Needs Patients. *Journal of Developmental and Behavioral Pediatrics* 8:198–202.

Palfrey, J.S., J.D. Singer, D.K. Walker, and J.A. Butler. 1986. Health and Special Education: A Study of New Developments for Handicapped Children in Five Metropolitan Communities. *Public Health Reports* 101:379–388.

Parcel, G.S., P.R. Nader, and M.P. Meyer. 1977. Adolescent Health Concerns, Problems, and Patterns of Utilizations in a Triethnic Urban Population. *Pediatrics* 60:157–164.

Resnick, M., R.W. Blum, and D. Hedin. 1980. The Appropriateness of Health Services for Adolescents: Youth's Opinions and Attitudes. *Journal of Adolescent Health Care* 1:137–141.

Richmond, J.B., and M. Kotelchuck. 1984. Personal Health Maintenance for Children. *Western Journal of Medicine* 141:816–823.

Robert Wood Johnson Foundation. 1985. *Special Report: National School Health Services Program*. Princeton, N.J.

Select Panel for the Promotion of Child Health. 1981. Better Health for Our Children: A National Strategy, DHHS Publication No. 77-55071. Washington, D.C.: G.P.O.

Singer, J.D., and J.A. Butler. 1987. The Education for All Handicapped Children Act: Schools as Agents of Social Reform. *Harvard Educational Review* 57:125–154.

Singer, J.D., J.A. Butler, J.S. Palfrey, and D.K. Walker. 1986. Characteristics of Special Education Placements: Findings from Probability Samples in Five Metropolitan School Districts. *Journal of Special Education* 20(3):319–337.

Smith, A.N., and L.D. Goodwin. 1982. School Nurse Achievement Program, Part I: Program Development in Twelve States. *Journal of School Health* 52:535–538.

Stevens, N.H., L.G. Davis, and J.M. Gutting. Undated. How Does Your District Measure Up: Characteristics of Exemplary Districts for School Health Promotion. Eugene, Ore.: Health Education, University of Oregon.

Stone, E.J. (ed.). 1983. *Proceedings of the National Conference on School Health Education Research in the Heart, Lung and Blood Areas. Journal of School Health* 54(6):1–80.

U.S. Congress, Office of Technology Assessment. 1987. *Technology-Dependent Children: Hospital v. Home Care*. Washington, D.C.: G.P.O.

U.S. Department of Education. 1980. *Second Annual Report to Congress on the Implementation of Public Law 94-142: The Education for All Handicapped Children Act*. Washington, D.C.: Office of Special Education and Rehabilitative Services, U.S. Department of Education.

———. 1985. *Seventh Annual Report to Congress on the Implementation of The Handicapped Act*. Washington, D.C.: Office of Special Education and Rehabilitative Services, U.S. Department of Education.

U.S. Department of Health, Education and Welfare. 1979. *Healthy People: The Surgeon General's Report on Health Promotion and Disease Prevention*. Washington, D.C.: G.P.O.

Walker, D.K. 1989. Educational Options for Pediatric Home Care Clients. In W. Votroubek and P. McCoy (eds.), *Pediatric Home Care*. Rockville, Md.: Aspen Publications.

Walker, D.K., C.J.G. Clark, F.H. Jacobs, and S.L. Gortmaker. 1981. Parents' and Professionals' Views on Health Education Topics. *Massachusetts Journal of Community Health* 1:18–23.

Walker, D.K., A. Cross, P. Heymann, H. Ruch-Ross, P. Benson, and J.W.G. Tuthill. 1982. Comparisons between Inner-city and Private School Adolescents' Perceptions of Health Problems. *Journal of Adolescent Health Care* 3:82–90.

Walker, D.K., and F.H. Jacobs. 1984. Chronically Ill Children in School. *Peabody Journal of Education* 61:28–74.

Walker, D.K., J.B. Richmond, and S. Buka. 1984. Summary and Recommendations for Next Steps. In D.K. Walker and J.B. Richmond (eds.), *Monitoring Child*

Health in the United States: Selected Issues and Policies. Cambridge, Mass.: Harvard University Press.

Wold, S.J. 1981. *School Nursing: A Framework for Practice.* St. Louis: C.V. Mosby.

Zigler, E., and J. Valentine (eds.). 1979. *Project Headstart.* New York: Free Press.

IV
Integrating Funding and Services for Children

12

The Evolution and Future Role of Title V

Bernard Guyer, M.D., M.P.H.

For more than 50 years, Title V of the Social Security Act has served as the legislative foundation for maternal and child health (MCH) services in the United States. Title V established the infrastructure for MCH services at the state level, and encouraged innovation in MCH policies at the federal level. One persistent theme in its history has been the expectation that the programs established under Title V would redress the deficiencies of a fragmented American health care system in meeting the health needs of mothers and children. Thus Title V's successes reflect its ability to fill gaps in health care coverage, and its failures stem in part from the inadequacies of the health care system that are too fundamental or too large in magnitude for Title V to address effectively.

Throughout its history, Title V has been able to adapt to changes in political and socioeconomic circumstances. Under a variety of conditions the program has assured that the special needs of mothers and children received political considerations. It has become a tradition of Title V to turn public sentiment for women and children into practical programs. But here too, Title V was essentially reactive, responding to changing needs but not directly addressing the more fundamental problems of our health care system.

A basic thesis of this chapter is that this traditional role of Title V must be redefined and strengthened to protect the health status of women and children in a future era when national health insurance may provide universal access to health care.

The History of Title V

Maternal and Child Health Services in the United States have gone through three major formative periods: the years from 1912 to 1935, during which federal programs such as the Children's Bureau, the Sheppard-Towner Act, and Title V of the Social Security Act were created; the 1960s, when amendments to the Social Security Act created Medicare (Title XVIII), Medicaid (Title XIX), and new Title V programs; and the 1980s, when further amendment to the Social Security Act created a Maternal and Child Health Services (MCH) Block Grant, which shifted control from federal to state governments.

The Early Years: 1912-1935

The roots of Title V are found in the children's welfare movement, and particularly in the Children's Bureau, created by Congress in 1912. This agency was directed to investigate and report "upon matters pertaining to the welfare of children and child life among all classes of our people and shall especially investigate the questions of infant mortality, the birth rate, orphanages, juvenile courts, desertion, dangerous occupations, accidents and diseases of children, employment, [and] legislation affecting children in the several states and territories" (Children's Bureau, 1956).

The Children's Bureau's broad mandate was pursued through a series of reports on such critical issues as infant mortality and child labor, and ultimately resulted in the passage of the Maternity and Infant Act of 1920 (the Sheppard-Towner Act), which provided grants-in-aid to assist state health agencies to establish and improve services to promote the health of women and children. The legislation expired in 1929 and was not renewed by the Congress. However, during the eight years of its existence, the Sheppard-Towner Act was associated with the creation of child health (hygiene) units in 47 states; the expansion of birth registration from 30 to 46 states; and the establishment of large numbers of child health centers and public health nursing services throughout the United States (Lesser, 1985). Many of these remained after the Act expired. Moreover, this experience enabled the Children's Bureau to later introduce children's health into the national agenda in the midst of a national economic depression, embodied as Title V of the Social Security Act in 1935 (Schmidt, 1974).

The inclusion of a Maternal and Child Health program in the Social Security Act represented a recognition by the president and the Congress that the federal government had a responsibility for the promotion and protection of the well-being of children as well as other dependent groups. This reflected two judgments. First, there was a widespread conviction that special measures for the protection of children were an essential part of a program of economic security (Lesser, 1985). Second, disparities in maternal mortality across the country and lack of access to specialty care for handicapped children were cited as evidence of a need for federal action.

Title V built on the experiences of the Sheppard-Towner Act to create a state capacity to develop systems of care for women and children, including handicapped children. The language of the Act—to enable states to "extend and improve" services—reflected a perceived need to build systems that could assure quality services.

Under Title V, states were funded on a formula basis (some of which was matched by state funds), to establish service units in state health departments for maternal and child health.[1] Through these state MCH units, clinical services were established including well-baby clinics, school health programs, immunization clinics, public health nursing services, nutrition and health education programs, and clinical programs for crippled children. Programs were to be comprehensive, and encouraged to be multidisciplinary, with measures for case finding, diagnosis, treatment and hospitalization, and after care. Prevention was emphasized as a part of all maternal and child health and crippled children's programs. For example, the act specified that services were to be provided to children who were crippled or "who are suffering from conditions which lead to crippling."[2]

Although the act required no means testing, states generally adopted the eligibility criteria used for public assistance. However, some services under the act were always considered to be free of charge, especially diagnostic services. In addition to service provision, the act stimulated service planning by requiring that state plans be developed and approved by the Children's Bureau before funding.

The early Title V programs clearly made health care more accessible to children, particularly specialty and preventive services. In an era before health insurance was available to the average working family, Title V represented the sole source of public funding for outpatient health care and for many children. Particularly during the years of World War II, the Emergency Medical and Infant Care (EMIC) program, administered by the Children's Bureau, provided a comprehensive system of medical, nursing, and hospital care for the prenatal, maternity, postpartum, and infant care for the wives and children of young armed services men who had come to live in military camps. By 1948, EMIC had served 1.5 million women and children, making it the largest single public health program ever undertaken in the United States (Lesser, 1985).

These accomplishments should not mask the limitations of Title V initiatives. The Social Security Act was a political compromise that backed away from more comprehensive proposals. Provisions establishing a minimum level of family subsistence were struck from the act, and pressure from organized medicine led to the elimination of proposals for a comprehensive national health insurance program (Schmidt, 1974). Title V never had the resources to address more than a small fraction of the needs that would have been met had these provisions been retained.

The Social Security Amendments of the 1960s

The Kennedy and Johnson administrations brought a nationwide reexamination of the responsibilities of the federal government for civil rights, education, social welfare, economic opportunity, and health. Among the consequences of this review were major pieces of federal legislation, including amendments to Title V and the creation of two new titles to the Social Security Act—Title XVIII (Medicare) and Title XIX (Medicaid).

Title V was sequentially expanded to address policy makers' concerns with particular health needs and populations. The concerns of President Kennedy for mental retardation resulted in amendments to Title V and new resources for maternal and child health programs. The 1963 Amendments (P.L. 88-156) authorized funds for the creation of Maternal and Infant Care (MIC) projects that would provide comprehensive care to pregnant, low-income women and their infants to address those conditions likely to lead to retarded development. By 1969, the federal government had funded 53 MIC projects serving over 100,000 women and infants nationwide (Lesser, 1985).

In 1964 a program of project grants to provide funds for comprehensive care for children and youth (C&Y) living in areas of high concentrations of poverty was proposed, and finally enacted at the same time as the creation of the Office of Economic Opportunity's Neighborhood Health Centers. By 1969, 58 C&Y projects, some closely tied to MIC projects and Neighborhood Health Centers, served 335,000 children nationwide (Lesser, 1985). Further amendments in the late 1960s and early 1970s expanded Title V to fund neonatal intensive care, family planning, and dental care. States were required to fund at least one of each of these types of projects.

The major legislation expanding access to health care for low-income populations was not through Title V amendments, however, but through the creation of the Medicaid program, which tied eligibility to existing public assistance programs such as AFDC. Since Title XIX was viewed primarily as a welfare program, relatively little attention was initially paid to the links with the medical care system. Legislative language addressed the need for cooperation between Title V and Title XIX agencies, but implementation of interagency agreements was difficult. At both the federal and state levels, Title V and Title XIX agencies had widely divergent philosophies and, in most states, were located in separate departments (Foltz, 1978, 1980).

Several policy themes emerge from this era. First, access into the health care system for the poor and other disadvantaged groups became the major focus of federal policy. The creation by Congress of separate categorical health programs for such disadvantaged groups as children with hemophilia, sickle cell anemia, and lead poisoning further reflected this emphasis on access.

Second, there was a shift in the orientation of federal policy. The federal government took a greater role in establishing and funding broad programmatic goals, but left to the states the responsibility for implementation, documentation, and data collection. State Title V plans, for example, were no longer submitted to the federal agency (Hutchins, personal communication). Oversight of state child health programs generally appears to have weakened during this era (Altenstetter and Bjorkman, 1974; Silver et al., 1976; Foltz, 1980).

Third, the proliferation of new programs benefiting children was accompanied by a loss of influence by Title V agencies over the formulation and implementation of policy. In 1970 Title V was taken out of the relatively independent Children's Bureau, which had reported directly to the Social Security Administrator, and placed at a lower level of the federal bureaucracy within the Public Health Service. New programs for community health centers, family planning, migrant health and health planning were deliberately administered through federal regional offices—not the states—because of the belief that states were unresponsive to needs, especially those of minority groups (Hutchins, personal communication). These different lines of authority led to conflict between the state Title V agencies and the newly mandated agencies (Miller, 1986).[3]

In summary, the influence and effectiveness of Title V waned during the post-World War II period and particularly during the important social welfare developments of the 1960s. Federal intent for child health policy was "ambiguous" with conflicting and overlapping mandates in the major legislative initiatives and divergent interpretation of the laws by federal agencies (Foltz, 1978). Faced with uncertain federal policies, inadequate funding to address legislative mandates and little federal oversight, states failed to develop programs to their full potential (Silver et al., 1976).

The Maternal and Child Health Services Block Grant

While the Great Society programs reflected a mixture (albeit sometimes a seemingly conflicted one) of state and federal responsibilities, the "New Federalism" policies of the Reagan presidency represented an unambiguous reduction in both federal oversight and financial support for Maternal and Child Health (MCH) programs.

The initial Reagan Administration proposals would have created Block Grant health and social welfare programs, grouping together up to 40 formerly categorical programs, with state discretion to reallocate funds among these services. These proposals for generic Block Grants proved unacceptable to Congress, however, which adapted the Administration's objectives to a set of more narrowly focused block grants, including one for maternal and child health that provided continuity for the existing state MCH programs (Omenn and Nathan, 1982; Iglehart, 1983).

The Title V/MCH Block Grant created a consolidated health program combining funding from several categorical programs, including Title V formula grant for MCH/CC services and Supplementary Security Income for Disabled Children's Program. The 1981 Omnibus Budget Reconciliation Act (PL 97–35) that created the MCH Block Grant enumerated several goals for the states: (1) to assure that mothers and children, especially those with low income or limited availability of health services, were provided access to quality health services; (2) to emphasize preventive measures, such as those to reduce infant mortality and prevent handicapping conditions, and to promote the health of mothers and children through primary pediatric and prenatal care; (3) to provide rehabilitative services to blind and disabled children eligible for Supplemental Security Income (SSI) under Social Security; and (4) to provide comprehensive services to handicapped children.

Several provisions were established to preserve continued support for MCH programs. State Title V programs were protected by requirements that the state health agency administer the consolidated programs. Transfers of MCH Block Grant funds to other health functions were specifically prohibited, although funds could be transferred in from other Block Grants. But eliminating federal regulations formerly attached to each categorical program created considerable discretion for the states. Although they were required to provide a "fair method" for the distribution of Block Grant funds and to make plans available for public comment, no federal regulations were written to interpret these provisions. In fact, the federal government initially resisted requests from the states for clarification of Title V requirements, although some federal guidance has since emerged.

Ironically, the threat to Title V programs engendered by the politics of Block Grants led to a strengthening of the national constituency for MCH programs through the reorganization of the Association of MCH/CCS Programs and the creation of the National MCH Resource Center. Thus, while federal funding for the MCH Block Grant was initially reduced by approximately 18 percent in the first year, this effect was partially mitigated by the availability of federal project funding for the categorical programs (GAO, 1984). Congress has since authorized and appropriated annual increases in funds and many state legislatures have more than offset federal cutbacks with increased funding (GAO, 1984).

Generally, states continued to give priority to the basic MCH/CCS programs while reducing funding for special projects and some of the consolidated health programs such as lead screening and sudden infant death syndrome programs. In general, the states surveyed responded to less federal regulation by standardizing administrative practices and improving planning and budgeting, but reduced efforts to provide reports on the program (GAO, 1984).

In summary, while the Block Grant approach removed some of the ambiguity that existed in federal child health policy, it did so at the price of removing the federal government from an active role in setting a national child health policy. While several states are experiencing an exciting expansion of MCH programming and growth in the MCH constituency, others are struggling through major fiscal constraints. The failure to assure a national standard for child health and health services results in wide disparities of programming. Title V has been left as a loosely affiliated group of state agencies, each searching to fulfill its ambitious mandate at the state level, and a federal office that has attempted to influence MCH policy through its discretionary demonstration, research and training funds.

The Current Organization of Maternal and Child Health Services under Title V

The Organization of MCH at the Federal and State Levels

Originally, the Children's Bureau had been located in the Department of Commerce and Labor, and the chief of the Children's Bureau was appointed by the President with the advice and consent of the Senate. In the 1940s the Children's Bureau was transferred to the Department of Labor and finally, to the newly formed Department of Health, Education and Welfare in 1953 (U.S. Department of Health, Education and Welfare, 1956). Currently, at the federal level, the Children's Bureau structure has evolved into a Bureau of Maternal and Child Health (BMCH) located in the U.S. Department of Health and Human Services. This evolution represents a closer integration of MCH with other public health services but, at the same time, has demoted MCH through several layers of bureaucracy from the top levels of federal decision making. The MCH Block Grant neither prescribes the structure of the federal office nor provides for its funding. Within BMCH, a professional staff has provided leadership through use of the 15 percent of funding set aside for training, research, and special demonstration programs. It also supervises the professional staff located in 10 regional offices around the country. BMCH promotes interagency collaboration at the federal level and has a close working relationship with public, professional, and voluntary agencies.

The relationship between the federal BMCH and the state MCH/CC programs has been simplified under the MCH Block Grant. The intent of the block grants was to shift authority to the states, and this has been accomplished. BMCH has no authority over the 85 percent of the block grant funds that are distributed on a formula basis. Federal review of states' expenditure plans is largely perfunctory, except for review of civil rights, affirmative action or illegal expenditures. Even the ability of the federal MCH agency to provide technical assistance and interpretation of the law was severely restricted by early policy decisions of the Secretary of Health and Human Services (Hutchins, personal communication), though subsequently, these functions of the federal Bureau have been strengthened.

The organization of MCH agencies at the state level reflects the original Title V concept as modified by more than 50 years of evolution and reorganization. In all 57 states and territories, MCH units are located within state Public Health Departments, usually under the umbrella of a larger Bureau of Community or Personal Health Services. MCH is thus located at a bureaucratic level somewhat removed from the highest levels of state health policy making. In contrast to the federal case, however, these state MCH units are often large in terms of budget and staffing, combining federal MCH Block Grant, Family Planning, and WIC funds with state MCH appropriations. The visibility and potential political influence creates the potential for conflict between commissioners of public health and their MCH directors (Daugherty, 1986). The elimination of Title V regulations through the Block Grant have weakened the ability of state MCH Directors to protect the Title V funds from "infringement" by health department administrators.

State MCH/CC service delivery systems vary across the country.[4] In some states most direct services are decentralized to local/county health departments and the state MCH office takes only an advisory or consultative role. This is most common in the South, the Midwest, and the West, and significant Title V funds are expended on the direct care personnel located in these local health departments. In a few states responsibility for direct services is centralized. This is common in several New England states that have no county health departments; for example, in Massachusetts a large centralized MCH unit provides services primarily through contracts with private, nonprofit community health providers, neighborhood health centers, and hospitals. Most states lie between these extremes.

There has been no systematic study relating the structure of state MCH agencies to their performance. In the decentralized systems, however, bureaucratic constraints appear to significantly limit innovation. In these states, state MCH and federal Title V funds are heavily committed to civil service personnel in county health departments making programmatic changes and incorporation of new disciplines relatively difficult. Program development requires the cooperation of county health officials as well as redeployment and retraining of existing personnel. States that contract with the nonprofit sector for delivery of direct care, find innovation to be somewhat easier (Guyer, 1984). On the other hand, these states lack the public sector infrastructure represented by the county health departments and thus may have greater difficulty targeting services to appropriate low-income clients.

The Relationship of MCH to Other Federal Programs

The organizational and operational relationship of Title V to other federal child health and welfare initiatives, including Medicaid, Special Education for the Handicapped, the Supplemental Food Program for Women, Infants and Children (WIC), Head Start, and family planning are extremely important but have received inadequate attention. In general, there have been only limited and inconsistent efforts to link Title V to these other programs. This has, however, varied somewhat by program and state. Some of these initiatives, such as WIC and family planning programs, have had closer ties to Title V because they are administered through state or local health departments that are also responsible for Title V programs (Berkenfield and Schwartz, 1980). Others, such as Medicaid and Head Start, are administered by different agencies than is Title V at both federal and state levels, leading to limited coordination and cooperation. Even for these latter programs, though, there seems to be growing interest and potential for cooperation with Title V. Various proposals for administrative integration of Title V and Medicaid have been considered in recent years (Yordy, 1981) and a new proposal for coordinating the programs is currently being discussed by representatives of state Title V and Medicaid agencies. New federal legislation (P.L. 99-457) extending special education services to younger children, from birth to three years old, may provide more opportunity for coordination of educational and health programming for early intervention programs.

Title V and the Financing of Maternal and Child Health Care

While Title V has focused primarily on the infrastructure of MCH/CC services, it has also played an historic role as a direct care provider and third-party funder of health care services. In this latter function however, it has been eclipsed by the advent of private and public health insurance schemes and the growth of the private practices of pediatrics and obstetrics. Title V currently pays for less than two percent of total expenditures for children's health care. But while small in absolute magnitude, Title V funding may prove an important means of filling gaps in the existing array of public and private insurance programs.

Although 90 percent of American children have some health insurance coverage (Butler et al., 1985; National Centers for Health Statistics, 1985), the limitations of this coverage have been extensively documented in other chapters in this volume and elsewhere. Private insurance policies may lack coverage for specific services like maternity care (Gold and Kennedy, 1985), limit coverage for handicapping conditions through exclusions or preexisting conditions, or impose ceilings on coverage that leave families underinsured for large hospital bills associated with serious childhood conditions or long-term disabling and handicapping conditions (Knox, 1986).

This is particularly true for parents taking low-paying jobs that come without benefit packages or with only limited health benefits (Massachusetts Human Services Coalition, 1985). In recent years there has been an increasing proportion with uninsured or underinsured children (Swartz, 1986).

Medicaid coverage of services tends to be more comprehensive, but studies have documented wide disparities in states' Medicaid coverage of maternity care (Gold and Kenney, 1985), eligibility tends to be restricted to only a fraction of children in low-income households (Rymer, 1986) and states are increasingly establishing ceilings on coverage that leave beneficiaries unprotected if their children are chronically or seriously ill.

Title V agencies *partially* address these needs because they have the administrative and financial flexibility to allocate funds to explicitly fill gaps. Currently, though, they lack the financial resources and legislative mandate to close the gaps completely. This potential for Title V as a remedial financing program could be more fully developed. To assess the potential for this approach, relative to those discussed in other chapters, it is useful to first review some of the strengths and weaknesses of existing Title V programs.

Strengths of Title V/MCH Agencies

The Title V program has exhibited, though not always fully exploited, four areas of strength: political support, state infrastructure, expertise in child health, and institutional flexibility.

Title V has been politically popular because programs that address the health care needs of women and children are easily conceptualized and justified. Its mission, although vague, is targeted to a vulnerable population group. Title V has thus retained its bipartisan congressional support for more than 50 years. This support has been reinforced because Title V is a part of the Social Security Act, legislation with a powerful political constituency and supportive Congressional committees.

Title V has also attracted a constituency among service providers, advocates for children, groups of parents concerned with particular childhood diseases, voluntary organizations, and state bureaucrats. At numerous recent junctures when Title V's future was uncertain, public support from this constituency has earned continued Congressional support.

Second, Title V has been responsible for the creation of an infrastructure of publicly financed MCH services. In 1984, according to reports from 41 states' health agencies, the MCH Block Grant and state matching funds accounted for approximately 10 percent of all state and local health agency revenues and 13 percent of funds devoted to personal health services (Public Health Foundation, 1986). When USDA WIC funds (excluding food dollars) are added, state and federal MCH funds account for about 25 percent of all funds for personal health services. Thus, MCH funds support a significant proportion of public health agency personnel.

Third, state MCH agencies contain a reservoir of expertise concerning the clinical problems of women and children and the services needed to address those problems. The strong clinical and programmatic base has resulted in significant innovations in state service delivery with a strong emphasis on prevention; nearly 70 percent of state MCH funds are devoted to preventive health services (Public Health Foundation, 1986).

Fourth, the institutional flexibility inherent in Title V has allowed it to serve as an umbrella agency with a broad mission that clearly focuses on the health care needs of women and children without necessarily being constrained by other concerns, such as cost containment. Numerous programs have been grouped together at the state and local level because they all fit under the broad mandate and mission of Title V programs. As noted earlier, links have developed between Title V and the WIC and family planning programs.

Although the weight of authority has shifted with time, Title V has always been a joint federal/state program with the legislative flexibility to adapt programming to the particular needs of local populations, service providers and bureaucracies. Title V has had the ability to use its limited financial resources to leverage the system and fill gaps in health care. While most studies of health care financing identify Title V dollars as only a minor component of "other" federal sources, these studies often overlook the ways in which Title V supplements the system. For example, many states support infant screening programs for PKU and hypothyroidism with Title V dollars; these services are provided without charge to families and contribute little to health care costs because they are regionalized (providing economies of scale) and kept outside the fee-for-service system.

Further, the populations most likely to depend on Title V-funded services today are those who fall into the gaps of the health care financing system, such as the working poor who seek care from community health centers and county health department clinics. Two important cases illustrate this important role for Title V: services for handicapped children (as well as their families) and initiatives to reduce infant mortality.

Title V has provided a broad scope of services for a relatively small proportion of handicapped children. In most states, Title V has paid for specialist medical care services, including hospitalization, for children whose families are uninsured or underinsured. Similarly, the benefits under Title V have extended to prostheses, wheelchairs and other therapeutic equipment, home care services, therapies, and family support through respite—services excluded under many insurance policies. As more families may find themselves underinsured in the future, they may turn increasingly to Title V agencies for these services.

The recent recognition of disparities in infant mortality and low birthweight among minority and poor populations in the country has led a large number of states to examine the gaps in prenatal, maternity, and infant care. Title V agencies have taken a prominent role in the analysis of these gaps in the service system and are being looked to, frequently, as the agency expected to implement corrective strategies.

Weaknesses of Current Title V Arrangements

Despite these important contributions, Title V's performance has never lived up to the grand expectations of its framers. This can be attributed to several factors, including insularity and parochialism within the program, the "ambiguity" of federal child health policy, failure to use information for advocacy, and inadequate funding.

Title V's insularity resulted in missed opportunities to better integrate its infrastructure with other major public health initiatives. As already noted, in the 1960s, Medicaid was enacted and structured without input concerning the special health care needs of mothers and children. Unlike 1935, when the leaders of the Children's Bureau influenced the framing of the Social Security Act, Title V officials appear to have had little influence on the Medicaid legislation. For example, Title V programs could have become the state agency administering the EPSDT provisions of Medicaid (Klerman, 1981). Because it was not, states failed to tap Title V expertise in developing standards for quality of health care or long-run goals for Medicaid. Nor to date has there been much linkage to the Special Education for the Handicapped (P.L. 94-142) programs for disabled school children or to other state and federal programs providing mental health services for children.

Even today, when concerns about uncompensated hospital costs and the uninsured are the subject of state commissions and task forces, the parties to these discussions include hospitals, insurance companies, state Medicaid agencies, and consortia of employers and labor unions, but not Title V. In many states, Title V remains absent from these discussions despite the fact that a large proportion of the uninsured generating uncompensated acute hospital care costs are women and children (Swartz, 1986).

Title V has also been criticized for fostering a kind of parochialism that has distrusted community level participation and resisted integration with other community-based programs. Maternal and child health as a field has been accused of traditionalism, of separating curative from preventive services, of promoting professional elitism by equating academic credentials with quality and of resisting family-centered care (Klerman, 1981). The federal and state Title V agencies have limited further the programs considered to be the legitimate domain of public health/MCH, ignoring the vast growth of the private sector of health care—hospitals, primary care providers, and HMOs.

A second criticism of Title V has focused on the unevenness of program administration. This is due, in part, to the "ambiguity" of federal child health policy (Foltz, 1978) and weak federal oversight during the last 30 years (Altenstetter and Bjorkman, 1974; Klerman, 1981; Rosenbaum, 1983). Gross disparities in the services available to indigent mothers and children have emerged between state programs and for specific populations within states. In part, these disparities represent a lack of planning, and in some cases discriminatory practices, but above all, the absence of adequate supervision by the federal MCH program. State health departments that administer Title V were not kept under close scrutiny in terms of their use of Title V funds or subjected to clear federal standards of performance.

Third, over the course of 50 years, Title V agencies at the state and federal levels gradually abandoned the important focus of the Children's Bureau on continuously documenting the health and welfare status of mothers and children. This weakness may have been among the most important reasons for the decline in the prominence of Title V as advocate and for the decrease in fiscal support. No systems for monitoring MCH health status were developed, few convincing studies were carried out, and even the managerial aspects of Title V activities were inadequately documented.

Finally, perhaps the single most important factor affecting the ability of Title V programs to carry out their mandate over the years has been the eroded value of Title V appropriations. While Title V programs have never been adequately funded to fulfill the broad mandate, inflation in health care costs experienced since the late 1960s has seriously cut the purchasing power of Title V funds. Taking inflation into account, the 1984 appropriation of $399 million had the purchasing power of only $128 million in 1967 dollars. For Title V to have maintained a constant purchasing power over this period of time, Congress should have appropriated $1.2 billion in 1984—three times the actual appropriation. Thus, while the focus on budget cuts since the Block Grant has dominated recent policy discussions, it is clear that Title V resources have been continuously eroding over the last 20 years (Magee and Pratt, 1985).

The failure of Congress to increase funding to keep pace with inflation probably reflects the reduced emphasis of MCH administration on information gathering and advocacy. It also is a result of administrators maintaining a narrow definition of the appropriate purview for Title V. As Title V has become narrowly defined, resources have been captured by other agencies, particularly community health centers and providers of specialty health care (Klerman, 1981; Rosenbaum, 1983).

The combination of these historical strengths and weaknesses have left Title V a relatively small federal program, relegated to a minor role in the federal health bureaucracy, unable to set a national health policy for mothers and children. At the same time, reports of Title V's impending demise (Budetti, Butler and McManus, 1982; Butler, 1982) have proven overly pessimistic. Although the transition to the Block Grant appears to have led to greater variation among states, it also to some extent bolstered support for the program at the state level. More than half the states responded to cuts in federal funding with increases in state spending (GAO, 1984). The Block Grant requirements for increased public participation led most states to hold public hearings and many states to establish advisory groups.

Adapting Title V's Functions to the Future

In planning for Title V's future role, it is useful to use as a starting point the four interrelated functions of a maternal and child health agency first described by Martha May Eliot: information and research, standard setting, technical assistance and provision of services (Eliot, 1956). Each of these functions encompasses a set of opportunities for future reform.

The recommendations presented here represent a composite of best practices from selected states and some useful general approaches that could be more broadly adopted.

Information, Evaluation, and Research

The failure to provide information and carry out research has been the area in which Title V agencies have most deviated from the tradition of the Children's Bureau, and the area where the greatest opportunities have been lost. In recent years, the data gathering and disseminating institutions of government have been seriously undermined by budget cuts. Title V agencies, however, seem to have abandoned these functions long before, and are only now beginning to see the value and power of information. A goal of Title V in the future must be to use its unique place in the bureaucracy and its access to data to advocate for women and children in policy decisions. In order to rebuild this function, Title V agencies at the federal, state, and local level must think about information needs systematically.

Influencing policy formation. Among the more basic information services to be provided by a Title V agency are the regular, routine publication of those data uniquely available to public agencies. Vital statistical annual reports are usually too obscure and detailed for policy makers. Source books of official data—such as those produced recently by the Children's Defense Fund (Hughes et al., 1986), the New Mexico Title V agency (1986), and the Massachusetts Title V agency (MDPH, 1986)—can powerfully influence the political environment.

Beyond vital statistics lie a series of regularly available data sets which hold promise for exploring health status outcomes and health care utilization and resources. These data sets include the Uniform Hospital Discharge Data Set (UHDDS) derived from the hospital discharge summary and used, increasingly, by third-party payers. State Medicaid Management Information Systems have rarely been tapped by MCH agencies despite the fact that Medicaid is the largest payer for services for low-income children. Title V agencies have also been successful at developing new MCH data sets such as the Maternal and Child Health Information Network (MATCH) in Ohio and the Integrated Maternal and Child Health Information system in Rhode Island.

Special studies by Title V agencies provide opportunities to influence policy making, much as the Children's Bureau's studies of infant mortality or child labor fundamentally altered the federal system in the early part of this century. Task forces and special commissions can provide the vehicle for assembling the agents of change. In Massachusetts these mechanisms were used in 1985 when a Task Force on the

Prevention of Low Birthweight and Infant Mortality developed a report, *Closing the Gaps,* that led to the creation of a major state initiative on infant mortality (MDPH, 1985). Earlier, in 1983, the Massachusetts MCH agency mounted a survey of childhood nutritional status as a response to the rising recognition of malnutrition (Guyer et al., 1985–86); again, a special study led the legislature to a major initiative on child nutrition (Atkins, 1985).

Perhaps the most important area for special study and research by MCH agencies today is the evaluation of the impact of cost-containment efforts and new health care financing proposals on the health status and health care utilization patterns of mothers and children. As the problems of the uninsured and underinsured are examined by other agencies of government, representatives of labor and industry, and professional groups, the needs of women and child dependents, especially high-risk groups such as sick neonates and multiply handicapped and developmentally delayed children must be represented.

Dissemination of information and communication with constituencies are inextricably linked to these information functions of Title V agencies. Not only do MCH units have access to unique data sets, but they are particularly placed in the bureaucracy at an interface between the sources of these data, policy makers in the various levels of the government, providers of health care services, and clients of MCH programs. These groups form the constituency for MCH and must be kept informed. Too few state MCH units have made efforts to fulfill this communication function through the publication of newsletters, articles, or video materials. The work of the Region IV MCH Data Network based at the University of North Carolina provides a model of data sharing among the southeastern states that will lead to better data from each of the states and a more uniform picture of MCH in the region (Peoples-Sheps, 1986).

Increasing Title V accountability. Because of the general failure of MCH agencies to count services provided or recipients of those services, accountability for services provided under Title V has been questioned. These simple counts are essential for Congress and state legislators who wish to justify the appropriation of dollars by reporting on populations served. Yet these data are rarely or irregularly available. Only recently have data been available that link services provided to recipients and, ultimately, outcomes (ASTHO Foundation, 1985).

Strengthening planning and needs assessment. Planning and needs assessment are based on the quantitative description of maternal and child health status. The language of the MCH Block Grant requires states "to describe populations, areas and localities in need of MCH services" and to provide a "fair method for distributing funds" to those populations and areas. Thus, the federal mandate provides a unique opportunity to use the basic planning document of the MCH/Title V agencies, the Report of Intended Expenditures (RIE), to document the current state of health and the patterns of services, and to demonstrate where services are available (Guyer et al., 1984).

Needs assessment must be seen by Title V agencies as a dynamic, innovative activity—which adapts the focus of MCH programs to the changing conditions of family life. Thus, in recent years the Title V agency in Massachusetts undertook needs assessment/planning activities for early intervention services for young, developmentally at-risk children, birth to three years of age, and their families (Evans et al., 1985). In addition, a desire to reexamine the structure of a traditional crippled children's clinic system led to the creation of Project Serve (1985).

Standard Setting

Standards of care represent statements of preferred clinical practices. These can take the form of legislative statutes, which constitute the most binding but typically most narrow, administrative regulations, or procedural guidelines. By virtue of their location within state public health agencies, Title V programs have the legal authority to set standards of health care for facilities and providers, and have traditionally done so through their licensure functions. In many parts of the country over the past 20 years, for example, Title V agencies have been involved in the regionalization of perinatal care, utilizing hospital licensure authority and collaboration with professional groups (Ryan et al., 1977). In most cases, however, these Title V standard-setting activities have been *reactive*. Obstetricians and neonatologists, for instance, took the lead in promoting regionalized care for mothers and newborns. Title V could assume a more active role in promoting appropriate care for women and children. Toward this end, the scope of standard setting in Title V agencies could be expanded to include the practices of third-party payers.

The primary means by which Title V agencies have influenced service delivery has been through the regulatory function of the states' departments of public health. In Massachusetts, for example, Pediatric Nursing Homes (PNHs) were created in the 1970s to provide residential/ institutional care for multiply handicapped children with significant medical nursing needs. The original PNHs were licensed by the state health department using the geriatric nursing home regulations to determine the service package. This pattern of care, however, was clearly inadequate to serve the needs of young children at various developmental levels (Glick et al., 1983). Therefore, the Title V agency reviewed PNH care and organized the clinical expertise to rewrite these regulations. Specific licensure regulations were used to raise the standard of care by increasing available hours of nursing and therapy, creating new services, integrating educational programs and increasing opportunities for parental involvement.

Another example occurred in South Carolina. Clinical standards developed by the Title V agency were used to develop a Medicaid waiver that required risk assessment, special services for high-risk women and directing high-risk populations into care at designated perinatal centers. This latter example is particularly important because it shows the potential influence of Title V on the expenditure of public funds through Medicaid (McManus, 1986).

Another important opportunity for Title V agencies, though less fully exploited in the past, is the potential for influencing private health insurance benefits through state legislatures and insurance commissions. In Massachusetts, specific legislation was developed to assure coverage for special foods for children with phenylketonuria (PKU) by insurance companies. The use of mandated benefits has been an important strategy for increasing coverage for preventive care, such as routine screenings and immunizations (Flint, 1986).

In the future, standard setting may become increasingly important as larger numbers of providers are prepaid and thus given a financial incentive to reduce the number of services provided. The clinical expertise of Title V agencies can be used to create prototype service packages and clinical protocols for at-risk populations.

Finally, Title V programs can use their standard-setting/regulatory function to encourage the creation of new systems of care. Particularly, in an era when concepts of competition and the market economy are heavily influencing the structure of health care, these planned, centralized functions are of great importance. The outstanding example of the benefits of an organized system of care using centralized planning is the existing regionalization of perinatal care and of certain specialty chronic disease care, e.g., hemophilia, congenital cardiac disease, and juvenile rheumatoid arthritis. The benefits of regionalization and planned service networks will also be reaped for pediatric intensive care, pediatric emergency care services, and some long-term care.

Technical Assistance

Technical Assistance represents a common activity of central MCH offices at both federal and state levels. The provision of expert advice and skills has its roots in the activities of the Children's Bureau and builds heavily upon the information and standard-setting functions. To be fully effective, this function must be approached with greater imagination and flexibility.

For example, while the use of multi-disciplinary clinical teams was an innovation promoted by Title V, these teams were rather rigidly defined as consisting of specific clinical disciplines—physicians, nurses, social workers, nutritionists, and physical therapists. As Title V agencies recognize changing roles and populations, new skills must be brought to bear. Early childhood educators should be part of the Early Intervention team. Childhood injury prevention will require collaboration with police, fire, and other public safety professionals as well as traffic engineers. The disciplinary rigidity of Title V programs in the past must be broken down if Title V is to meet the shifting needs of America's children.

Provision of Services

Title V's role as a service provider is the area where the past provides the fewest guidelines for the future. Historically, the role of Title V as service provider has diminished, but its contemporary status varies greatly from one state to the next. The discussion that follows represents an effort to identify alternatives for a more consistent future role in this area. Possible goals for Title V activities include targeting particular populations, services, or general system management.

Closing the gaps. As long as there is no universal health insurance in the United States, Title V can be a source of funds to make care financially accessible to uninsured women and children. A good example of this strategy is the Massachusetts Healthy Start program (Hess, 1986). The recognition that a significant proportion of pregnant women were uninsured for pregnancy and maternity related services led the state legislature to create a limited health insurance scheme under Title V/MCH auspices to remove financial barriers to obtaining care.

There are a number of other groups that merit consideration as recipients of Title-V provided services. These include people living in rural areas, where county health departments provide the only access to low-income populations, as well as those in poor urban areas, where much of the primary care is delivered through community health centers.

Support for school health care and special programs for pregnant and parenting teens are a particularly important case. While these programs are experiencing a current resurgence of popularity—particularly as a site for provision of adolescent health care—they have had an extremely uneven course since their introduction in the early 1900s. Schools have not always welcomed the role as health facility; and private, organized medicine has objected to schools competing for patients. Yet it has always seemed logical that schools are an appropriate site to reach all children for routine health screenings like vision, hearing, spinal deformity, and for universal immunization. As the American family has changed in the 1980s, it now appears that schools may be an important site for health care for those children not likely to have access to more traditional health providers. These alternative health systems, however, must be integrated into the broader health system and Title V can take a leadership role in promoting these school health services (Gephart, Egan and Hutchins, 1984).

Encouraging innovative services. The ability of Title V agencies to use funds to create innovative services represents a strong tie to the tradition of Children's Bureau. Title V is able to be experimental in designing new categories of services, crossing some of the gray zones between medical and "nonmedical" areas and creating both new models and payment mechanisms. An example of this development is the Massachusetts Early Intervention (EI) program for young, developmentally at-risk children. Massachusetts created a new category of health care, established it in state law, developed program model standards, provided funds under contract to a network of programs, and developed reimbursement mechanisms (Meisels, 1986). It is clear that with a strong political base, EI in Massachusetts has established itself as an accepted health care service. Eventually private third-party reimbursement is anticipated, so that the state MCH funds will become an increasingly smaller proportion of the total. New federal legislation, P.L. 99-457, links early intervention services to the special education services, resulting in a nationwide expansion of EI (Gilkerson et al., 1987).

Another aspect of innovation in service delivery that can be fostered by Title V agencies involves a *continuum of care* linked through a case-management system. Several groups are likely to be most in need of case managers. Continuity is required for effective care of high-risk mothers from the identification of pregnancy through prenatal care and birth to the provision of early intervention and home visiting services to families of young infants. As noted in Chapter 2, case management ranks high among the needs of handicapped children and their families. The expertise, boundary-spanning nature and experience with both MCH and Crippled Children's programs make Title V agencies uniquely well suited to play this boundary-spanning role. Title V case managers have proven themselves effective in negotiating these needs through the service delivery system.

Supplementing minimal services. Title V funds have been used to supplement inadequate health care coverage to assure that for certain eligible populations, i.e., women, children, and the handicapped, a parallel system will exist to overcome those inadequacies. Where third-party payers have limited benefits for various handicapping conditions, Title V will purchase supplementary services, e.g., buy wheelchairs, pay for needed home care, etc. Ironically, this policy approach often serves the best interests of the insurance carriers who offer only minimal coverage to potential high-cost users as well as the families who have access to Title V services.

The supplementing role of Title V has great political popularity, however. Legislators can seek specific health care services for specific, highly visible constituents and usually get satisfaction. Advocacy groups can usually put pressure on the system to address some specific needy group. Unfortunately, implementation of these programs leaves Title V agencies vulnerable to criticisms of being duplicative, unfair, and uncoordinated.

It has also created situations in which Title V agencies, particularly crippled children's programs, provide services that conflict and compete with similar programs found in the private or nonprofit health sectors (Ireys et al., 1985). Each state must therefore review its delivery of care to determine which services are outdated and could be provided elsewhere (Project SERVE, 1985).

One type of service that may most require Title V initiatives involves *newly recognized areas of preventive health,* e.g., childhood injury prevention, nutrition, and prevention of adult chronic diseases. First, injury and violence are the leading causes of childhood mortality, leading causes of morbidity, and long-term disability, and the greatest cause of productive years of life lost. Strategies for injury control encompass efforts to change behaviors and practices of families and children, regulation and enforcement of safety practices, and efforts to engineer the environment to eliminate injury hazards. MCH agencies must become part of coalitions around the country to implement these control strategies. Second, assessment of childhood nutritional status, development of nutrition surveillance systems and strengthening the links between MCH and WIC programs must remain a high priority. Finally, among the most important future areas of public policy will be the prevention of adult chronic diseases in early life. Controversies remain about the strategies for addressing the roles of obesity, cholesterol, exercise, salt, etc., in these patterns. MCH agencies will need to become parts of broader coalitions to address these issues.

Unifying state responsibility for MCH. Services for children and youth are currently delivered through multiple state agencies. Departments of Mental Health provide inpatient, outpatient, and long-term care services for mentally ill and retarded individuals. Welfare agencies administer income maintenance benefits and often, the Medicaid program. Social Service Agencies provide protective services and foster care. Rehabilitation agencies, Developmental Disability Councils, and commissions for the deaf and blind provide specialized services for specific populations. Health departments provide Title V, WIC, women's health and other programs. Consolidation of these programs into a single state agency for women and children would unify the focus on the population, create a large enough agency to have clout within state government, and would facilitate the interagency coordination that so frequently eludes state agencies. A major consolidation of this type would be opposed by the existing state agencies who stand to lose resources and responsibilities and, on principle, by those who would fear that creation of a new state agency would result in expansion of the state budget. As an alternative, the Title V program could act as an umbrella agency, coordinating the activities and initiatives of other state bureaucracies.

The Federal Role

If the preceding recommendation for state MCH programs are to be effectively implemented, the structure and mandate of Title V must be strengthened at the federal level.

Reorganize the federal MCH agency. At the federal level, the Maternal and Child Health Agency must be located at a sufficiently high level of the federal bureaucracy to have an influence on policy making in other branches of the Department of Health and Human Services. As previously noted, the first chiefs of the Children's Bureau were appointed by the President, reported directly to the Social Security Administrator, and interacted with officials just below cabinet rank. If Title V is to regain its influence, particularly in the formation of financing policies at the Health Care Financing Administration, the agency chief must have the independence, stature and authority to advocate for MCH policies.

The Select Panel on Child Health recommended a "Maternal and Child Health Administration" as a new agency of the Public Health Service in order to coordinate and consolidate authority for children in the Department of Health and Human Services (Select Panel, 1981; Yordy, 1981). That proposal was not implemented by the incoming Reagan Administration but should now be reconsidered. The recent elevation of MCH one level in the federal bureaucracy (Freedman, 1986) is unlikely to result in effective advocacy.

Strengthen federal oversight of MCH programs. Because MCH remains a state-based delivery system, federal law and regulations must assure equity across the states by strengthening the structure of state programs, guiding state and local agencies on issues of planning and services, and demanding accountability from these agencies. To assure consistency across the country, federal law and regulation must strengthen the required content of the RIE and establish general standards for MCH agencies. The Association for Maternal and Child Health Programs is currently developing a model RIE intended to promote consistency and completeness across the states.

To be more effective in its advocacy role, MCH should create a national data system that will provide an accurate picture of the health of women and children and can be used as a tool for agency accountability.

Finally, the federal MCH office should increase its efforts to identify and disseminate innovations in state MCH programs. The Title V experience, particularly under the MCH Block Grant, has shown that some states can serve as laboratories for development of innovative approaches to the health needs of mothers and children. These innovations in service delivery, management and financing contain practical lessons that may be transferable to other states facing similar problems under like constraints. Too often now, this potential is never exploited.

Conclusions and Priorities for Reform

Preston (1984) showed that the elderly have done better in reversing the health and social effects of poverty over the last 30 years than have women and children. In large part, these gains are attributed to government support, including the benefits of health care through Medicare. Preston argued that the Great Society programs of the 1960s approached the problems of the elderly differently than those of poor mothers and children. Medicare was enacted as a federally administered social insurance covering all the elderly regardless of income, thereby assuring access to health care. While further reforms in Medicare are needed, its success in assuring health care for the elderly is clear (Blumenthal et al., 1986). Medicaid, however, was enacted as a means-tested, state-based program with variability in eligibility and scope of services and federal-state cost sharing.

An effective program to promote maternal and child health must rest on a national commitment to universal access to health care for mothers and children and greater safeguards to provide for interstate equity. The experience of both Medicaid and Title V reveals the significant inconsistencies that emerge from a state-based program. The decline of perinatal health care services in Michigan following the economic crisis in the auto industry in the early 1980s is an excellent example of the latter concern (Walker et al., 1983).

A strong Title V will be an essential component of a health care system in which access to health care is more fully assured. Title V will need to continue to monitor the impact of such a system on the health status of mothers and children, set standards for the delivery of care, and provide innovative services. Above all, a Title V infrastructure will need to assure preventive and community-based services not generally provided by private medical practitioners.

The leaders of the Children's Bureau seized upon the calamity of the Great Depression to develop the bold concepts which served the needs of mothers, children and the handicapped for 50 years. We must now provide the leadership to structure the current ferment over inequities in access to health care, the plight of the uninsured, and the crisis in health care financing to design a system that will meet the needs of mothers, children and the handicapped for the next 50 years.

Notes

1. In this sense, Title V has always been a "Block Grant" program.
2. Since this chapter was written, "crippled children's services" have been renamed "services for children with special health needs." The other term is used in its historical context.
3. These tensions grew after 1970, when federal funding failed to keep pace with inflationary health care costs (Coburn, 1981).
4. In 45 states and territories, CCS programs are found in the same organizational unit of the state public health department as MCH, but often under a separate director; the remaining 12 states have CCS located in state university medical schools or in another agency of state government (Ireys et al., 1985).

Acknowledgments

I wish to thank Vince Hutchins, Cathy Hess, John Butler, George Silver, Pam Drumheller, and particularly Mark Schlesinger for their careful reviews and thoughtful comments on various drafts of this chapter.

References

Altenstetter, C., and J.W. Bjorkman. 1974. The Impact of Federal Child Health Programs on State Health Policy Formation and Service Delivery: The Case of Connecticut. *Health Policy Project Working Papers,* Report No. 2. New Haven: Yale University School of Medicine.

ASTHO Foundation. 1985. Services for Mothers and Children. *Public Health Agencies 1983*, Vol. 3. Kensington, Md.: Association of State and Territorial Health Officials Foundation.

Atkins, C.G. 1985. Building a Political Consensus around Childhood Nutrition. *Zero to Three: Bulletin of the National Center for Clinical Infant Programs* 5(3):10–11. Washington, D.C.

Berkenfield, J., and J.B. Schwartz. 1980. Nutrition Intervention in the Community—The "W.I.C." Program. *New England Journal of Medicine* 302:579–581.

Blumenthal, D., M. Schlesinger, and P.B. Drumheller. 1986. The Future of Medicare. *New England Journal of Medicine* 314:722–728.

Bowen, O.R. 1986. First Report on the Consolidated Federal Programs Under the Maternal and Child Health Services Block Grant Act. From O.R. Bowen, Secretary of Health and Human Services to the U.S. Congress.

Brenner, R.H. 1974. Development of Federal-State Programs in the New Deal and World War II; Maternal and Child Health and Crippled Children Services in the Social Security Act. *Children and Youth in America*, Vol. 3. Cambridge, Mass.: Harvard University Press.

Budetti, P.R., J. Butler, and P. McManus. 1982. Federal Health Program Reforms: Implications for Child Health Care. *Milbank Memorial Fund Quarterly/Health and Society* 60(1):155–181.

Butler, J.A. 1982. Speech to the Association of Directors of State MCH/CC Programs. Washington, D.C.

Butler, J.A., W.D. Winter, J.D. Singer, and M. Wenger. 1985. Medical Care Use and Expenditure among Children and Youth in the United States: Analysis of a National Probability Sample. *Pediatrics* 76:495–507.

Children's Bureau. 1956. *Your Children's Bureau: Its Current Program*. Children's Bureau Publication No. 357. Washington, D.C.: DHEW.

Coburn, A.F. 1981. *Implementation and Federal Child Health Policy*. Thesis, Florence Heller Graduate School for Advanced Studies in Social Welfare, Brandeis University, Waltham, Mass.

Cohen, W.J. 1986. Commentary: Jubilees of Social Security. *Monday Comments, CHPC-SEM Newsletter*, No. 29 (February 10). Detroit.

Daugherty, J. 1986. State Hampered Model Care Plan. *Detroit Free Press*, June 8, p. 11A.

Dutton, D.B. 1981. Children's Health Care: The Myth of Equal Access. *Better Health Care for Our Children: A National Strategy. The Report of the Select Panel for the Promotion of Child Health, Volume IV— Background Papers*, pp. 357–440. DHHS Publication No. 79-55071. Washington, D.C.: G.P.O.

Eliot, M.M. 1956. Foreword to *Your Children's Bureau: Its Current Program*. Children's Bureau Publication No. 357. Washington, D.C.: DHEW.

Evans, F.B., F. Jacobs, and K. Kastorf. 1985. Conducting an Early Intervention Needs Assessment in Massachusetts. *Network News: A Technical Newsletter of the Region IV Network for Data Management and Utilization* 1(2):13–14. Chapel Hill: University of North Carolina.

Flint, S. 1986. Florida Mandates Coverage of Pediatric Preventive Care. *Child Health Financing Report* 3(4). American Academy of Pediatrics.

Foltz, A.M. 1978. *Uncertainties of Federal Child Health Policies: Impact in Two States*. NCHSR Research Digest Series, DHEW (PHS) Publication No. 78-3190. DHEW, National Center for Health Services Research.

———. 1980. Care and Carelessness in Federal Child Health Policy. *Journal of Public Health Policy* 1(2):141–149.

Freedman, S.A. 1986. *Creation of a Bureau of Maternal and Child Health.* Proposal to the Assistant Secretary for Health. Letter from the Institute for Child Health Policy, July 28. Gainesville, Fla.

Gephart, J., M.C. Egan, and V.L. Hutchins. 1984. Perspectives on Health of School-Age Children: Expectations for the Future. *Journal of School Health* 54:11–17.

Gibson, R.M., and D.R. Waldo. 1982. National Health Expenditures, 1981. *Health Care Financing Review* 4(1):1–35.

Gilkerson, L., A.G. Hilliard, E. Schrag, and J.P. Shonkoff. 1987. Commentary on P.L. 99-457. *Zero to Three: Bulletin of the National Center for Clinical Infant Programs* 6(3):13–17. Washington, D.C.

Glick, P., B. Guyer, B. Burr, and I.E. Gorbach. 1983. Pediatric Nursing Homes; Implications of the Massachusetts Experience for Residential Care of Multiply Handicapped Children. *New England Journal of Medicine* 309:640–646.

Gold, R.B., and A.M. Kenney. 1985. Paying for Maternity Care. *Family Planning Perspectives* 17:103–111.

Government Accounting Office Report. 1984. *Maternal and Child Health Block Grant: Program Changes Emerging Under State Administration.* Report to Congress by the Comptroller General of the United States. GAO/HRO 84-35.

Guyer, B., M. Allen, R. Coffin, W. Hollinshead, E. Siker, and J.C. Serrage. 1982. The Maternal and Child Health Service Block Grant: Implications for Pediatricians in New England. *New England Pediatrician* 4(1):1–12.

Guyer, B., L. Schor, K.P. Messenger, P. Prenney, and F. Evans. 1984. Needs Assessment under the Maternal and Child Health Services Block Grant. *American Journal of Public Health* 74:1014–1019.

Guyer, B., C.A. Wehler, and M.T. Anderka. 1985–86. Anthropometric Evidence of Malnutrition among Low-Income Children in Massachusetts in 1983. *Massachusetts Journal of Community Health* 2:3–9.

Hess, C. 1986. Healthy Start. *Massachusetts Medicine* 2:47–48.

Hughes, D., K. Johnson, J. Simons, and S. Rosenbaum. 1986. *Maternal and Child Health Data Book.* Washington, D.C.: Children's Defense Fund.

Hutchins, V. 1987. Associate Director, Bureau of Maternal and Child Health and Resources Development, U.S. Department of Health and Human Services. Personal communication with the author.

Iglehart, J.K. 1983. The Reagan Record on Health Care. *New England Journal of Medicine* 308:232–236.

Ireys, H.T., R.J.-P. Hauck, and J.M. Perrin. 1985. Variability among State Crippled Children's Service Programs: Pluralism Thrives. *American Journal of Public Health* 75:375–381.

Jacobs, F.H., and D.K. Walker. 1978. Pediatricians and the Education for All Handicapped Children Act of 1975 (P.L. 94-142). *Pediatrics* 61:135–137.

Klerman, L.V. 1981. Title V—The Maternal and Child Health and Crippled Children's Services Section of the Social Security Act: Problems and Opportunities. In *Better Health for Our Children: A National Strategy. The Report of the Select Panel for the Promotion of Child Health. Volume IV—Background Papers,* pp. 609–641. DHHS Publication No. 79–55071. Washington, D.C.: G.P.O.

Knox, R.A. 1986. Insurance System Puts Parents of Chronically Ill in Financial Bind. *Boston Globe,* December 14, p. 33.

Lesser, A.J. 1985. The Origin and Development of Maternal and Child Health Programs in the United States. *American Journal of Public Health* 75:590–598.

McManus, M. 1986. Medicaid Services and Delivery Settings for Maternal and Child Health. In R. Curtis and I. Hill (eds.), *Affording Access to Quality Care: Strategies for State Medicaid Cost Management,* pp. 95–125. Washington, D.C.: National Governors' Association and Center for Health Policy Research.

Magee, E.M., and M.W. Pratt. 1985. *Fifty Years of U.S. Federal Support to Promote the Health of Mothers and Children and Handicapped Children in America.* Vienna, Va.: Information Sciences Research Institute.

Massachusetts Department of Public Health. 1985. *Closing the Gaps: Strategies for Improving the Health in Massachusetts Infants.* Boston: Task Force on Prevention of Low Birth Weight and Infant Mortality.

———. 1986. *The Health of Women and Children in Massachusetts: A Source Book of Data.* Boston: Commonwealth of Massachusetts.

Meisels, S.J. 1986. A Functional Analysis of the Evolution of Public Policy for Handicapped Young Children. *Educational Evaluation and Policy Analysis* 7:115–126.

Miller, C.A. 1986. Keynote address to the Annual Meeting of the Association for MCH/CCS Programs. April. Washington, D.C.

National Center for Health Statistics. 1985. *Insurance Coverage and Ambulatory Medical Care of Low-Income Children: United States, 1980.* Series C, Analytic Report No. 1., DHHS Publication No. 85-20401. Washington, D.C.: G.P.O.

New Mexico Health and Environment Department (NMHED) and The New Mexico Health Systems Agency. 1986. *The Health of Mothers and Infants in New Mexico: Infant Mortality, Low Birthweight Babies, Teen Pregnancy and Related Topics.* Santa Fe, N.M.

Omenn, G.S., and R.P. Nathan. 1982. What's Behind Those Block Grants in Health? *New England Journal of Medicine* 306:1057–1060.

Peoples-Sheps, M.D. 1986. *Network News. A Technical Newsletter of the Region IV Network for Data Management and Utilization* 2(2):1–3. Chapel Hill: University of North Carolina.

Preston, S.H. 1984. Children and the Elderly in the United States. *Scientific American* 251(6):44–49.

Project SERVE. 1985. *New Directions: Serving Children with Special Health Care Needs in Massachusetts.* Boston: Massachusetts Health Research Institute.

Public Health Foundation. 1986. *1984 Public Health Chartbook.* Washington, D.C.: Association of State and Territorial Health Officials.

Rogers, D.E., R.J. Blendon, and T.W. Moloney. 1982. Who Needs Medicaid? *New England Journal of Medicine* 307:13–18.

Rosenbaum, S. 1983. The Maternal and Child Health Block Grant Act of 1981: Teaching an Old Program New Tricks. *Clearinghouse Review,* August/September:400–414.

Ryan, G.M., A.H. Pettigrew, S. Fogerty, and C.L. Donahue. 1977. Regionalizing Perinatal Health Care in Massachusetts. *New England Journal of Medicine* 296:228–230.

Rymer, M. 1986. Medicaid Eligibility Options. In R. Curtis and I. Hill, (eds.), *Affording Access to Quality Care,* pp. 1–29. Washington, D.C.: National Governors' Association and Center for Health Policy Research.

Schmidt, W.M. 1974. How Children Got into the Act. In R.H. Brenner (ed.), *Children and Youth in America,* Vol. 3. Cambridge, Mass.: Harvard University Press.

Select Panel for the Promotion of Child Health. 1981. *Better Health for Our Children: A National Strategy.* DHHS Publication No. 79-55071. Washington, D.C.: G.P.O.

Silver, G.A., C. Altenstetter, J.W. Bjorkman, M. Chen, and A.M. Foltz. 1976. *Impact of Federal Health Policies in the States of Connecticut and Vermont.* Final

Report to National Center for Health Services Research on grant HS 00900 (National Technical Information Service, Springfield, Va., 22161, 1976, PB262 959).
Swartz, K. 1986. Number and Characteristics of the Uninsured in the United States. In M.B. Sulvetta and K. Swartz (eds.). *The Uninsured and Uncompensated Care; A Chartbook.* National Health Policy Forum. Washington, D.C.: George Washington University.
U.S. Department of Health, Education and Welfare. 1956. *Your Children's Bureau: Its Current Program.* Children's Bureau Publication No. 357. Washington, D.C.: DHEW.
U.S. Department of Health and Human Services. 1986. *Health United States 1986.* DHHS Publication No. 87-1232. Washington, D.C.: G.P.O.
Walker, B., J. Chabut, M. Poland, and J.R. Taylor. 1983. *The Impact of Unemployment on the Health of Mothers and Children in Michigan; Recommendations for the Nation.* Lansing: Michigan Department of Health.
Wallace, H.M., H. Goldstein, and A.C. Oglesby. 1974. The Health and Medical Care of Children Under Title 19 (Medicaid). *American Journal of Public Health* 64:501–507.
Wise, P.H., M. Kotelchuck, M.I. Wilson, and M. Mills. 1985. Racial and Socioeconomic Disparities in Childhood Mortality in Boston. *New England Journal of Medicine* 313:360–366.
Yordy, K.D. 1981. Federal Administrative Arrangements for Maternal and Child Health. In *Better Health for Our Children: A National Strategy. The Report of the Select Panel for the Promotion of Child Health. Volume IV—Background Papers,* pp. 659–706. DHHS Publication No. 79-55071. Washington, D.C.: G.P.O.

13

Little People in a Big Policy World: *Lasting Questions and New Directions in Health Policy for Children*

Mark J. Schlesinger, Ph.D., and Leon Eisenberg, M.D.

This chapter represents our attempt to integrate the ideas developed in earlier chapters with those presented at the associated conference "Children in a Changing Health Care System," held in November 1986 at the Kennedy School of Government at Harvard University.[1] Our thinking in this area has benefited from the contributions of both the discussants at the conference and the other participants. Although we did not seek an explicit consensus at the conference, we believe that our recommendations reflect the general tenor of the discussion as well as the concerns and vision of many of the participants. The agenda for policy reform presented in this chapter represents our attempt to strike a balance between the optimal and the feasible, embodied as specific reforms that could be implemented over the next five years. As with all compromises, they will leave some readers unsatisfied. Almost certainly these proposals would not be wholeheartedly endorsed by some who attended the conference or, indeed, by all of the authors of earlier chapters. We believe, however, that the philosophy of reform and specific proposals presented here represent a realistic and politically sustainable strategy for improving the health of American children.

A decade ago, many in Congress had grown concerned about the health and well-being of America's children. To provide them with better information and direction for their policymaking, they established a Select Panel for the Promotion of Child Health. In the closing months of the Carter Administration this group issued its report, *Better Health for Our Children: A National Strategy* (1981). With almost 600 pages of recommendations and analysis,[2] spanning several volumes, this report is unparalleled in the breadth and depth of its assessment of children's health care and the prospects for constructive reform. It thus serves as an important touchstone for our current thinking and efforts.

The Select Panel suggested that existing programs for children's health care were flawed in several ways. They did not adequately finance the medical care needed by pregnant women and children, offered services in a fragmented and duplicative manner, and were unable to assure appropriate accountability. These shortcomings were felt most heavily by low-income families. Mothers and their children in these households were significantly less likely to have health insurance, a regular source of medical care, or adequate prenatal care. To remedy these problems, the Select Panel proposed a large number of reforms. Prominent among these were changes in Medicaid eligibility (basing eligibility on family income, rather than welfare status, and requiring that all states raise eligibility to the federal poverty line), increased enrollment of children in organized systems of care (such as HMOs and community health centers), changes in provider practices and payment that would encourage more comprehensive primary care, prenatal care, and mental health care for children, as well as a revised and expanded role for Title V programs, with an increased emphasis on planning and quality assurance for children's health services.

Some of these goals have been at least partially met. The Omnibus Budget Reconciliation Act (OBRA) of 1986 gave states for the first time the authority to set Medicaid eligibility for pregnant women and young children independent of AFDC criteria, severing the link between health coverage and welfare. As of 1987, 25 states had expanded Medicaid eligibility above AFDC levels, 22 of them to 100 percent of the federal poverty line (Burwell and Rymer, 1987). Enrollment of low-income families in organized systems of care has also increased. Between 1980 and 1986, the proportion of Medicaid recipients enrolled in HMOs grew from 1 to 10 percent (Anderson and Fox, 1987). Infant mortality rates continued their decline, with the goals established by the Surgeon General for average infant mortality for the year 1990 now seemingly in reach (Public Health Service, 1986).

But for each of these accomplishments, there were several setbacks. The adequacy of prenatal care and the prevalence of low-birthweight babies have improved little, if at all; in some states and for some groups of mothers the situation appears to be worsening (Public Health Service, 1986). These failures are being felt most by families already at highest risk for poor health outcomes. As of 1984, the proportion of black women who received late or no prenatal care was twice that of white women (Hughes et al., 1987). Among black teenagers, inadequate prenatal care was three times as common as for the average American mother. There has been at best limited adoption of the methods of provider reimbursement recommended by the Select Panel; as discussed by Horgan and Flint (Chapter 7), the new methods that are emerging hold as many pitfalls as promises for children's health care. Instead of doubling Title V funding, as advised by the Select Panel, federal contributions were significantly reduced. Federal funds were also repackaged as a block grant, though the panel had explicitly recommended against this.

Even the "successes" were somewhat mixed. Medicaid eligibility was separated from welfare only after years of decline in the inflation-adjusted levels of AFDC eligibility. As a result, even with the expansions following OBRA in 1986, a smaller proportion of children living in poverty are covered by Medicaid today than were covered in 1980 (Burwell and Rymer, 1987). Although infant mortality is falling, this country is doing worse than other developed nations in reducing infant deaths. In the late 1970s, the United States ranked sixteenth among developed countries, as of 1985, it had dropped back to nineteenth (Hughes et al., 1988). Nor have overall reductions infant mortality in this country closed the gap between blacks and whites. In recent years, infant and maternal mortality rates among minorities have leveled-off and in some parts of the country have begun to increase (Public Health Service, 1986; Hughes et al., 1988).

Equally perturbing, the 1980s have seen several new threats to children's health care that were not foreseen by the Select Panel. The adequacy of private insurance coverage for children has been significantly eroded. Three ongoing trends contributed to this decline. As an increasing proportion of employment was in low-paying jobs with limited benefits in the service sector, the number of adults and their dependents without health insurance as a fringe benefit increased by about one-third (Sulvetta and Swartz, 1986). To control costs, employers required higher deductibles and copayments on the policies that they did offer, effectively eliminating insurance coverage for much of children's primary health care. A growing number of employers self-insured, which under ERISA provisions exempted them from state regulations that had required coverage of well-child and mental health care benefits for dependents (Polchow, 1986).

These trends have significantly increased financial barriers to maternal and children's health care. Women without health insurance now account for 40 percent of all births, and at least one-quarter of these women receive inadequate prenatal care (General Accounting Office, 1987). Between 1982 and 1986, the percentage of American children without a regular source of health care almost doubled, growing from 5.8 percent to 9.9 percent (Robert Wood Johnson Foundation, 1983, 1987). Over this same period, the proportion of children without a physician visit in the previous year increased by 50 percent (Robert Wood Johnson Foundation, 1983, 1987). Financial barriers are most likely to restrict access for children from low-income families, who will likely receive fewer eye and ear exams, treatment for infections and care for injuries (Lohr et al., 1986). These are among the services which the Select Panel had identified as already inadequate at the start of the decade (Select Panel, 1980).

A second unanticipated problem has been the emergence of administrative restrictions on insurance coverage. Nine states currently restrict the number of hospital days covered by Medicaid, six limiting coverage to 15 days or fewer per year (Rosenbaum and Hughes, 1986). Though children are only infrequently hospitalized, many of the most severely ill would exceed these limits (Payne and Restuccia, 1987). A dozen states limit Medicaid coverage in terms of the number or total expenditures for prenatal visits, several explicitly prohibiting coverage early in pregnancy (Rosenbaum and Hughes, 1986). Although less is known about the nature of restrictions in private insurance plans, the use of similar administrative controls has increased significantly during the 1980s (Gabel et al., 1987).

Finally, the growth of entrepreneurialism in both private and government-operated health care settings has far exceeded that anticipated by the Select Panel. *Better Health for Our Children* called for increased participation by the local community in the governance of health care facilities and the delivery of services. This was intended to enhance community support for children's health care and to make providers more responsive to children's health needs that were best understood by the local residents. But entrepreneurial medicine has instead made providers more responsive to the purchasing power of large insurers, public programs, and employer groups. Defined increasingly by values common to commercial enterprise, health care facilities are becoming less sensitive to broader community interests and less inclined to promote community participation in governance (Jones et al., 1987; Schlesinger, 1987). The needs of children from low-income families—who are less likely to be insured or otherwise enfranchised within the health care system—are thus more likely to be neglected.

Some of the failures of the Select Panel report can be attributed simply to bad timing. The advent of the Reagan Administration changed, at least temporarily, popular and political perceptions about the appropriate role of the federal government. Burgeoning deficits clamped a vise on federal coffers that might otherwise have funded proposed expansions of Title V or Medicaid. A recession in the early 1980s led to sharp increases the number of Americans living in the poverty, revealing new gaps in the safety net of social programs and overburdening government-operated health care facilities. The changing political climate was reflected in new expectations of private health care providers, accelerating trends for commercialization of American medicine.

But the fate of the Select Panel's recommendations cannot be wholly written off to unfortunate happenstance. We believe that the track record of the past decade, for both the Select Panel's proposals and the health care system generally, reveals important lessons for maternal and child health policy in the future. It is our intent in this final chapter to identify some of the more important of these lessons. From this base, we will then formulate a set of proposed policies that can address the most important emerging problems for maternal and child health care and do so in a manner that is compatible with ongoing trends in health care and feasible in the political climate of the foreseeable future.

The issue that is perhaps most fundamental, and thus an appropriate starting point, is one that the Select Panel did not directly address at all. By Congressional mandate (P.L. 95-626), this panel was directed to "formulate specific goals with respect to the promotion of the health status of children and expectant mothers in the United States [and] develop a comprehensive national plan for achieving these goals." But this formulation presumes that it is appropriate to think in terms of initiatives specific to children, that a sensible "child health policy" can be created distinct from the policies shaping the health care of other Americans. This is not in fact obvious. It merits discussion because a better understanding about *why* children's health care deserves special attention provides some important insights into *how* such initiatives should be designed. Issues identified by exploring this question will serve as the basis for three sets of reforms: those intended to improve financial access to children's health services, reforms intended to improve the quality of those services, and reforms designed to reshape the mission and improve the effectiveness of the public programs that provide a "safety net" for children from disadvantaged households.

The Merits of a Separate Maternal and Child Health Policy

Most Americans believe that we have a societal responsibility for the well-being of our children. This is motivated as much from a sense of collective self-interest as from any altruism toward others. Many increasingly perceive a need to "invest" in children to provide for a productive workforce in the future. This viewpoint has led to reports on child health care that are labeled "Investing in the Future" (Office of Technology Assessment, 1988) or recommendations for educational reform that are referred to as "investment options for the educationally disadvantaged" (Committee on Economic Development 1988).

But generally favorable attitudes toward services for children do not always translate into support for particular policies or programs, nor do they guarantee that all children will be judged equally good investments. Nor does a general concern for children's welfare provide much guidance for a distinct child health policy. To establish a clearer sense of what might constitute an appropriate health policy for children, one must really consider three different, though related, questions.

- What is it that is unusual about children or their health care needs that merits special consideration by policy makers?
- Given the diverse needs of children of different ages and in different socioeconomic circumstances, is it possible to construct a sensible and consistent national policy?
- Can one formulate an effective set of policies directed toward children when they receive much of their care from providers who also treat other patients and whose practices will therefore be shaped by policies and incentives designed for other groups with different health care needs?

These are not questions with easy answers. But how they are answered will in large part determine which specific reforms to the financing and delivery of children's health care are most desirable or most feasible.

The Special Needs of Children and Public Policy

The case is often made that health policy toward children should be shaped by particular needs that distinguish children from other groups. In the preceding chapters, for example, various authors noted that:

- Many of the most significant health problems of children and adolescents (including malnutrition, substance abuse, learning and behavior problems) tend to be multiply determined and not exclusively biological. As a result, they tend to be neglected by the medical care system because they can be less directly engaged by physicians alone, requiring coordination with other community programs and assessment of the social, financial and psychological resources within children's families.
- Although children less frequently require institutional care than do adults, for a number of conditions they have very long stays. For others there is much higher variance in length and method of treatment than for adults. As a result, methods of provider payment appropriate for adults' health care may create inappropriate incentives when applied to younger patients.
- Children from families with limited financial resources have special health needs to ensure adequate development, but at best episodic

ties to providers, threatening the continuity and availability of appropriate services.
- Effectively addressing many of the health care needs of children requires that providers be willing and able to collaborate with parents and other significant persons in the children's environment.
- The health care problems of children (with the exception of infants in need of neonatal intensive care) are less likely than those of adults to result in death, making it more difficult to assess the incidence of child health problems or the effectiveness of interventions. Children's health care needs thus require less technology-intensive and expensive interventions, making them appear less essential to those for whom the importance of health problems is synonymous with their cost.

All these observations are accurate. They reflect assessments of the weaknesses within our health care that date back at least a decade (Silver, 1978; Select Panel, 1980). These concerns should be reflected in reform of health care financing and delivery systems. But they do not in themselves provide a sufficient rationale for a separate health policy for children because they also apply to other Americans. If many of the health problems of children require interventions broader than medical treatment, the same is true for millions of chronically ill elderly (Butler and Newacheck, 1981). If existing methods for paying providers are inadequate for some children, they are equally inappropriate for a variety of medical conditions among adult patients (Horne et al., 1984). Families provide an important source of care not only for children, but also for many disabled adults (Doty, 1986). The same trends that are creating greater financial barriers for access to care by children are also affecting other members of their families (Freeman et al., 1987).

If health policy were shaped exclusively by health care needs, there would thus seem to be little reason to formulate a separate set of policies for children. Although the limitations of existing arrangements need to be addressed, children could benefit from general reforms designed to meet the needs of all Americans.

If children do have special claim to policy makers' attention, it is less because their needs are different than because their needs are not as fully represented under the arrangements that determine how health services in this country are financed and delivered. In the absence of remedial policy, children may thus be excluded, directly or indirectly, from the benefits of reforms that aid their parents or grandparents.

This is most clearly evident for private insurance. As noted by Rosenbaum (Chapter 5), private health insurance in the United States is for the most part provided as a fringe benefit of employment. As with other fringe benefits, the provisions of these policies emerge through labor-management negotiations. No one represents children at these negotiations. Consequently, their benefits tend to be less complete—as of 1985, 20 to 25 percent of children who had parents covered by employer-based insurance were not themselves covered. As employers increase their efforts to bargain down health care costs, it is likely to be the coverage for dependents that is the first to give.[3] This is particularly true for those services, such as inpatient mental health care, where children's services use a disproportionate share of the resources (Evelyn, 1988).

Problems of inadequate representation for children are exacerbated by other considerations. If insurance fails to cover preventive care for employees, and they are therefore less healthy or fit, the company bears much of the cost in terms of job absenteeism, lower employee morale, and reduced productivity on the job (Behrens, 1987). But the same is not true for the employees' children. Since children need somewhat different types of preventive coverage from that of adults, even if they are eligible for the same services as their parents, they will be excluded from some care they require. It was precisely these concerns that led states to mandate coverages such as well-child benefits in private plans (Polchow, 1986). But, as noted earlier, as more companies self-insure, they circumvent these regulatory requirements.

Similar concerns emerge when employees choose among a number of private insurance plans. As competition among insurers continues to intensify, they will be under increased pressure to offer benefits that attract enrollees while holding down costs and premiums. This will lead to reductions in some coverages and expansions in others. Without adequate regulation to guarantee minimum benefits for the services that children need, parents may inadvertently select plans that fail to provide adequate coverage. And as noted by Taylor and colleagues (Chapter 2), once children have developed a serious chronic condition—there are several million such children in the United States—it may be impossible for parents to switch plans or jobs without having treatment excluded from coverage as a "preexisting condition" (Hobbs et al., 1985).

For all these reasons, children's health needs may be inadequately reflected in the private insurance coverage available to most families. In our assessment, these potential inadequacies merit action by policy makers. But the same factors that lead to inadequate private insurance coverage may also limit the effectiveness of government intervention. To the extent that children are less adequately represented than are other groups in Congress or state legislatures, appropriations for programs targeted to their needs will suffer commensurately (Silver, 1978; Sugarman, 1987). At least at the state level, this problem appears quite serious, as illustrated by experience with Medicaid over the past ten years. Children have received a steadily declining share of Medicaid revenues during this period (Burwell and Rymer, 1987). And there is considerable variation among states in the extent to which children's interests are represented and protected (see Chapter 6 and 12). Between 1975 and 1985, for example, the inflation-adjusted value of AFDC benefits was increased or held roughly constant in eight states, but in nine other states fell by more than 40 percent (Burwell and Rymer, 1987).

Children's interests are thus not adequately represented in either public or private sectors. This can have important consequences for the financing and delivery of their health care. Educating policy makers, labor leaders, and business executives about these failings will undoubtedly help change attitudes to some extent. To provide a reliable base for future action, however, changing attitudes must be reinforced by changing institutions, reforms that more closely link the well-being of children to that of other age groups. Constructing such policies, however, requires confronting several other difficult issues.

Consistent Policies and Diverse Needs

Even if we agree that children, as a group, merit special consideration by policy makers, it is not at all obvious that children can or should be treated as a homogeneous group by policy makers. Children have a wide variety of unmet health needs (Sugarman, 1987). Those deemed most important for adolescents are very different than those affecting younger children. As Taylor and colleagues noted, the most needed additional service for chronically ill children may be case management, though other groups of children may be more in need of developmental monitoring or periodic health screening programs. Children from low-income households frequently require a more intensive and comprehensive array of health services than their counterparts from middle-class families (Klerman, 1988).

This complexity is exacerbated by a heterogeneous health care system. For children treated by prepaid health care providers, the most pressing policy concerns involve the potential for undertreatment of some illnesses. For those under fee-for-service care, the greater threat may involve excessive treatment, often for the very same services that might be underprovided under prepaid auspices (Chapter 8). As a result, policy makers may be required to formulate policies that work in diametrically opposed directions, depending on the reimbursement arrangements under which childrens' health care is provided.

Social and economic considerations complicate the picture still further. The same socioeconomic factors that affect children's access to health services also mediate the relative performance of different systems for financing and delivering childrens' health care. The same level of cost sharing that will lead to prudent purchasing by middle-income families will create financial barriers to needed care for children from low-income households (Lohr et al., 1986). Organizational arrangements, such as HMOs, may provide less adequate care for children and mothers with limited income and education than they do for other enrollees who are better off (Chapter 8).

Given this complexity and diversity, health policy for children will almost inevitably lack the elegance or clarity that we might desire. It is difficult to devise reforms that are simple and coherent but that mesh neatly with existing arrangements for financing and delivering health care, which are neither simple nor coherent. These same factors raise more fundamental questions about whether it is in fact sensible to speak at all of a health policy for children in the generic sense, or whether constructive policy making in this area must focus on particular subgroups of children, such as those who are very young, those without private insurance, those who are chronically ill, or those from low-income households.

This is in part a question of public management, in part one of political strategy. The administrative challenge lies in the distribution of responsibility for public programs and policies that affect children across a variety of state and federal agencies and a number of Congressional committees. Private insurance regulation, Medicaid program decisions, characteristics of school health programs and Title V fund allocations rest primarily at the state level and all in different departments. Budgets for many of these programs, though, are determined in large part by the federal government. Initiatives to address gaps in insurance or Medicaid coverage can emerge from either state or federal government. It is certainly difficult to define a clear health policy agenda for children when decisionmaking is so decentralized and fragmented. The question for policy makers is how this handicap can be most effectively surmounted or circumvented.

To address this "disarray of programs and policies" the Select Committee proposed in 1980 that the federal government create a Maternal and Child Health Administration to provide a focus for maternal and child health issues and policy making within the Department of Health and Human Services. It also suggested that a National Commission on Maternal and Child Health make periodic reports to Congress and the Administration. Neither of these changes occurred. The continuing lack of central direction, in the assessment of the authors of several chapters, has impeded the development of an effective national policy for maternal and child health. Disparities and inequities have grown greater as Congress authorized greater latitude for state-based programs and as states have lost their ability to regulate insurance coverage due to employers' shift to self-insurance.

But the debate over a new federal agency or commission is to some extent misleading. The fundamental issue here involves the extent to which our nation can accept differences in treatment for children covered under different insurance plans or living in different states. In our assessment, these disparities must be narrowed. The interstate variations in Titles V and XIX must be reduced. Although state discretion has allowed expansion of benefits for some groups, it has also allowed benefits for other children to be progressively eroded over time, leaving some with extremely inadequate access to health care. Neither the ideological appeal of states' rights nor the potential benefits of state-level experimentation can justify the inequities that currently exist in Medicaid eligibility and coverage provisions, nor the inadequacies of the MCH/Title V programs in a number of states. More consistent national standards can and must be established for these programs. And we believe that they can be established without inhibiting the efforts of some states to establish more generous programs for their citizens.

The strategic political questions for MCH policy involve how much or how best to combine the political fortunes of those women and children who readily generate public sympathy with others who have less popular support. Historically, eligibility established under various parts of the Social Security Act was defined broadly, with a strong presumption of equal treatment for all who were eligible for benefits. In recent years, however, states have been given greater latitude in such programs to offer greater benefits to some children, while cutting back for others. In Chapter 12, Guyer describes how the inclusion of Title V funds in the MCH block grant led to a shift in resources, with the politically popular crippled children's services maintaining a larger share of declining budgets than did other MCH programs. During this same period, there was a significant shift in Medicaid resources from older to younger children. The Omnibus Budget Reconciliation Act in 1981 embodied severe cutbacks in eligibility for teen-aged recipients. In contrast, beginning with the Deficit Reduction Act of 1984, Congress initiated a sequential expansion of Medicaid eligibility for pregnant women and young children (Chapter 6).

There may be convincing reasons for targeting services to particular age groups. Certainly the benefits of more adequate prenatal care have been clearly demonstrated, as to a lesser extent have various services for young children (Select Panel, 1981; Shadish, 1981; General Accounting Office, 1987). But the shifts in public resources during the 1980s go beyond any measurable differences in the relative needs or efficacy of treatments for children of different ages. Increasingly, tax dollars appear to be available only to those children whose needs can be effectively packaged and sold in the political marketplace. This raises an alarming specter—that children whose health care needs are less apparent or more controversial, such as those involving pregnancy, substance abuse or mental illness, will receive a progressively smaller share of future public dollars.

We believe that maternal and child health programs would be more soundly and fairly based if they consistently treated the needs of all children. We are also mindful, however, that under the current political and budgetary climate the political appeal of pregnant women and infants may not protect the interests of other children, as was true for the Medicaid program throughout the late 1970s and early 1980s (Burwell and Rymer, 1987). Based on this experience, we conclude that if policy makers are more adequately to address the needs of all children, they must rebalance the political equation by establishing common standards of financial access to health care between children and older Americans.

At the same time, policy must reflect children's lesser ability to pursue that health care. There must be greater direction from the federal government and a renewed emphasis on adequate minimal standards for programs that finance or deliver health services. To prevent those children whose needs may be less graphic or whose services more controversial from losing ground in this process, different strategies and programs must be developed to assure access to needed services.

Children in an Adult Health Care System

Whatever the merits of health programs or policies designed to meet the needs of children, history makes clear that many of the changes in the health care system that significantly affect children are driven primarily by concerns about the cost, quality, or accessibility of services for their parents or grandparents. This occurs in part because insurance is typically purchased for families, not children. Consequently, as employers increased the use of HMOs, PPOs, and other managed care arrangements for their employees, children were drawn into these systems (Gabel et al., 1987). Policy initiatives developed for older groups of patients can also "spillover" to affect children. This can occur even though policy makers explicitly excluded children from the original reforms. As discussed by Horgan and Flint, when Medicare adopted its DRG payment system, it exempted pediatric hospitals out of concern that a system designed for the elderly would not accurately reflect resource use by younger patients. Within 3 years, though, a dozen states had developed DRG payment systems for their Medicaid programs that emulated arrangements adopted by Medicare (Payne and Restuccia, 1987). Many children were affected by these reforms.

The links between health care reform for children and adults can create opportunities as well as risks. For example, some observers believe that children would benefit if insurers paid physicians in proportion to the time spent in patient care, since this would favor the time-intensive services that many children need and increase the financial rewards of pediatric practices (Chapter 7). Very similar arguments have been made for having Medicare employ a relative-value system for older patients (Blumenthal and Hsiao, 1988). Due to their complicated conditions and multiple pathologies, the elderly also require a significant commitment of time by health professionals to ensure accurate diagnosis and adequate treatment (Rowe, 1985). At a time when there are growing concerns about future intergenerational conflicts over scarce public resources, it is noteworthy (and somewhat reassuring) to establish that there are indeed some potential policy changes which would benefit both older and younger Americans.

We know of no practical way to insulate children from most of these interactions. For better or worse then, the quality and accessibility of children's health care, as well as the efficacy of government initiatives designed to further these goals, will depend to a large extent on policies and practices developed for older generations. Those who would protect children's interests must guard against undesirable spill-over effects. Those who would improve children's well-being should seek initiatives that also improve health care delivery and financing for older patients. An effective health policy toward children cannot therefore be limited to a single agency or committee with this as its concern. It must instead be reflected in a sensitivity toward children's needs on the part of policy makers concerned with all aspects of health and human resources.

A Plan for Children-Oriented Health Reforms: Principles and Policies

We develop here a set of reforms with a dual focus—one that emphasizes establishing shared standards among groups of children and adults to ensure adequate financial access, with a more child-specific strategy to assure that children receive appropriate services of adequate quality. Particularly with regard to issues of financing, it is thus tempting to look for system-wide reforms. Confronted by the complexity of existing arrangements for financing and delivering services, a unified approach looks very appealing. It is natural to think in terms of improving children's health coverage in the context of a national health insurance program that would enroll all Americans.

But though the popular appeal of national health insurance once again appears to be growing, it is unlikely to be feasible in the near future. Moreover, the forms of national health insurance that are compatible with American politics and preferences are less likely to involve a uniform national program than the integration of a set of more narrowly-defined coverages, incorporated under some common standards. Consequently, in discussing strategies of reform below, we have focused on more incremental approaches to improving the quality and accessibility of children's health care.

Even if reform is incremental, it can and should be shaped by a more general set of principles and a more far-reaching vision. The reforms detailed below are premised on three basic principles:

- it is a public responsibility to ensure that all children are afforded access to needed health care services, whatever their family-status;
- public policy should give greatest priority to those services that are inadequately provided and those children who are underserved by private markets; and
- the circumstances and needs of children are sufficiently diverse that inflexible rules and regulations will inevitably compromise the quality of children's health care.

These principles are implicit in the writings and proposals of many child health advocates. It is important that they be made explicit and clear to those who are not specialists in children's health care, both so that they understand the full implications of these principles and so that they can be made aware of the extent to which ongoing changes in the health care system and health policies have violated these norms. The proposed reforms described below also reflect several more pragmatic considerations. Based on our review of the unmet needs and emerging concerns in the health care of America's children, we have identified five additional criteria that we believe should guide future public policy initiatives.

First, the rationale for a health policy unique to children rests less on their special health needs than on questions of how adequately those needs are expressed or considered by decision makers. Reform proposals must therefore explicitly address this issue at both the service delivery and policymaking levels. Our earlier discussion suggests that, perhaps most important, the financial accessibility of children's health care must be more closely linked to that received by other age groups, whose interests may be more fully represented in these deliberations. In addition, programs must be expanded that augment and improve parents' ability to seek health services on their children's behalf. Mechanisms must be established to ensure that children's access to health care is assured even when their parents do not actively pursue it. Quality assurance programs must be sensitive to the special health needs of those children at high risk for poor health care, whose families will typically be least able to assess inappropriate health care or effectively voice their complaints.

Second, although most children's health advocates have focused on Medicaid to improve financial access to health care, benefits provided children under private insurance may now be of greater importance. The high costs of care have encouraged employers to cut back on health benefits, and dependents are likely to bear the brunt of this cost. It is no longer sufficient to assume that if employees have adequate insurance, their dependents will be equally well covered. Public action is required to assure that children's insurance benefits are not eroded over time. Consequently, initiatives to improve children's access to health care must address both private and public insurance.

Third, a growing number of children in both public and private insurance programs are enrolled in managed care arrangements. Under these systems, administrative practices and bureaucratic requirements play an important role in determining the provider's willingness or ability to offer particular services. This can lead to arbitrary denials of benefits or reductions in treatment. As a result, reform proposals must look beyond questions of eligibility and coverage to assess the impact and implications of these administrative constraints.

Fourth, since much of the policy that affects children's health care is made by state governments, it is important to consider how much latitude to allow states in formulating programs. Greater latitude is typically justified on the grounds either that citizens in different states favor different types of public spending or that state discretion permits greater experimentation and innovation. But discretion also potentially creates inequities. For some programs, or for particular aspects of those programs, the benefits of state discretion are outweighed by the liabilities of unequal treatment. We identify below what we believe to be the most important sources of these inequities, and how they might be reduced.

Fifth, although there is growing public sentiment for expanding services to children, this enthusiasm does not apply equally to all children or all health needs. Those whose needs are least obvious (or least photogenic) as well as those in need of more controversial services or services that are not narrowly biological, will be the last offered additional public and private funding. We must design programs and institutions that safeguard the welfare of these less popular groups of children.

These principles and standards are reflected, albeit imperfectly, in the specific proposals presented below. These are grouped into three categories: those addressed to issues of financial access, those designed to assure more adequate care once children have been brought into the health care system, and those intended to revamp and reinvigorate government-provided services.

Assuring financial access to maternal and child health care. Both public and private bases for financing children's health care have eroded over the past decade. The ratio of children in poverty to those receiving Medicaid declined from 95 percent in the mid-1970s to 80 percent in the mid-1980s, reaching a low point of 74 percent in 1983 (Burwell and Rymer, 1987). Although 27 states have since expanded eligibility for pregnant women and infants, this has for the most part simply regained ground lost in previous years (Rosenbaum et al., 1988). There has been a corresponding decline in private insurance coverage, resulting in a 20–25 percent increase in the number of uninsured children between the late 1970s and mid-1980s.

Policies to assure reasonable financial access must therefore address two objectives. First, safeguards must protect against further erosion of coverage under Medicaid and private insurance. Second, insurance coverage must be extended to the millions of pregnant women and children who are currently uninsured. We propose here reforms that we believe can accomplish both these ends, though the reforms in themselves will be somewhat controversial.

As noted earlier, changing Medicaid eligibility during the 1980s has significantly shifted public resources toward young children and the elderly and away from older children and their parents. These reallocations were exacerbated when states were permitted to cover services for only particular Medicaid-eligible groups. Fifteen state Medicaid programs currently reimburse day treatment for patients with dementia, paying for remedial, habilitative and psychosocial care. Yet developmentally disabled children in these states who have the exact same functional impairments are not covered by Medicaid for these services, because they are classified as educational and not medical needs (Rosenbaum, 1988). In our assessment, these distinctions have produced unacceptable inequities. Six-year-old children living just below the poverty line are no less deserving of public support than are their infant siblings, yet the majority of American states today deny Medicaid to the former while granting it to the latter (Rosenbaum et al., 1988). An older family receiving SSI has no stronger claim to society's resources than one eligible for AFDC, yet in most states the income at which one becomes eligible for Medicaid under SSI is significantly above that for AFDC. Individuals with equal impairment and equal financial resources should have equal access to remedial services, whatever their age or family status.

We therefore propose that all age-based differences in eligibility and service coverage under Medicaid be eliminated. All families, young and old, should be judged by the same standards in determining their need for publicly subsidized health care. In the same way that SSI eligibility is "indexed" to adjust for inflation, so too should AFDC eligibility levels.

There are clearly strong ethical arguments in favor of more equal treatment of Americans in low-income households whatever their age (Cohen, 1980; Freeman, 1983). Nonetheless, this proposal is likely to be controversial, in part because it reverses a strategy that has been successfully pursued by child health advocates over the past five years. These advocates have been successful at incrementally expanding Medicaid coverage precisely by making distinctions according to age, by singling out those groups that are the most politically appealing (e.g., infants and young children) or for whom the strongest case can be made for the societal benefits from expanded insurance (e.g., prenatal care) (Hughes et al., 1987).

This approach has been effective in expanding Medicaid eligibility during an era of severe federal budget constraints. Its advocates would argue, moreover, that it presages additional incremental expansion, with Congress successively authorizing, and states establishing, expanded eligibility for additional categories of older children. But another scenario appears more likely. With politically attractive children already covered, it will become increasingly difficult to achieve additional expansion. This is particularly true for teenagers, whose greatest health needs involve mental health care, substance abuse counseling and family planning, hardly the services to inspire a supportive majority in Congress or state legislatures.

The lessons of history are clear. Medicare was seen by many of its proponents as the first step on the road to national health insurance (Marmor, 1970). The elderly, the group that was widely perceived at the time as the "deserving poor," seemed an appropriate starting point. Twenty-five years later, the next steps have yet to be taken. Incremental expansion by age thus does not seem a promising avenue to a broad-based and equitable program of public insurance.

Eliminating age distinctions will also be controversial for a second reason. There are those who interpret the recent history of Medicaid as an example of how children's interests suffer when they share a program with other, politically more powerful, groups. "Medicaid is perhaps unique among public programs in that it is the only major assistance program in which the elderly and children compete for resources. Our analyses show that, over the past decade, the aged and disabled have fared better than have poor children and families in gaining access to Medicaid-covered services" (Burwell and Rymer, 1987, p. 41).

It is indisputable that spending on elders' health care is taking a progressively larger share of Medicaid's resources. But we believe that is a mistake to conclude that this is *because* elders and children are part of a single program. These resource shifts have occurred not because the two groups have shared a program but because they have had too little of the program in common, because states have had the flexibility to set eligibility standards separately for different age groups. Hence, while the eligibility standards for AFDC-based Medicaid have declined 30 percent in inflation-adjusted dollars over the past decade, income standards under SSI have actually increased 10 percent in real terms (Burwell and Rymer, 1987). It is these differences that have produced current inequities, and it is these differences that the reforms proposed here would eliminate.

The limitations of private health insurance for children are similar to those of Medicaid. Dependents may not be eligible for coverage under employer-based policies or may not be subsidized at the same rate as employees' coverage. Services under dependent coverage may be more restricted than those for employees and in many cases are not well-adapted to the special health care needs of children.

One strategy to remedy these failings would have government regulate insurance coverages, mandating certain minimum benefits for dependent coverage. States have traditionally played this role. As of 1986, for example, 25 states required that private insurance include coverage of newborns and several states mandated well-baby coverage (Polchow, 1986). But these state mandates are becoming less effective as more companies self-insure, which under ERISA provisions puts them outside the authority of state insurance regulations. The federal government could assume this role and establish its own set of minimum benefits. But this would require the creation of a new federal authority and additional regulations, neither of which would be greatly favored in the current political climate. It could also lead to significant delays. There are legitimate differences over what constitute appropriate minimum benefits for children's health care. Attempts to resolve these differences to allow for uniform national standards would almost certainly be contentious and inevitably time-consuming.

These limitations of direct regulation argue for a different approach to protect private insurance benefits for children. We propose here a strategy comparable to the one recommended for Medicaid reform that focuses on eliminating age-related inequities. The federal government should require, for employer-based insurance policies to be exempted from federal taxes, that these policies pay out at least a minimal proportion of their benefits in the form of coverage for dependents. This would protect dependent benefits by linking their value to the value of health benefits for employees. It would do this without excessive or intrusive regulation. There is precedent for establishing requirements of this sort on employees' fringe benefits. Similar rules were adopted toward somewhat different ends as antidiscrimination requirements on cafeteria benefit plans, first established in 1978 and expanded as part of the Tax Reform Act of 1986 (Fox and Schaffer, 1987).

We anticipate that these reforms that more closely link children's welfare to that of older individuals will stem the recent erosion of public and private health care coverage. Stabilizing benefits under private insurance and Medicaid is, however, only the first step in addressing financial access to children's health care. It is also essential to expand insurance to those currently without any coverage. Short of enacting comprehensive national health insurance, there are two possible strategies for more incremental reform—the first building on existing employment-based coverage, the second reconfiguring the Medicaid program.

Equally thoughtful and well-meaning policy makers support each of these approaches. In an interesting juxtaposition of political stereotypes, Senator Kennedy, a Democrat, introduced to Congress legislation building on employer insurance, while Senator Chaffee, a Republican, proposed an expansion of Medicaid. As of spring 1988, several states were experimenting, or considering experiments, based on each model. While either approach has its own strengths and weaknesses, we believe that expanding and reconfiguring Medicaid eligibility holds greater immediate promise for improving children's health care.

First and foremost, the coverage provided under Medicaid better fits the needs of children than does a typical private policy. Employer-based insurance plans increasingly incorporate substantial annual deductibles, which leave most outpatient care for children effectively uncovered (Chapter 5). It is not unusual for annual deductibles to be set at several hundred dollars. This is as large as total yearly health care costs for many children (Rymer and Adler, 1987). Few private policies cover the services included in Medicaid's EPSDT program, services that have been shown to be important for many low-income children (Hughes et al., 1988; Klerman, 1988; Schorr, 1988). Second, Medicaid expansion avoids some of the implementation issues that would face employer-based approaches. Employers that do not now offer health insurance as a fringe benefit are generally small and thus unable to obtain large-group discounts (Chollet, 1987). To make insurance more affordable for these companies, some form of state-wide or area-wide pooling arrangements would need to be created, undoubtedly with a public subsidy. This function could filled by Medicaid, without creating any new programs. Third, employer-based insurance provides coverage only indirectly for children. Medicaid coverage, on the other hand, could be made available for children whatever the insurance status of their parents.

We are mindful of Medicaid's limitations, particularly the significant interstate disparities in the program. These can, however, be straightforwardly addressed by requiring more uniform program administration (Chapter 6), some aspects of which will be discussed later in this chapter.

We therefore propose expanding Medicaid eligibility in two stages. In the first stage, all states would be required to extend Medicaid coverage to all families with incomes at or below the federal poverty line. States wishing to retain more generous eligibility could do so, but would be required to extend this eligibility to noninstitutionalized individuals of all ages. There seems to be no convincing rationale for allowing states latitude in minimal standards of eligibility. There is no great potential for innovation or experimentation, expanded eligibility is straightforward and clearly needed. Nor would such requirements impose great burdens on states, even those with the most restricted tax bases (Davidson et al., 1986). We estimate that the added costs to state and federal government for this required coverage would be about ten billion dollars annually.

About half the nation's uninsured children would be covered under these provisions (Sulvetta and Swartz, 1986). To make insurance affordable for the rest, states should be required to offer Medicaid coverage to all other residents for a sliding premium based on family income and enrollee age (Wilensky, 1987). Many children could be covered under these insurancelike arrangements, even with relatively moderate public subsidies. In 1985, 3.1 million uninsured children were in families with incomes twice the poverty line or above (Chollet, 1987). Many of these families could afford a moderately priced insurance policy. And an age-based premium would, for many children, be relatively inexpensive. Medicaid utilization statistics reveal that in 1980 children between the ages of 5 and 14 had average annual health expenditures of under $500 even in states with high health care costs, and considerably lower in other states (Rymer and Adler, 1987).

Realistically, these initiatives will not overcome all financial barriers to health care for children. Not all uninsured families will feel that they can afford to pay premiums for Medicaid, even at subsidized rates. And past experience with Medicaid suggests that even those who are eligible for coverage at no cost will not all take advantage of this opportunity—statistics collected by the Congressional Budget Office indicate that only about half of all eligible children actually receive Medicaid benefits. Nonetheless, this approach seems to offer a sensible and cost effective means of significantly increasing financial access to health services. We propose later other reforms to offset its liabilities.

A Medicaid reform strategy has other benefits as well. Given the option to purchase Medicaid coverage for an income-adjusted premium, welfare recipients would no longer be faced with the prospect of losing affordable health insurance for their children when they take a job. This would eliminate what is currently a significant disincentive for those on AFDC to seek employment. A sliding-scale premium for Medicaid could also be integrated with proposals requiring that employers offer health insurance as a fringe benefit. Companies could simply "buy into" the Medicaid program for their employees, with Medicaid providing the large group risk-pooling that would make coverage more affordable. This would be more straightforward and administratively feasible than the complicated "pooling" arrangements that states now sponsor for small business. It would reduce the concerns now expressed about the costs of employer mandates for small business, since government would be sharing in the cost of insuring low-income workers.

Assuring more adequate health care for children. Overcoming initial financial barriers is only the first step in improving maternal and child health care. Even after patients gain access to a provider, the appropriateness and quality of the services they receive is by no means assured. As health care providers operate in an increasingly price-competitive, cost-pressured environment, they will be encouraged to squeeze ever-greater efficiency out of the delivery system. Inevitably, there will be instances where, in the process of cutting fat, they also excise muscle and bone. We simply know too little about the efficacy of many procedures and practices to avoid this trade-off, and this is a price we all will pay for lower health care spending. But it is vitally important that we guard against cost saving measures that impose unreasonable or disproportionate costs on children.

The most obvious problematic arrangements are the ceilings on hospital and prenatal coverage that have become features of the Medicaid programs of some states. These limits are inherently arbitrary and unfair. It is certainly true that they affect only a relatively small number of women and children. But these are the children who are most severely ill and the mothers who are most at risk of bad outcomes from pregnancy. These are the last groups who should bear the burden of reducing health care spending. They already face the greatest burdens from ill health. Enhancing access would almost certainly improve their health and reduce burdens on their families. These ceilings and limits on coverage under Medicaid should be prohibited by federal law.[4]

Though details about private insurance coverage are less readily available, similar provisions are a part of some private policies (Chapter 5). These too should be prohibited. The principal challenge is how to do this. ERISA restrictions on regulation of self insured plans make effective prohibitions difficult at the state level. Ceilings on coverage could be prohibited for policies to remain exempt from federal taxes. But it may be infeasible, and perhaps unwise, to introduce such detailed requirements into the federal tax code. If Congress is unwilling to amend ERISA to permit states at least limited oversight over self-insured plans, it must substitute direct federal regulation of insurance benefits. There is no clear case for preferring federal to state intervention, but some regulation is both essential and inevitable.

To the extent that explicit ceilings on coverage are prohibited, it is likely that private insurers, employers, and Medicaid administrators will turn increasingly to various forms of managed care to brake the rise of health care expenditures. As a result, children will increasingly be receiving their health care in organized delivery settings, many in which practitioners are prepaid. This seems a generally positive trend. For most children these plans will provide acceptable, and in some cases improved, health care. But these same arrangements may lead to inadequate care for specific groups of children. Unattended malnutrition, anemia, lead poisoning, chronic illnesses and impairments do not cost the health plan—or the health care system—as much as they cost the social service, juvenile justice or education systems. Consequently, the financial incentives within a managed care setting may leave these children undertreated, relative to the societally-optimal level of care. Care may even be less adequate than under the existing fragmented fee-for-service systems, because providers will no longer have financial incentives to provide this care and because some families will be unable to lead their children through the administrative hurdles built into most managed care systems.

Three strategies can be pursued to protect the quality of care for these groups of children. The first would exempt them, and possibly their families, from enrolling in managed care settings. Wisconsin, for example, allows Medicaid-covered children with chronic illnesses to be held out of mandatory HMO enrollment. This policy however, is currently the exception—most states with mandatory HMO enrollment of AFDC/Medicaid eligibles do not exempt special populations.

A second strategy would involve more complete and comprehensive quality assurance programs for children enrolled in managed care settings. Quality assurance is a growing concern for all purchasers of managed care (Eisenberg and Kabcenell, 1988; Luft, 1988). There is also growing awareness that plans that deliver good quality care for some enrollees may be less effective for others (Luft, 1988). This concern has encouraged increased government oversight of care in HMOs (Schlesinger and Drumheller, 1988). Congress has required that the Health Care Financing Administration (HCFA) expand the purview of Medicare's Professional Review Organizations to monitor quality in HMOs that enroll Medicare beneficiaries. But no comparably targeted programs of quality assurance have been developed for children. This apparent inequity is attributable in part to states' slow development of quality assurance mechanisms within their Medicaid managed care programs (Anderson and Fox, 1987). It also reflects differences in financing mechanisms for children's and elder's health services. The elderly have care paid primarily through a unified national program, which can be readily assigned responsibility if quality problems develop. In contrast, children's health care financing is fragmented among an array of public and private coverages, with no clear locus of authority and responsibility.

A third strategy for addressing the challenges of managed care for children would be to foster plans that specialized in the care of enrollees with chronic illnesses and impairments of various types. The prevalence of these conditions among children is sufficiently low that most HMOs or other managed care arrangements will not normally develop the capacity to effectively care for children with these special needs. Even if policies were created to encourage more specialized plans, only in relatively large urban areas could specialized plans be sufficiently large to be cost-effective. Specialized managed care could be made more widely available, though, if plans enrolled chronically ill enrollees of all ages. This approach offers substantial potential benefits. The service needs of chronically ill elders are not that different from those of developmentally disabled children. Indeed, integrating chronically impaired populations of various ages may promote innovations in treatment, bringing together providers who would otherwise be segregated by the age of their patients and promoting cross-fertilization of thinking and treatment practices.

There currently exist no age-integrated, specialized care plans of this sort. Federal regulations for HMO participation in Medicare and Medicaid discourage such specialization, by requiring that a substantial share of the HMOs enrollees be privately insured (Bonnano and Wetle, 1984). But the recent experience of age-integrated case management programs run by several states appears promising. Both Wisconsin's Community Options Program and New York's Nursing Home Without Walls provide case management for a number of disability groups ranging from the very young to the very old. This integration has in fact encouraged borrowing of treatment philosophies and techniques developed for some age groups and successfully applying them to others. It also broadens the base of political support for these special populations, groups that may otherwise be neglected because they a relatively small number of residents in any given state or locality.

Each of these three approaches has its limitations. One could require that Medicaid enrollees or private insurance families have the option to avoid joining a managed care plan. But even with such restrictions, families will inevitably face financial incentives or other inducements to enroll in such plans. It is easy to mandate that quality assurance programs in HMOs pay particular attention to children's health needs. But those needs most likely to be neglected, involving chronic illnesses and impairments, are also those for which there are the weakest professional norms defining appropriate treatment (Schlesinger, 1986). This raises questions about the ability of quality assurance programs to adequately protect the children about whom we are most concerned. Finally, although age-integrated programs are probably feasible, and in some senses beneficial, they also raise the specter of the disabled being segregated from the rest of the population, potentially cared for through plans that are progressively starved for funding as public resources are diverted to larger and politically more powerful groups.

Given these weaknesses, it will be necessary to pursue a combination of strategies to protect the quality of children's health care. Following Wisconsin's example, managed care programs should give families the option being exempted if their child has special health care needs. HCFA should be authorized to finance development of age-integrated HMOs specializing in the care of the chronically ill and impaired. Perhaps most important, states should be mandated to develop more adequate systems of quality assurance for children enrolled in managed care settings. At a minimum, these should cover all Medicaid enrollees. But because many children will be enrolled in HMOs under the auspices of private insurance, it would also be useful to extend quality assurance monitoring to these populations as well. This argues for placing quality oversight in some state agency other than that administering Medicaid. One plausible candidate would be the office of Maternal and Child Health within the Department of Public Health. This agency could be authorized to develop quality assurance protocols in collaboration with representatives from the Medicaid program, private insurers, and employers. Such a program would be required to have oversight over Medicaid managed care programs. Private insurers or employers could also purchase quality assurance monitoring from this state agency to cover their beneficiaries enrolled in managed care plans.

The public sector: Reweaving the safety net. The health care needs of children that are most likely to be neglected today are often those that are the least obvious. They come in the form of visits too long postponed, of subtle anemias that inhibit learning, of too many visits to harried and overworked physicians who lack the time and attention to accurately diagnose a complex problem or manage its treatment. If we are successful at expanding insurance coverage to children, this will be even more true. Problems with access will no longer be concentrated among children who can be readily identified as uninsured. Instead, as insurers increasingly move to prospective payment, the children denied adequate treatment will be those with illnesses that are more costly than average, those requiring unusually complex or time-consuming care.

The growing subtlety of these problems does not make them less important. Because private providers will not be willing or able to meet all the health needs of America's children, even when they are insured, it is essential that we maintain a vital array of public health institutions. But to successfully address the emerging problems of children's health, this safety net of public services will not simply have to be bigger or stronger, but be designed in a different pattern, with a different weave. To this end, we propose strengthening three functions of the public sector: case management, outreach and system management.

For a number of reasons, there is now an increasing need for agencies that can help parents manage their children's health care. Many emerging children's health problems can only be addressed through a combination of medical and social services, typically provided in a variety of settings under the auspices of a number of different agencies. As noted by Taylor and colleagues (Chapter 2), case management ranks foremost among the needs expressed by the parents of chronically ill children. But it is also a need of many other families. A third of all low-income women who received inadequate prenatal care, for example, attributed this failure to their inability to identify a provider who was willing to offer that care (General Accounting Office, 1987).

Historically, parents have relied on providers to help them negotiate the health care system. However, as providers of health and social services become increasingly entrepreneurial, competitive, and pressured to reduce use of services, the financial interests of these providers will diverge from the best interests of the children and their families. Even if providers avoid overt conflicts of interest, families will still be forced to question the reliability of information and advice they receive. They may also require advocates to help them obtain the care they need in an administratively constrained, cost-limited health care delivery system.

A second function of the public sector that must be strengthened involves its capacity for outreach—its ability to ensure that those in need receive the benefits to which they are entitled and the health care they require. An unacceptably large number of women and children currently receive insufficient care simply because they are unaware of their options. Forty percent of low-income women in this country with inadequate prenatal care did not fully understand their need for care or the services that were available in their community (General Accounting Office, 1987). More than half the women and children eligible for Medicaid do not in fact receive Medicaid-covered services, at least a quarter of these because they do not know that they qualify for benefits (Dobson et al., 1986; General Accounting Office, 1987). The failure to provide more aggressive outreach, such as home nursing visits, is one of the principal differences between the maternal and child health care system in the United States and its more successful counterparts in Western Europe (Miller, 1987). Ironically, though a strong outreach component is a hallmark of the most innovative and successful demonstration projects in this country, outreach services are the first to be cut when programs come under financial pressure, in large part because they are not reimbursed by public or private insurers (Schorr, 1988).

Finally, public agencies must develop a greater capacity to provide "system management" to complement more individualized case management. The fragmentation in the financing and delivery is costly and reduces its effectiveness. Although it can be largely overcome through case management, case management in itself adds to the costs of maternal and child health, without delivering any additional services. In some cases, it is less costly to address fragmentation by changing the system, rather than adapting individuals to that system.

> We need a systems manager—some entity that will help community providers piece together delivery systems where they are needed (e.g., helping a local clinic build up its obstetrical capacity through negotiation and recruitment assistance). We need an entity that will negotiate with related authorities (e.g., school boards, Medicaid agencies, social service agencies and institutions) for reforms that will allow smoother integration among a range of health financing and service delivery programs. For example, in most states, special education and Medicaid agencies have noncomplementary protocols for conducting developmental assessments through [P.L.] 94-142 and EPSDT. This means that special education diagnostic centers give no weight to the findings from an EPSDT developmental assessment. Conversely, Medicaid may not pay "special ed" people for performing the developmental assessment component on an EPSDT child simply because they are employed by an education agency rather than as a staff of a medically directed clinic. (Rosenbaum, 1988)

Although children's health needs have always been complex and the delivery system complicated, ongoing changes in the health care system have increased the need for system management. As health care providers face increased financial pressures, they are encouraged to "dump" patients, shifting high-cost patients to other systems of care (and sources of payment). Without effective efforts to build bridges among service providers, a growing number of children will fall through the cracks. Those most at risk will be children from families with parents who are only marginally connected to providers of care or places of employment, and thus less likely to have a access to sources of reliable advice and guidance.

We are certainly not the first to propose such reforms (Silver, 1978). In response to its concerns about the complexity and diversity of the U.S. health care system, the Select Panel (1981) called for increased "capacity for outreach," "coordination of services," and "continuity of care." But there has been little progress toward these ends over the past decade. We attribute this failure in part to the strategy of implementation proposed by the Select Panel, one that relied on control by the providers of primary care. For a variety of reasons, these providers are ill-suited, individually and institutionally, to act as managers or provide outreach. Physicians are often poorly trained assume these roles. Public clinics, a major source of care for low-income children, typically operate under budget constraints so severe that they are not only unable to afford outreach services, they also have little incentive to bring additional patients into an already overcrowded, underfunded setting.

For these reasons, we recommend that case management and outreach functions be centered in an agency outside the direct medical delivery system. Children with special needs could be integrated into case management programs designed to address the needs of the disabled and impaired of all ages, such as the Community Options Program mentioned earlier in the chapter. We propose that case management and outreach services for other children and pregnant women be assigned to Title V agencies. Combined with the quality assurance functions described earlier, these reforms would place these agencies in the forefront in representing the interests of children in this country. To serve this role effectively, Title V agencies would have to broaden their focus beyond their traditional role as service providers for narrowly-defined groups of severely impaired children. They would be required to develop the capacity to address the needs of all children in all parts of their states.

In some senses, this new mission would require a transformation that would make Title V agencies more like their counterparts at the other end of the age spectrum—state units on aging created under the Older Americans Act of 1965 and incorporating area agencies under 1973 amendments. Like these agencies for the elderly, state Title V authorities would need to develop local or area offices, with the capacity to provide outreach, information and case management in each area.

The track record of state and area agencies on aging has been somewhat checkered. Nonetheless, they have proven widely effective in focusing the attention of policymakers on the needs of their clients: "the potential importance of the Older Americans Act arises not from the volume of funding for its social programs, but from its definition of national goals for the aged and creation of a state and local network for planning, advocacy and delivery" (Newcomer et al., 1983). And in the states where this aging network has been most fully developed, their performance offers an impressive display of how service systems can be effectively shaped, even when financing and delivery systems remain fragmented.

These changes would be made in the structure and function of Title V agencies. At least equally important as these institutional reforms, however, are changes in the philosophy underlying public programs for women and children. Many of these services have their origins in the welfare programs of various eras. They thus carry with them a stigma and strong public pressure to give up services as soon as is financially feasible. Many applaud this arrangement, believing that it reduces the prospects of welfare dependency among low-income families. But even if one accepts this goal and this assessment, one must also recognize some attendant costs. Case managers cannot effectively manage care if their clients episodically disappear from their purview whenever family income climbs a dollar above some threshold, only to reappear a short time later when unmet needs and health care costs drive their income again below the eligibility level. Outreach functions far less effectively if agencies become more concerned with tests for income than with tests for unmet health needs.

For these reasons, even if we continue to provide some services on a means-tested basis, case management and outreach functions should be made available to all children. If families have questions about their children's health insurance coverage or health care needs, there should be a single agency in the community to which they can turn and upon which they can rely, whatever their economic circumstances and however they would pay for the care that the case manager recommends. Rather than thrust out the door as soon as legally permissible, clients should be encouraged to stay in contact with their case manager. They should view him or her as a resource, someone to whom they can turn before their situation becomes untenable.

Although the proposed reforms to support case management and outreach require major changes in approach and institutional arrangements, the goal of system management remains in many ways the most challenging. Public agencies have limited leverage over a largely private service delivery and financing system. Cooperative agreements between public and private providers hold some promise, but they are also likely to remain difficult to establish in an era of intense competition to attract patients (Schlesinger, 1987). Thus, although we believe that system management should be included in the mandate of Title V agencies, realistically the results are likely to be somewhat limited.

One aspect of system management, however, holds greater promise—improving the ties between the education and health care systems. These links are of growing importance. As Medicaid eligibility has been expanded by income in recent years, it has been correspondingly narrowed by age, so the benefits of expanded eligibility rest largely with preschool children, leaving their older siblings without insurance coverage. As the employer-based insurance system becomes a less reliable source for financing the health care of dependents, schools, with their near-universal participation (at least through the middle grades), become on obvious alternative. As more severely impaired children are incorporated into mainstream education, schools also become a means of reaching these groups with special needs.

These needs can be most effectively addressed through an expanded system of school-based health clinics. Though no panacea for children's health needs, school-based clinics provide a mechanism for providing those services (including counseling and substance-abuse treatment) and reaching those children (including pregnant teenagers) least effectively served by the other reforms discussed here. Certainly there will be barriers to this expansion. School-based clinics can be controversial, particularly if they include family planning services. Public opinion, however, appears to be growing more supportive of school-based initiatives, reflecting a growing uneasiness over the consequences of continued neglect of these older children, including high rates of school-age pregnancy and its attendant costs in terms of social dependency. The specter of AIDS may encourage parents to be increasingly receptive to health-related initiatives that incorporate sex education and family planning.

Among the greatest impediments to more effective school-based health services have been the lack of strong leadership from either the schools or health providers, limited resources, and continued tensions between departments of education and public health (Walker et al., Chapter 11). To overcome some of these barriers, we propose that federal legislation funding community health centers be amended to require that they set up satellite clinics in schools in low-income underserved areas. Placing these clinics under the authority of CHCs will avoid adding to the burdens of school administrators. They could be run with greater flexibility, including at hours when classes were not in session.

To ensure adequate funding for these programs, the clinics should be accorded a special form of "presumptive eligibility" for Medicaid, with all students in the school made eligible for Medicaid-covered services at the school-based clinic. This presumptive eligibility would avoid the social stigma of documenting low family income. It would thus encourage access by teenagers, who are at an age when they are particularly sensitive to social stigma and peer pressure. If these school-based clinics were appropriately targeted to low-income neighborhoods, the costs of serving a small number of children from households above the poverty line would be offset by the administrative costs avoided by not documenting eligibility on an individual basis.

These proposed changes call for a significant reorientation in the public service system for children. Inevitably, gaps will remain even if all are implemented. Combined with the other reforms proposed above, however, they ensure that children will have better access to needed health services, even if they are from households where their parents are less able to act as effective advocates on their behalf. We believe that this is the appropriate role for the public sector and a responsibility that must be met.

Conclusion: Children's Health and Our Future

We have laid out an agenda for health policy reform that is designed to be sensitive to the needs of America's children. Underlying this plan was an effort to resolve two important issues. The first involves the extent to which one can address the special health needs of children without segregating them into separate programs. There are certainly some important differences in the health care needs of children and the average adult. These are often neglected by existing health programs as well as proposed reforms. But designing special programs for children, separately financed and administered, runs the risk of creating policies and programs that fail to address the broader forces shaping children's health care and that lack a sufficiently broad political base to assure future public support.

In developing this proposal, we have tried to strike a balance between these concerns, opting for a broader base in financing and service delivery, combined with a more specialized set of initiatives that would monitor adequacy of care. The need for a broad political base argues strongly for reforms that more closely link the financing of children's health care to that for adults. The need to establish a sufficient population base for programs to serve special needs entails designing those programs so that they integrate enrollees of all ages. But these integrative programs must be balanced by initiatives developing case management, service management, and quality assurance focused specifically on children. To promote public accountability, it seems sensible to integrate these functions within a single agency.

Related to this issue is a second, involving a tension between health policies common to all children and those that focus on children with special needs. Past public policy has often taken the second approach, concentrating either on children with unusually severe illnesses (e.g., the CCS program) or those from economically disadvantaged families (e.g., the OEO's Neighborhood Health Centers). These have been laudable and effective programs. But increasingly, the problems that merited this initially targeted approach are spreading to other groups of children. If in the past it was the most severely ill children who were likely to be undertreated, today the threat of inadequate care is common to a variety of children with chronic conditions who received their care in prepaid health plans. If it was formerly those without insurance who were most likely to be denied access to care, they are increasingly being joined by children whose care under various forms of prospective payment is not adequately reimbursed to cover the costs incurred by providers. The problems faced by low-income and severely ill children have not necessarily declined—over the past decade they have in fact probably grown. They are, however, no longer unique. Consequently, the reforms detailed in this chapter have attempted to meet the needs of these traditional target groups while also reaching beyond to those children, predominantly covered under employer-based insurance, who we have in the past simply assumed would receive adequate care.

These underlying issues are not unique to either health policies or policies for children. They are common to a wide range of public programs where the services provided must to some extent be tailored to the needs of the individual recipient. They are common to all government interventions designed to serve groups whose interests are not well-represented through either the private market or the political process. The approaches to reform that are described here may thus have implications for a wide range of public policy. These may be particularly applicable to the design of social insurance programs, such as Medicare. Such programs must strike a delicate balance between universal participation—and thus broad-based political support—and a sensitivity to the differing needs of those they serve. The strategy detailed in this chapter involves broad uniform standards of eligibility and financial participation, but a more narrowly focused system of quality assurances and services for those with special needs. We believe that this appropriately resolves the tensions inherent in social insurance programs and could be successfully pursued in a variety of other contexts.

This chapter's discussion of maternal and child health has been far from exhaustive. Many more specific health care problems, including questions of appropriate treatment of mental illness in children, the consequences of child abuse, and the implications of the growing AIDS epidemic, were not explicitly considered. There were some broader considerations, such as the legal and social influences on health care use, that were also not discussed in great detail. The authors of previous chapters make a number of important observations on these and other matters. Their omission here should by no means be considered a judgment about their relative importance. It was our intent in this chapter to map out a strategy of reform that was broader than these more specific problems, but focused primarily on reforms within the health care system.

Not all that was proposed here will be readily enacted. But we believe that these proposals are politically realistic, that they represent goals that could be achieved over the course of the next five years. Though we have tried to be sensitive to current concerns over federal deficits, some of the recommendations presented here do call for more government spending. In each case, we believe that this additional spending is justified by both the short- and long-term returns to society.

In the longer term, the problems that we have identified and the reforms that we have proposed virtually all justify the development of a universal national health insurance program. Issues of equity, such as those that emerged in this chapter, can be most effectively addressed through open debate and discussion about the norms our society favors in its health care system. The fragmentation and complexity that hampers efforts to ensure children's health can best be overcome through a financing system that deals more inclusively with health services. None of our more specific proposals should hinder the eventual development of more comprehensive reforms. Indeed, we believe that those who would design such a program need to consider exactly the issues that we have discussed here.

Underpinning all these recommendations is a belief that effective health policy reform must be based on an understanding of both children's health needs and an awareness of how factors outside the health care system can affect the providers' ability to meet those needs. We are encouraged by what we perceive to be a gradual national reawakening to the importance of assuring a healthy start for our children and for future generations. But we are not content to assume that public attitudes will continue to develop along these lines. It is essential that we foster institutions that promote awareness of the needs of different age groups and encourage a concern for intergenerational equity.

National policy in recent years has all too often been characterized by neglect of children's health, along with education, shelter, and other basic needs. And while we have been looking the other way, what many believed to be a sound system for financing and delivering children's health care has been eroding. It has not eroded too far to be restored and improved. But it has gone too far for us to afford any further neglect. The time has come to see clearly and to act on that vision, to meet the needs of children and their families—and thus the needs of our nation.

Notes

1. This conference, and the research presented there, was generously supported by the Office of Maternal and Child Health of the U.S. Department of Health and Human Services.
2. The report also included another 1200 pages of background papers and statistical tables.
3. This pattern is not limited to the United States. In Japan, where employment-based insurance has been integrated within a multi-part national health insurance system, dependents covered under employer-based plans face significantly higher copayments than do workers (Steslicke, 1987).
4. Ceilings on coverage for inpatient care generally evolved during an era when hospitals were reimbursed on the basis of costs, and such restrictions were considered desirable to limit lengths of stay and unnecessary hospital days. As Medicaid shifts to prospective payment (such as payment based on DRGs) for hospitals, however, financial incentives will be created to limit lengths of stay. Ceilings on coverage thus are becoming superfluous as well as inequitable.

References

Anderson, M.D., and P. Fox. 1987. Lessons Learned from Medicaid Managed Care Approaches. *Health Affairs* 6(1):71–86.

Behrens, R. 1987. Health Promotion in the Workplace. In J. Meyer and M. Lewin (eds.), *Charting the Future of Health Care,* pp. 133–148. Washington, D.C.: American Enterprise Institute.

Blumenthal, D., and W. Hsiao. 1988. Payments of Physicians under Medicare. In D. Blumenthal, M. Schlesinger, and P.B. Drumheller (eds.), *Renewing the Promise: Medicare and Its Reform,* pp. 115–132. New York: Oxford University Press.

Burwell, B.O., and M.P. Rymer. 1987. Trends in Medicaid Eligibility: 1975 to 1985. *Health Affairs* 6(4):30–45.

Butler, L.H., and P.W. Newacheck. 1981. Health and Social Factors Relevant to Long Term Care Policy. In J. Meltzer, F. Farrow and H. Richman (eds.), *Policy Options in Long-Term Care,* pp. 38–77. Chicago: University of Chicago Press.

Cohen, H. 1980. *Equal Rights for Children.* Totowa, N.J.: Littlefield, Adams, and Co.

Davidson, S.M., J. Cromwell, and R. Schurman. 1986. Medicaid Myths: Trends in Medicaid Expenditures and the Prospects for Reform. *Journal of Health Politics, Policy, and Law* 10(4):699–728.

Dobson, A., J. Scharff, and L. Corder. 1986. First Six Months of Medicaid Data. *National Medical Care Utilization and Expenditure Survey,* Series B, Descriptive Report No. 1. DHHS Publication No. 85-2029. Office of Research and Demonstrations, HCFA. Washington, D.C.: G.P.O.

Doty, P. 1986. Family Care of the Elderly: The Role of Public Policy. *Milbank Memorial Fund Quarterly* 64(1):34–75.

Eisenberg, J.M., and A. Kabcenell. 1988. Organized Practice and the Quality of Medical Care. *Inquiry* 25(1):78–89.

Employee Benefit Research Institute. 1987. *Government Mandating of Employee Benefits, An EBRI-ERF Policy Forum,* Washington, D.C.

Evelyn, R. 1988. Corporations Grow Fearful of Mental Health Costs. *Psychiatric Times/Medicine and Behavior* January:27.

Fox, D.M., and D.C. Schaffer. 1987. Tax Policy as Social Policy: Cafeteria Plans, 1978–1985. *Journal of Health Politics, Policy, and Law* 12(4):609–644.

Freeman, H.E., R.J. Blendon, L.H. Aiken, S. Sudman, C.F. Mullinex, and C.R. Corey. 1987. Americans Report on Their Access to Health Care. *Health Affairs* 6(1):6–18.

Freeman, M.A. 1983. *The Rights and Wrongs of Children.* London: Frances Pinter Publishers.

Gabel, J., C. Jajich-Toth, K. Williams, S. Loughran, and K. Haugh. 1987. The Commercial Health Insurance Industry in Transition. *Health Affairs* 6(3):46–60.

General Accounting Office. 1987. *Prenatal Care, Medicaid Recipients and Uninsured Women Obtain Insufficient Care.* Report to the Chairman, Subcommittee on Human Resources and Intergovernmental Relations, Committee on Government Operations, House of Representatives, September. Washington, D.C.

Hobbs, N., J.M. Perrin, and H.T. Ireys. 1985. *Chronically Ill Children and Their Families.* San Francisco: Jossey-Bass.

Horn, S.D., R.A. Horn, and P.D. Sharkey. 1984. The Severity of Illness Index as a Severity Adjustment to Diagnosis-Related Groups. *Health Care Financing Review* Annual Supplement:33–46.

Hughes, D., K. Johnson, S. Rosenbaum, J. Simons, and E. Butler. 1988. *The Health of America's Children.* Washington, D.C.: Children's Defense Fund.

Jones, S.B., M.K. DuVal, and M. Lesparre. 1987. Competition or Conscience? Mixed-Mission Dilemmas of the Voluntary Hospital. *Inquiry* 24(2):110–118.

Klerman, L., and M.B. Parker. 1988. Improving the Health of Infants and Young Children in Poverty. Unpublished Paper for the National Resource Center for Children in Poverty, New York.

Lohr, K.N., R.H. Brook, C.J. Kamberg, G.A. Goldberg, A. Leibowitz, J. Deesey, D. Reboussin, and J.P. Newhouse. 1986. Use of Medical Care in the Rand Health Insurance Experiment: Diagnosis- and Service-Specific Analyses in a Randomized Controlled Trial. *Medical Care* Supplement 24:9.

Luft, H.S. 1988. HMOs and the Quality of Care. *Inquiry* 25(1):147–156.

Miller, C.A. 1987. *Maternal Health and Infant Survival.* Washington, D.C.: National Center for Clinical Infant Programs.

Newcomer, R.J., Benjamin, A.E., and C.L. Estes. 1983. The Older Americans Act. In R.J. Newcomer and C.L. Estes (eds.), *Fiscal Austerity and Aging, Shifting Government Responsibility for the Elderly,* pp. 187–205. Newbury Park, Calif.: Sage Publications.

Office of Disease Prevention and Health Promotion. 1988. DHHS, PHS. *Disease Prevention/Health Promotion: The Facts.* Palo Alto: Bull Publishing.

Office of Technology Assessment, U.S. Congress. 1987. *Healthy Children: Investing in the Future.* OTA-H-345. Washington, D.C.: G.P.O.

Payne, S.M.C., and J.D. Restuccia. 1987. Policy Issues Related to Prospective Payment for Pediatric Hospitalization. *Health Care Financing Review* 9(1):71–81.

Polchow, M. 1986. *State Efforts at Health Care Cost Containment: 1986 Update.* Washington, D.C.: National Conference of State Legislatures.

Public Health Service. 1986. *The 1990 Health Objectives for the Nation: A Midcourse Review*. Washington, D.C.: Office of Disease Prevention and Health Promotion, DHHS.
Robert Wood Johnson Foundation. 1983. Updated Report on Access to Health Care for the American People. *Special Report* Number 1.
Robert Wood Johnson Foundation. 1987. Access to Health Care in the United States: Results of a 1986 Survey. *Special Report* Number 2.
Rosenbaum, S., and D.C. Hughes. 1986. Financing Maternity Care. Presented at the Bush Institute Conference on Prenatal Care, May 27-28, Washington D.C.
Rosenbaum, S., D.C. Hughes, and K. Johnson. 1988. Maternal and Child Health Services for Medically Indigent Children and Pregnant Women. *Medical Care* 26(4):315–332.
Rosenbaum, S. 1988. Personal communication.
Rowe, J.W. 1985. Health Care of the Elderly. *New England Journal of Medicine* 312(13):827–35.
Schlesinger, M. 1986. On the Limits of Expanding Health Care Reform: Chronic Care in Prepaid Settings. *Milbank Memorial Fund Quarterly* 64(l2):189–215.
Schlesinger, M. 1987. Paying the Price: Medical Care, Minorities, and the Newly Competitive Health Care System. *Milbank Memorial Fund Quarterly* 65 (Supplement 2):270–296.
Schorr, L.B. with D. Schorr. 1988. *Within Our Reach: Breaking the Cycle of Disadvantage*. New York: Anchor Press, Doubleday.
Select Panel for the Promotion of Child Health (To the U.S. Congress and the Secretary of Health and Human Services). 1981. *Better Health for Our Children: A National Strategy*. Vol. 1, DHHS. Washington, D.C.
Shadish, W. 1981. *Health Care Financing Grants and Contracts Report*. Office of Research, Demonstrations, and Statistics, HCFA. April. Washington, D.C.
Silver, G. 1978. *Child Health: America's Future*. Rockville, Md.: Aspen Publications.
Steslicke, W. 1987. The Japanese State of Health: A Political-Economic Perspective. In E. Norbeck and M. Lock (eds.), *Health, Illness, and Medical Care in Japan*. Honolulu: University of Hawaii Press.
Sugarman, J. 1987. Memo to the President on Human Services and Welfare Policies for Children, Youth and Families. *Youth Policy* 9(12):9–12.
Sulvetta, M.B., and K. Swartz. 1986. *The Uninsured and Uncompensated Care: A Chartbook*. Washington, D.C.: National Health Policy Forum.
Wilensky, G. 1987. Viable Strategies for Dealing with the Uninsured. *Health Affairs* 6(1):33–46.

Index

Page numbers in italic denote tables.

Abortion, 51, 53, 61
Access to health care: effects of Medicaid, 195; effects of organizational changes, 184, 199, 200; for low-income children, 327–28; socioeconomic factors, 333–34
Acquired Immune Deficiency Syndrome. *See* AIDS
Acute illness: in national survey, 22; prevalence of, 7; restricted activity from, 9; use of hospital and ambulatory services, 10
Admission practices and per case payments, 165
Adolescents. *See* Teenagers
Adopted children, Medicaid for disabled, 117
Adoption Assistance and Welfare Act, 125
Adoption, expenditures for federal program, *76*
Advocacy: for children, in school, 266; for families, 32; public financing for, 46
Aid to Families with Dependent Children: benefits, 333; eligibility, 222, 326; and Medicaid, 134, 151, 300; recipients and expenditures, *135*
AIDS: daycare for children with, 246–47; financing for health care, 41; and public providers, 233; school health education for, 275; and substance abuse, 13
Alcohol, 13, 15, 276, 277
Alcohol, Drug Abuse and Mental Health Administration, 278; block grant, 73
All payers system and hospital payment, 172–73
AMA (American Medical Association): and school health, 268; surveys, 82, 185, 192, 205

Ambulatory services, *10*, 217
American Medical Association. *See* AMA
American Public Health Association, reports of health education, 275
American School Health Association, study on health education, 275
Anatomy and physiology education, 277
Association for the Care of Children's Health, 28–29
Association of Maternal and Child Health/Crippled Children Services programs, reorganization of, 302–3
Asthma: frequency in low-income children, 12; importance of services, 33; as national survey condition, 23; persistence into adulthood, 13; prevalence, 6–7; restricted activity days, 8–9; use of hospital and ambulatory services for, 10
Audiologists, in public schools, 282

Balanced dual system, 236–37
Bed disability days, 8, *9*
Behavioral problems, 6, 196–97
Behavioral risks for health conditions, 12–13
Birth weight, low. *See* Low birth weight
Births, by state, 230
Blue Cross/Blue Shield, 35, 163
Body dynamics courses, 276
Brookline Early Education Project, 249–50, 254
Burden of illness for children, distribution and hospitalization of, *8*
Bureau of Maternal and Child Health, and health demonstration programs, 286

Capitation rates, for high users of services, 17
Capitation systems, 169, 174–75

361

Care coordination, within traditional payment system, 170
Case-managed systems, 170–71
Case management: for disabled students, 287; and HMOs, 346–48; and Preferred Provider Organizations, 171; public financing of, 46; vs. system management, 350–51; and Title V, 316; as unmet need, 333
Ceilings, on insurance coverage, 345–46
Centers for Disease Control, 73, 278
CHAMPUS (Civilian Health and Medical Program of the Uniformed Services), 70, 72–73
Child abuse, expenditures for federal program, 76
Child care, 75, 243–60
Child deaths, frequency in low-income children, 12
Child Health Assurance Program, effects on Medicaid eligibility, 136
Child health programs, 69, 257
Child health supplement condition groups, 23
Child Health Supplement to the National Health Interview Survey, 6–7, 18, 21–24
Child labor, Children's Bureau studies of, 311–12
Child poverty. See Low-income children
Child savers, 49, 51, 53
Child Support Enforcement Amendments (Public Law 98–378), 114
Child welfare services, 76
Children and Youth projects, 219, 221, 300
Children with Special Needs, study of school health education, 279
Children's Bureau, 297, 311–12
Children's Defense Fund: as child advocates, xv; and Early and Periodic Screening, Diagnosis and Treatment, 143; source books, 311; survey of federally funded programs, 228
Children's health care, 336–37
Children's Medicaid Program, 153
Chronic illness: and capitated systems, 174; costs, 29, 34, 37–38; education and socialization for children with, 30–31; and families, 28–34; and high-cost users of medical care, 5; HMOs for, 188; increase in, 4; and isolation strategy, 201–2; managed care for, 38–40; in national survey, 22; out-of-pocket expenses, *34;* prevalence, 7; regionalization of care, 314; restricted activity days, 8–9; use of hospital and ambulatory services, 10
Civilian Health and Medical Program of the Uniformed Services (CHAMPUS), 70, 72–73
Classification systems for children's hospitalization, 173
Clinic services, Medicaid coverage of, 140
COBRA (Consolidated Budget Reconciliation Act of 1985), 136–38, 151
Cognitive services, 168
Coinsurance and deductibles by type of insurance, *108*
Collaborative Study of Children with Special Needs, 272
Commodities, expenditures for, 75
Community health centers: establishment, 221; expenditures, 73; funding for, 230–31; as public provider, 215, 216; use of, 218
Community health education, 277
Community mental health centers, 80, 215, 216
Community Options Program, 347, 351
Community resources, for chronic illness, 33
Community services for children, 19
Compensation strategy, 203–4
Competition: effects on Medicaid, 195; between health care services, 193–98; price-based effects, 199–200
Congenital anomalies, due to low birth weight, 11–12
Consent laws, reforms, 52–56
Consolidated Budget Reconciliation Act of 1985 (COBRA), 136–38, 151
Consumer health education, 277
Contraceptives, 53, 220
Conversion strategy, 202–3

Cost containment, for health insurance, 110
Cost-sharing, 106–9, 111
CPR education, 277
Crippled children programs, 74, 192
Crippled Children's Services, 222, 228–29. *See also* Programs for Children with Special Health Care Needs

Data: collection, 18–19, 266; publication, 311–12
Daycare, 245, 246–47, 250–56, 257, 259
Deductibles, by type of coverage, *108*
Deficit Reduction Act, 136, 335
Dental care: 103, 250, 268; insurance, types of coverage, *101;* Medicaid coverage of services, 140; screening, 252
Dentists, expenditures, 77–78, 80
Department of Defense, 215
Department of Education, Agriculture and Transportation, 278
Department of Health and Human Services, 215, 278
Dependent coverage, employer contribution, *99*
Diagnosis Related Groups (DRGs): classification system, 173; "creep," 165; effects on public providers, 232–33; hospital prices, 163; New Jersey experience, 165; problems with, 166
Diagnostic services, coverage for, 103, 140
Disabled, block grants for, 302
Disabled students, school health professionals for, 284
Discharge, premature, and prospective payment, 165
Disease education, 277
Disease rate, 16
Division of Maternal and Child Health, 303–4
DPT immunization for school, 268
Drug education, 277
Drugs, prescription, insurance coverage of, 103, 140
Dumping, patient, 223, 351

Early and Periodic Screening, Diagnosis and Treatment (EPSDT): and Children's Defense Fund, 143; as compensation strategy, 204; effects of institutional affiliations, 192; expanded benefits, 144; federal funding and number of children in, 260; problems with, 142; and school health, 281; and Title V, 308
Early childhood programs, federal funding for, *260*
Education for All Handicapped Children Act, 279–80, 281–85
Education: for children with chronic illness, 30–31; through daycare, 254–55; first aid, 276–77; growth and development, 277
Elementary and Secondary Education Act, 280
Emergency feeding, expenditures, 75
Emergency Medical and Infant Care program, 299
Emergency services: expenditures, 80; outpatient, covered by private health insurance, 103; percent of children using, 217; state Medicaid coverage for hospital, 140
Employer Retirement and Income Security Act (ERISA): impact on state regulation, 113–16; and insurance coverage ceilings, 346; promotion of employer self-funding, 124
Employer-provided insurance: children covered by, 70, 90; expansion of, 43; family coverage, 98; as fringe benefit, 96; regulation of, 120–22; subsidies for, 98–99; tax incentives, 112
Employment status and insurance coverage, 95
Entitlement legislation, 53
Entrepreneurial medicine, 328
Environmental education, 276–77
ESEA Chapter 1, effects on school health care, 288
European Economic Community, child care policies, 256
European health policy, 20–21
Expenditures for health care: calculations, 86–88; charitable contributions, 71–72; on children,

Expenditures for health care—
continued
344; dentists, 77–78; family contribution, 67; funds for, 68; hospitalization, 77–78; medication, 77–78; physicians, 77–78, *80;* by program, *72–73;* public and private, *78;* trends, by program, *73*

Fair Labor Standards Act, 116–17
Family-centered care, 28–34
Family planning, 73, 216, 219
Family policy, European, 256–59
Family violence, expenditures on, 76
Federal health research programs, 76
Federal Interagency Day Care regulations, 248
Federally funded programs, survey of, 228
Fee-for-service: AMA survey of physicians, 82; effects on length of physician visit, 187; effects on mental illness treatment, 206; modified payment, 164–68; physicians' payment, 163–64; and Preferred Provider Organizations, 171; vs. prepaid solo practice, 186–87
Financial aid, for chronic illness, 33
Financial counseling, financing for, 46
Follow Through programs, 280
Food stamp expenditures, 75
For-profit corporations, 191–92, 193–94
Foster care, 52, 76
Fragmentation of services, 19–20
France, child care policy, 256–57
Fringe benefits: and employer-provided insurance, 91–92, 96; plans, 100–106

Genetic disease testing, 228–29
Germany, child care policy, 258–59
Great Society Programs, reductions in, 279–80
Group practices, 186–87

Handicapped children: and capitated system, 174; early education program for, 260; nursing homes for, 313–14; school health programs for, 281–85; Title V funding for services, 308

Handicapped education (Public Law 94–142), 76
Headstart: developmental assessment at, 254; expenditures, 76, 80; federal funding for, 260; health monitoring, *250;* and Maternal and Child Health program, 305; number of children, 244; and social integration, 255; success of, 260
Health Care Financing Administration, and quality assurance, 347
Health clinics, percent of children using, 217
Health conditions in children, *5, 6, 7, 9;* prevalence, 4, 21–24
Health counseling of teenagers, 272
Health education: certification, 277; effectiveness, 286–87; number of hours taught, *278;* number of students, 276; in schools, 266, 275–79; states requiring, *277;* and system management, 353
Health financing program, 119–20
Health insurance: benefits limitations, 104; children covered by, *70;* for chronic illness, 34–40; cost containment by employers, 110–11; coverage, *97,* 111, 345–46; deductibles and coinsurance, *108;* dental coverage, *101;* employer survey, 94; expansion of 42–44; high risk exclusions, 106; improved benefits, 339; limitations on dependent coverage, 99–100; minimum benefits, 342–43; national, 337–38; outpatient mental health coverage, *102;* pooling systems, 118; state programs for, 43; status of children, *93;* and teenagers' legal rights, 56; traditional and case management, 170; trends, 110–12; vouchers, 122–23. *See also* Employer-provided insurance; Medicaid; Private health insurance
Health maintenance organizations (HMOs): as alternative payment system, 163; as capitated system, 169; and case management, 346–48; and chronic illness, 35, 38–40, 188; effects on mental illness treatment, 206; effects on patient referrals, 192–93; employer-provided, 102,

Index 365

104; enrollment in, 102; and isolation strategy, 201–2; for low-income children, 187–88; Medicaid enrollment in, 232; and multihospital systems, 190; organizational forms, 161; and the public sector, 216; and school health programs, 289
Health Organizer Model, 267–69, 270
Health policy for children, 59–61, 204–6
Health providers, use of services by children, *217*
Health reforms, 337–57
Health status, measurement of, 15–16
Hearing care, insurance coverage of, 103
Hearing impairment: heterogeneous symptoms, 27; importance of services, 33; as national survey condition, 23; risk of persistence, 13–14
Hib vaccine, 252
High users of medical services, 15, 16–17
High-risk children: definition of, 184; effects of competition on, 196; effects of organizational changes, 198–99, *200;* and integrated practices, 186; quality assurance programs for, 338–39
Hill-Burton Act: for facility construction, 220; and facility reductions, 231–32; for low-cost services, 216
Home care, 39–40, 44
Horizontal integration, 190
Hospital-based incentives and physician payment, 192
Hospital payment, 172–75; cost-based, 163; per case, for acute care, 173; prospective payment systems, 164
Hospital Survey and Construction Act. *See* Hill-Burton Act
Hospitalization: days, for children, *8;* expenditures, 35, 77–78, 79; rates, 3, *4*
Hospitals: closures, 223–24, coverage ceilings, 345–46; coverage of inpatient services, 103; number of public providers, 216; public, with deficits, 223; restrictions in stay, 328; unprofitable, and institutional affiliations, 191; use of, *10*
House Select Committee on Children, xv

Immunizations: delayed, frequency in low-income children, 12; expenditures, 73; monitoring of, 250, 252; for school, 268, 285
Income: health insurance coverage by, *97;* and health insurance premium payment status, *99;* and maximum benefits, *105;* of physicians, *194;* type of insurance coverage and type of services covered, *103*
Income-adjusted premiums for Medicaid, 344–45
Indemnity plans, 109–10
Independent Practice Associations (IPAs): effects on patient referrals, 192–93; growth of, 185–86; HMO as, 161
Indian Health Service, 72–73, 215
Indigent mothers and children, and Title V, 309
Infant Health and Development Program, 246
Infant mortality: block grants for, 302; Children's Bureau studies of, 298, 311–12; decline of, 326–27; Title V funding for, 308
Infectious disease, 73, 245–46
Information collection groups, 218, 311–12
Institutional affiliations, 189–95
Institution care, 52
Insurance. *See* Health insurance
Insurance premium payment status and family income, *99*
Insurance premiums, 98
Insurance reimbursement, for disabled students, 284–85
Integrated ambulatory practices, 199–200
Integrated Maternal and Child Health Information System, 311
Integrated practices, benefits, 186
Integrated services, need for, 349–54
Intensive care facilities, pediatric and neonatal, 225–27

Intergovernment Health Policy Project, 141
Intergroup relationships courses, 276
Intermediate Care Facilities for mentally retarded, 140
Investor-owned facilities, 227
Isolation strategy, 201–2

Kennedy/Waxman plan, 117, 121
"Kiddie libbers," 49–50, 52–53

Lead levels in blood, elevated,
Lead poisoning, 6, 12, 15, 228–29
Legal issues, 49–61
Local health clinics, expenditures, 80–81
Local health departments, number of public providers, 216
Local health expenditures, by program, 74
Longevity, as measure of health status, 15–16
Low birth weight: frequency in low-income children, 12; increased risk of health conditions, 11–12; percent of children, 7; prevalence, 326; and substance abuse, 13
Low-income children: access to health care, 327–28; effects of competition on, 196; food stamp expenditures for, 75; frequency of health problems, *12;* and health care policy, 183; as high users of services, 17; increase in, 89; increased risk for health conditions, 11; insurance status, 92–93; insured by HMOs, 187; to Medicaid recipients, ratio, 340; percentage of, 15; unmet needs, 333; use of public services, 217
Low-income families, and cost-sharing, 107

Mainstreaming, 257, 282–84
Managed care, 38–40, 346–48
Managed care systems, Medicaid enrollment in, 232
Marketing expenditures, 195
Massachusetts: Early Intervention Program, 316; Health Start Program, 315; insurance laws, 35–36
Maternal and Child Health (MCH): benefits of separate policy, 329–30; block grants, 73, 228, 297–99, 301–3, 307; current organization, 303–5; funding for, 228–30, 305–6, 340–45; Information Network (MATCH), 311; reduction in support, 301; relationship with federal programs, 305; state expenditures, 74; states' roles, 304–5; technical assistance, 314–15. *See also* Title V of the Social Security Act
Maternal and Infant Care (MIC) projects: creation of, 300; standards for, 219; and Title V, 221
Maternity and Infancy Act, 221, 297–98
Maternity services, state, users of, 230
Maximum benefits of private health insurance, *105*
Medi-Cal program and conversion strategy, 203
Medicaid: beneficiaries in HMOs, study of, 38; benefits, 123–24, 139–40; and case management, 170–71; and chronic illness, 40; as compensation strategy, 204; creation of, 297, 300; disabled recipients, 117, 149; and DRGs, 163; effects of competition, 195; eligibility, 134–39, 353–54; eligibility for pregnant women and infants, 340; enrollment in Headstart, 75, 250; expansion of, 43–44, 118–19, 173; expansion of eligibility, 343–45; expenditures, 72–73, 78; fees, 145, *147,* 167; financing for low-income families, xi; funding for community health centers, 221; history of, 132–34; and HMOs, 188, 193; and isolation strategy, 201–2; Management Information Systems, 311; and MCH programs, 305; need for surveys, 18; optional services, *140,* 141; out-of-pocket expenses, 69; participation rates, 151; patients in prepaid plans, 232; payment, 138, *150,* 160; and physicians, 144–47; vs. private health insurance, 91; and the public sector, 216; purpose of, 131–32; recipients

and, 133, *135;* reduction in education, 279; reductions in eligibility, 222; reforms, 148–55, 340–42; restrictions, 145, 328; and risk reduction, 20; and school health program, 290; as source of health care financing, 67, 68; state expenditures, 74; state fees, 146; states' roles, 133–34; Suffolk County Demonstration, *148;* and Title V, 308; trends in, 69, 141–44

Medical care price index, 69

Medical screening and treatment, in Headstart, 250

Medically indigent, insurance for, 118

Medically Needy Program, 44

Medicare: creation of, 297, 300; exemptions, 189; expenditures, 73; and hospital prospective payment, 172; and isolation strategy, 201–2; vs. Medicaid, 319–20; prospective payment and premature discharge, 165; Professional Review and quality assurance, 347; and the public sector, 216; trends in expenditures, 69; use of DRGs, 163

Medication, 14, 77–78

Mental health care: covered by private health insurance, 103; effects of competition, 196; outpatient, insurance coverage of, *102*

Mental health education, 277

Mental health policy for children, 60

Mental health programs, expenditures, 74

Mental illness treatment, risks, 206

Mental impairment, 9, 22

Mental retardation: as a disabling condition, 28; importance of services, 33; Medicaid benefits for, 139–40; as a national survey condition, 23; prevalence, 6; restricted activity days for, 8

Migrant Health Centers: expenditures, 73, 80; funding for, 230–31; as a public provider, 215–16; use of, 218

Mixed system reimbursement, 174

Mortality rates, decline in childhood, 3

Multifacility systems, 189–93, 199–200

Municipal Health Services Program, 235

National Association of Children's Hospitals and Related Institutions, 71

National Association of Community Health Centers, survey, 218

National Cancer Institute, 278

National Center for Health Statistics, surveys by, 18–19

National Education Association, 268

National Health Demonstration Programs, 285–87

National health policy, need for, 20–21

National Health Services Corps, 73, 81

National Heart, Lung and Blood Institute, 278

National Institutes of Health, 76

National Longitudinal Survey of Youth, 19

National Maternal and Child Health Resource Center, 302–3

National Medical Care Expenditure Survey (NMCES), 94; Health Insurance Employer Survey, 100

National Medical Care Utilization and Expenditure Survey, 94, 217–18

National Natality Follow-back Survey, 18–19

National Professional School Health Organization, 275

National Survey of Family Growth, 219

Needy families, expenditures for, 75

Neonatal intensive care facilities, 225–27

Neonatal intermediate care facilities, 225–27

Neonatal morbidity, 173

Neonatal mortality, 12

New Federalism policies, 301–3

New morbidity: definition, 272; physician supply, 289; school health program, 282

New paternalism, 58–59

Not-for-profit, nongovernment facilities, 226–27

Nurse practitioner model: and adolescent health issues, 289; description, 269; expenditures for, 270; and health demonstration projects, 286; resistance from school officials, 272

Nursery school, 243, 244

Nursing Homes Without Walls program, 347
Nutrition: child, expenditures for, 75; at daycare, 252–53; education, 277
Nutritional status of children, survey, 312

OBRA. *See* Omnibus Budget Reconciliation Act
Obstetrical care, Medicaid fees for, 146
Occupational therapy, 33, 140; in schools, 282
Office of Disease Prevention and Health Promotion, 277–78
Office of Economic Opportunity: comparison of public providers, 219; establishment of, 221; Neighborhood Health Centers, 300
Office of Special Education, 286
Office on Smoking and Health, 278
Office visits, Medicaid fees for, 146
Omnibus Budget Reconciliation Act (OBRA): and child health block grants, 302; funding cutbacks, 335; funding for maternal and child health, 228–29; and Medicaid eligibility, 135, 138, 326–27
Omnibus Budget Reconciliation Act of 1986 (SOBRA), 134–38, 151
Organizational changes: effects of, *199;* effects on health care delivery, 184; effects on high-risk children, *200*
Out-of-pocket expenses: by type of coverage, *69;* for chronic illness, *34;* for the uninsured, 68
Outliers, hospital payment for, 172
Outpatient service, covered by private health insurance, 103
Outreach services, 350–54

Parent Labor Law, need for, 261
Parent networks, 46
Patient referrals, 192–93
Payment, 164–65, 166–67, 168
Payment systems, 159, 161–64, 175; all payers system, 172–73; capitation systems, 169, 174–75; mixed system reimbursement, 174; physician payment, 163–64, 192; prospective payment systems, 172–74. *See also* Health maintenance organizations
Pediatric care, 224, *225–27;* nursing homes, 313–14
Pediatrician-to-children ratio, 159
Perinatal care, 11–12, 314
Personal care services, Medicaid coverage of, 140
PGPs (prepaid group practices), 161, 185–86
Physical and psychosocial problems, 17–18
Physical therapy: for chronic illness, 33; Medicaid coverage of, 140; in schools, 282
Physician payment: AMA survey of, 192; types of, 163–64
Physician prospective payment systems, 166–67
Physicians: expenditures by, 80; expenditures for, 77–78; income and visits per week, *194;* office, percent of children using, 217; outpatient services covered by private health insurance, 103
Physician supply: 158; children-to-physician ratio, *159;* and competition, 193–95; effects on school health care, 288–89; statistics, 194
Planned Parenthood, 216
Poor children. *See* Low-income children
Postneonatal mortality, frequency in low-income children, 12
PPOs, 171, 192–93, 232
Preexisting conditions, denial of benefits, 35
Preferred Provider Organizations (PPOs), 171, 192–93, 232
Pregnancy care: effects of competition, 195; insurance coverage of, 306; and uncompensated care, 173
Pregnant women, use of public services, 217
Premature infants, daycare for, 246
Prenatal care: adequacy of, 326–27, block grants for, 302; coverage ceilings, 345–46; effects of competition, 195; European, 20; and Preferred Provider Organization, 171; public vs. private providers, 219; survey of, 219

Index 369

Prepaid group practices (PGPs), 161, 185–86
Prepaid groups, effects on physician visits, 187
Prepaid managed health care, for high users of services, 17
Prepaid plans, effects on uninsured, 188–89
Prepaid Provider Organizations, effects on school health care, 288
Preventive services: block grants for, 302; in Europe, 20–21; insurance coverage of, 111; Medicaid coverage of, 140; payment for, 168; and Preferred Provider Organizations, 171; in schools, 266; and Title V, 317; utilization of, 109, 175
Private health insurance: assessment of, 94; children covered by, *70;* eligibility, 94–100; and employment status, 95; exclusion of children, 331–32; expenditures, 78, 90–91; failure to cover preventive care, 332; family income and premium payment status, *99;* government regulation, 112–19; incentives for, 117; limitations of, 35–38; and Medicaid, comparison, 91; out-of-pocket expenses, 69; services covered, *103;* state regulation of, 113–14
Private nursing, Medicaid coverage of, 140
Private practitioners and school health programs, 290
Privatization, 234–35
Program of Projects, 228–29
Programs for Children with Special Health Care Needs, 40–41, 45–47
Project SERVE, 34, 36–38, 47, 313
Prospective payment systems, 172–74
Prosthetic devices, Medicaid coverage of, 140
Provider payments, 158–76
Psychiatric hospital admissions and behavior problems, 196–97
Psychiatric inpatient services, Medicaid coverage of, 140
Psychiatric problems and substance abuse, 13
Psychologists, 80, 282
Public Health Foundation, 218
Public health insurance, 118–19, 123–24, 131–55. *See also* Medicaid
Public Health Service: management, 73; number of users, 229; as provider of inpatient services, 215
Public health, expenditures, 80
Public hospitals, reproductive and pediatric services, 224
Public Law 94-142, 76
Public Law 98-378, 114
Public policy affecting children's health care, xviii-xix
Public providers: comparison of, 219; history, 220–21; number of, *216;* policy options, 233–34; trends, 231–33
Public sector, definition, 215–16

Quality assurance program, 338–39, 346–48
Quality of care: effects of competition, 197; effects of for-profit corporations, 191–92; effects of organizational changes, 184, 199–200; and high-cost children, 174–75; in institutional affiliations, 192; in public sector, 218–20

Recreational opportunities, for chronic illness, 33
Regional IV Maternal and Child Health Data Network, 312
Regionalization of perinatal and chronic care, 314
Regionalized care and Title V, 313–14
Rehabilitation services, Medicaid coverage of, 140
Relative Value Scales (RVS), 167–68
Report of Intended Expenditures, 313
Report on Health Promotion and Disease Prevention, 275
Reproductive health services, in public hospitals, 224
Research: expenditures, *76;* value of, 311–12
Residential treatment centers, 80
Resource-based Relative Value Scale, 168
Respite care, funding of, 46
Rights and entitlements, for chronic illness, 32–33

370 Index

Risk: high, implications of, 14–15; increased, for health conditions, 11–13; of persistence, *14;* of poor health, 18–20; states, *15*
Robert Wood Johnson Foundation, 289
RVS (Relative Value Scales), 167–68

Safety education, 277
School health clinics, expansion of, 353–54
School health education, 266, 275–79
School health promotion, sponsoring agencies for, 278
School health services: competition with private practitioners, 272; confidentially, 57; definition, 265; expenditures, 80–81, 270; expenditures for, by state, *271;* future trends, 287–90; Great Society programs, 280–81; for handicapped children, 281–85; physician involvement, 283; problems with, 272–75; state expenditures, 74; types of, 267–69
School meals, expenditures, 75
School nurses: for disabled students, 284; expenditures by, 80; role in health organizer model, 267; role of, 274; state expenditures for, 74
School psychologists, expenditure by, 80
Schools: as child advocates, 266; for data collection, 266; medical requirements for, *268;* preventive services, 266
Screening services, Medicaid coverage, 140
Select Panel for the Promotion of Child Health, 159, 187, 325
Self-funded plans, employer-provided insurance, 115
Self-help groups, funding for, 46
Sex education, 276–77
Sheppard-Towner Act, 221, 297–98
Sick child care center 249
SIDS (sudden infant death syndrome), funding for, 228–29
Skill Nursing Facilities (SFNs), 139–40
Skimming, 165

SOBRA (Omnibus Budget Reconciliation Act of 1986), 134–38, 151
Social Security Act of 1936, xi
Social Services Block Grant, *76,* 222
Social workers, expenditures by, 80
Socialization of children with chronic illness, 31, 33
Sociodemographic risks, 11, 12
Socioeconomic factors for access to health care, 333–34
Sociology courses, 276
Solo practice: physicians, decline in, 185; prepaid vs. fee-for-service, 186–87
Special education for the handicapped, 305, 309
Special needs of children, 330–37
Special services for chronic illness, 44
Speech impairment, 6, 8, 23, 140
Speech pathologists, 282
Speech therapy, for chronic illness, 33
State and local government facilities for children, number of, 225–26
State expenditures for health care, by program, *74*
State health agencies, use of, 218
State health department clinics, expenditures, 80
State Health Department Maternity Services and Live Births, users of, *230*
State regulation of private health insurance, 113–14
State role in health care, 222–23, 339
Strategies for health system reform, 201–4
Subsidized meals, expenditures for, 75
Substance abuse, 13, 15
Sudden infant death syndrome (SIDS), funding for, 228–29
Suffolk County Demonstration, 148
Summer Feeding Program, expenditures, 75
Supplemental Security Income for Disabled Children's Program, 134, 228, 302
Supplementary services and Title V, 316–17
Support groups for chronic illness, 33

Support services, for chronic illness, 32–34
Surgery, outpatient, covered by private health insurance, 103
Sweden, child care policy, 257–58
System management, 350–51, 353

Task Force on the Prevention of Low Birth Weight and Infant Mortality, 311–12
Tax code, 116–17, 216
Tax Equity and Fiscal Responsibility Act of 1982 (TEFRA), 136
Tax incentives: for child care, 260; for employer-provided insurance, 112
Teenagers: admissions to private facilities, 196; births, frequency of, 12; with chronic illness, 31; drivers and alcohol-related accidents, 13; health care and Title V, 315–16; pregnancy, 219, 228–29, 289; rights, 53–56
TEFRA (Tax Equity and Fiscal Responsibility Act of 1982), 136
Tertiary centers, 166, 191
Title V of the Social Security Act: accountability, 312; decline of influence, 300–301; expenditures, 305–6; future, 310–19; history, 297–301; incorporation of provisions for pregnant women and children, 221; lack of monitoring, 309–10; Maternal and Child Health Services Block Grant, 40–41; partnership with Medicaid and Blue Cross/Blue Shield, 45–46; provision of services, 315–18; reductions in education, 279; reductions in interstate variation, 335; and regionalized care, 313–14; role of federal government, 318–19; special needs children, 40–41; standards, 313–14; states' role, 317–18; strengths, 306–8; supplementary services, 316–17; weaknesses, 308–10
Title X of Public Health Services Act, 219

Title XIX of Social Security Act, 154–55, 335. *See also* Medicaid
Title XX of Public Health Service Act, 219, 260; Social Services Block Grant, 76, 222
Transfer policies, effects of competition, 197–98

U.S. Surgeon General Report on Health Promotion and Disease Prevention, 275
Uncompensated care: and community health centers, 231; effects on public hospitals, 223; hospital expenditures, 71; increase in, 231–32; and neonatal morbidity, 173; number of facilities, 221; physician expenditures, 70–71; and pregnancy, 173
Uniform Hospital Discharge Data Set, 311
Uninsured: admission to government facilities, 217; effects of competition, 196; increase in, 91, 327; number of, 35, 96; Title V for, 315
Uninsured children: effects from prepaid plans, 188–89; and health care policy, 183; Medicaid for, 344–45; number of, 42–43, 340; socioeconomic status, 93
Union-provided insurance, children covered by, 70
United Nations Declaration of the Rights of the Child, 51
Unprofitable services, effects of for-profit corporations, 191–92
Usual, customary and reasonable (UCR) procedures, 163–64, 167
Utilization of public health care services, 217–18

Vertical integration of facilities, 190
Veteran's Administration, 73, 215
Vision problems: importance of services, 33; as national survey condition, 23; prevalence, 6; restricted activity days, 8

Well-baby care, 171
Well-child clinics, 81
Women, Infants and Children (WIC) program, xi; certification, 81; expenditures, 75; funds for, 307; and Maternal and Child Health Program, 305, 317
Worker's compensation, 73
Working mothers, 243
Working women, *244*